# DISTRESS TOLERANCE

# DISTRESS
# TOLERANCE

*Theory, Research,
and Clinical Applications*

Edited by
MICHAEL J. ZVOLENSKY
AMIT BERNSTEIN
ANKA A. VUJANOVIC

THE GUILFORD PRESS
New York        London

© 2011 The Guilford Press
A Division of Guilford Publications, Inc.
72 Spring Street, New York, NY 10012
www.guilford.com

Printed in the United States of America

This book is printed on acid-free paper.

Last digit is print number: 9 8 7 6 5 4 3 2 1

**Library of Congress Cataloging-in-Publication Data**

Distress tolerance : theory, research, and clinical applications / edited by Michael J.
Zvolensky, Amit Bernstein, Anka A. Vujanovic.
     p. ; cm.
   Includes bibliographical references and index.
   ISBN 978-1-60918-038-6 (hardcover : alk. paper)
   1. Psychology, Pathological.   2. Distress (Psychology)   I. Zvolensky, Michael J.
II. Bernstein, Amit.   III. Vujanovic, Anka A.
   [DNLM: 1. Stress, Psychological—physiopathology.   2. Stress, Psychological—
psychology.   3. Mental Disorders—physiopathology.   4. Psychophysiologic Disorders—
physiopathology.   5. Stress, Physiological.   WM 172 D614 2011]
   RC454.D55 2011
   616.89—dc22
                                                              2010025131

# About the Editors

**Michael J. Zvolensky, PhD,** is Richard and Pamela Ader Green and Gold Distinguished Professor in the Department of Psychology and Director of the Anxiety and Health Research Laboratory at the University of Vermont. His research program cuts across basic and applied work in the area of anxiety disorders. Specifically, his work is focused principally on examining vulnerability processes involved with the onset and maintenance of these disorders. Dr. Zvolensky has been especially involved in better understanding the role of cigarette smoking in the etiology and maintenance of panic psychopathology and, at the same time, the role that panic vulnerability factors may play in smoking cessation.

**Amit Bernstein, PhD,** is Senior Lecturer and Yigal Alon Fellow in the Department of Psychology and Director of the International Research Collaborative on Anxiety Laboratory at the University of Haifa, Israel. Previously, he was a postdoctoral fellow at the Center for Health Care Evaluation at the VA Palo Alto Health Care System and the Department of Psychiatry and Behavioral Sciences at Stanford University School of Medicine. Dr. Bernstein's research is focused on specific and transdiagnostic vulnerability and resilience processes underlying anxiety and related disorders, such as addiction.

**Anka A. Vujanovic, PhD,** is Staff Research Psychologist at the National Center for PTSD, Behavioral Science Division, VA Boston Healthcare System, and Assistant Professor in the Division of Psychiatry, Boston University School of Medicine. Dr. Vujanovic's research program focuses on cognitive–affective and behavioral risk and maintenance factors related to posttraumatic stress disorder and co-occurring posttraumatic stress and substance use disorders.

# Contributors

**Michael D. Anestis, MS,** Department of Psychology, Florida State University, Tallahassee, Florida

**Gordon J. G. Asmundson, PhD,** Department of Psychology, University of Regina, Regina, Saskatchewan, Canada

**Amit Bernstein, PhD,** Department of Psychology, University of Haifa, Haifa, Israel

**Marina A. Bornovalova, PhD,** Department of Psychology, University of South Florida, Tampa, Florida

**Richard A. Brown, PhD,** Department of Psychiatry and Human Behavior, Alpert Medical School, Brown University, Providence, Rhode Island

**R. Nicholas Carleton, PhD,** Department of Psychology, University of Regina, Regina, Saskatchewan, Canada

**Shauna L. Clen, BS,** Department of Psychology, Kent State University, Kent, Ohio

**Kelsey C. Collimore, MA,** Department of Psychology, University of Regina, Regina, Saskatchewan, Canada

**Stacey B. Daughters, PhD,** Department of Public and Community Health, University of Maryland, College Park, Maryland

**Erin L. Fink, BA,** Department of Psychology, Florida State University, Tallahassee, Florida

**David M. Fresco, PhD,** Department of Psychology, Kent State University, Kent, Ohio

**Elizabeth V. Gifford, PhD,** Center for Health Care Evaluation, VA Palo Alto Health Care System, Menlo Park, California; Department of Psychiatry and Behavioral Sciences, Stanford University School of Medicine, Stanford, California

**Kim L. Gratz, PhD,** Department of Psychiatry and Human Behavior, University of Mississippi Medical Center, Jackson, Mississippi

**Thomas E. Joiner, PhD,** Department of Psychology, Florida State University, Tallahassee, Florida

**Meghan Keough, MS,** Department of Psychology, Florida State University, Tallahassee, Florida

**Carl W. Lejuez, PhD,** Department of Psychology, University of Maryland, College Park, Maryland

**Teresa M. Leyro, BA,** Department of Psychology, University of Vermont, Burlington, Vermont

**Brett T. Litz, PhD,** National Center for PTSD, Behavioral Science Division, VA Boston Healthcare System, and Division of Psychiatry, Boston University School of Medicine, Boston, Massachusetts

**Thomas R. Lynch, PhD,** Mood Disorders Centre, College of Life and Environmental Sciences, Psychology, University of Exeter, Exeter, United Kingdom

**Douglas S. Mennin, PhD,** Department of Psychology, Yale University, New Haven, Connecticut

**Melissa Mitchell, MS,** Department of Psychology, Florida State University, Tallahassee, Florida

**Guy A. Mizon, PhD,** Mood Disorders Centre, College of Life and Environmental Sciences, Psychology, University of Exeter, Exeter, United Kingdom

**Daniel L. Peluso, MA,** Department of Psychology, University of Regina, Regina, Saskatchewan, Canada

**Christina Riccardi, MS,** Department of Psychology, Florida State University, Tallahassee, Florida

**Jessica M. Richards, BS,** Department of Psychology, University of Maryland, College Park, Maryland

**Norman B. Schmidt, PhD,** Department of Psychology, Florida State University, Tallahassee, Florida

**Edward A. Selby, MS,** Department of Psychology, Florida State University, Tallahassee, Florida

**April R. Smith, MS,** Department of Psychology, Florida State University, Tallahassee, Florida

**Jodie A. Trafton, PhD,** VA Program Evaluation and Resource Center, VA Office of Mental Health Services, Center for Health Care Evaluation, VA Palo Alto Health Care System, Menlo Park,

California; Department of Psychiatry and Behavioral Sciences, Stanford University School of Medicine, Stanford, California

**Matthew T. Tull, PhD,** Department of Psychiatry and Human Behavior, University of Mississippi Medical Center, Jackson, Mississippi

**Anka A. Vujanovic, PhD,** National Center for PTSD, Behavioral Science Division, VA Boston Healthcare System, and Division of Psychiatry, Boston University School of Medicine, Boston, Massachusetts

**Carl F. Weems, PhD,** Department of Psychology, University of New Orleans, New Orleans, Louisiana

**Patrick G. Welch, MA,** Department of Psychology, University of Regina, Regina, Saskatchewan, Canada

**Michael J. Zvolensky, PhD,** Department of Psychology, University of Vermont, Burlington, Vermont

# Preface

There has been rapid growth in research and theory on vulnerability processes for psychopathology. This work has been intellectually exciting, clinically and theoretically useful, and representative of a major point of scientific advancement in better understanding the nature and expression of mental disorders. Distress tolerance has emerged as a psychological construct of growing interest for clinical scientists and practitioners. It is theorized that distress tolerance may contribute to the development, maintenance, and therapeutic extinction of a variety of forms of psychopathology. Consequently, interest in distress tolerance has been driven by its theoretical potential to contribute to models of risk and resilience and related clinical implications and applications. Linehan's (1993) influential work on borderline personality disorder represents an early and important illustration of the clinical relevance of distress tolerance. Within this theoretical model, persistent unwillingness or inability to tolerate emotional distress is a central mechanism underlying borderline personality disorder symptoms. Linehan's dialectical behavior therapy, therefore, aims to promote therapeutic change in distress tolerance and related emotion dysregulation processes that may underlie borderline personality disorder. The field has since seen the proliferation of related psychosocial interventions similarly designed to promote tolerance for internal and external sources of distress, thus targeting vulnerability for psychopathology (e.g., Barlow, Allen, & Choate, 2004; Hayes, Strosahl, & Wilson, 1999; Orsillo & Roemer, 2005).

Despite clinical interest in the role of distress tolerance in the onset and maintenance of psychopathology and its treatment, a corresponding compilation of empirical and theoretical knowledge is lacking. As a result, it is difficult to discern (1) the scope of distinct conceptual models of distress tolerance and methodologies used to assess them; (2) the role(s) of distress tolerance in the onset and maintenance of various forms of psychopathology; (3) the possible impact of psychological symptoms on distress tolerance; and (4) the most effective methods for clinically translating our knowledge into efficacious prevention and treatment approaches.

The aim of the present volume is to systematically identify, aggregate, and synthesize information on the nature of distress tolerance and its relations to psychological symptoms and disorders. The book was designed to focus on distress tolerance research across a comprehensive range of foundational theoretical and clinical issues as well as psychopathology content areas. Chapters in Part I focus on theory, assessment, and conceptualization issues related to distress tolerance. In this first part of the volume, authors offer an initial nomological context and set of transdisciplinary perspectives to conceptualizing and studying distress tolerance and thereby provide an important foundation for contributions made in Part II.

Part II includes a series of chapters on the relations between distress tolerance and related processes and various forms of psychopathology. These chapters provide a theoretical basis for understanding distress tolerance–psychopathology associations and the clinical implications of this work for prevention/treatment.

Part III comprises a final chapter that synthesizes gaps in our knowledge base on research presented across Parts I and II and points to promising future directions in the study of distress tolerance.

The contributions to the present volume document that distress tolerance is an important construct to consider in developing new insights about the onset and maintenance of psychopathology as well as its prevention and treatment. At the same time, a number of formative questions remain regarding the nature of the construct, including its associations with other risk and protective processes and its exact roles in vulnerability for, and resilience to, psychopathology. These gaps in knowledge represent exciting domains for future study. We hope the present volume may serve as a catalyst for directing such work.

## REFERENCES

Barlow, D. H., Allen, L., & Choate, M. (2004). Toward a unified treatment for emotional disorders. *Behavior Therapy, 35*, 205–230.
Hayes, S., Strosahl, K., & Wilson, K. (1999). *Acceptance and commitment*

*therapy: An experiential approach to behavior change.* New York: Guilford Press.

Linehan, M. M. (1993). *Cognitive-behavioral treatment of borderline personality disorder.* New York: Guilford Press.

Orsillo, S. M., & Roemer, L. (2005). *Acceptance and mindfulness-based approaches to anxiety: Conceptualization and treatment.* New York: Springer.

# Acknowledgments

The idea for this book arose in part from the thoughtful suggestion of Jim Nageotte, Senior Editor at The Guilford Press. We would like to thank Jim for assisting us in the development of the conceptual framework for this volume, providing important feedback regarding the structure and organization of the volume, and supporting our efforts throughout the course of the project. We also wish to thank Guilford for providing us with the unique opportunity to bring together a diverse group of authors whose original contributions constitute the present volume.

We also would like to express our great appreciation to Carrie M. Potter, Research Technician at the National Center for PTSD, Behavioral Science Division, VA Boston Healthcare System, and Anka Vujanovic's Research Coordinator. Carrie provided invaluable assistance in preparing this volume for submission.

# Contents

## PART III. FUTURE DIRECTIONS

# PART I

# Theory, Assessment, and Conceptualization

# 1

# Historical Perspectives, Theory, and Measurement of Distress Tolerance

Michael J. Zvolensky, Teresa M. Leyro,
Amit Bernstein, *and* Anka A. Vujanovic

Researchers and clinicians have had a long-standing interest in elucidating the role of distress tolerance focused on aversive internal states (e.g., negative emotions, uncomfortable bodily sensations) in various forms of psychopathology (e.g., Frenkel-Brunswik, 1948, 1951; Hajek, 1991; Hajek, Belcher, & Stapleton, 1987; Linehan, 1993a, 1993b; Simons & Gaher, 2005). Many of these accounts are focused on distinct conceptualizations of distress tolerance among persons with, or at risk for, Axis I and II psychopathology (e.g., Gross & Muñoz, 1995; Lynch & Bronner, 2006; Mennin, Heimberg, Turk, & Fresco, 2002; Zvolensky & Otto, 2007). In the study of substance use and dependence, for example, intolerance of emotional and somatic sensations has been suggested to be a key explanatory mechanism underlying maintenance of use (Brown, Lejuez, Kahler, Strong, & Zvolensky, 2005; Chaney, Roszell, & Cummings, 1982; Otto, Powers, & Fischmann, 2005). In addition, distress tolerance has increasingly been viewed as an important construct in developing new insights about the onset and maintenance of psycho-

The first and second authors contributed equally to the present chapter and both should be considered lead author.

pathology as well as its prevention and treatment (Zvolensky & Otto, 2007). For example, interest in distress tolerance in the context of psychological disorders has been paralleled by the growth and dissemination of psychosocial interventions designed to promote greater degrees of emotional acceptance, mindfulness, and self-awareness (e.g., Barlow, Allen, & Choate, 2004; Hayes, Strosahl, & Wilson, 1999; Orsillo & Roemer, 2005; Linehan, 1993). Many of these psychosocial treatments have begun to show promising outcomes (e.g., Kabat-Zinn, Lipworth, Burney, & Sellers, 1987; Orsillo, Roemer, & Barlow, 2003; Ramel, Goldin, Carmona, & McQuaid, 2004; Roemer & Orsillo, 2002; Williams, Teasdale, Segal, & Soulsby, 2000).

Despite the promise of existing work on distress tolerance in regard to the study of psychopathology, there has not been a comprehensive review of the extant empirical literature focused on the construct. As a result, theoretical and empirical integration of distress tolerance work, or a broad-based perspective as to how this literature is shaping our understanding of psychopathology, is lacking. Thus, there are numerous conceptualizations, assessment tactics, and, presumably, inferences derived from extant bodies of distress tolerance research. Similarly, aforementioned treatments designed to target distress tolerance have approached this construct clinically in a variety of ways (e.g., Barlow et al., 2004; Linehan, 1993; Williams et al., 2000) because, in part, of varying conceptual perspectives on distress tolerance, its putative role(s) in psychopathology, and the optimal means to therapeutically engender change in the construct.

Overall, the lack of an integrative volume on distress tolerance impedes our ability to fully ascertain from the extant literature (1) the scope of distinct and overlapping conceptual models of distress tolerance and methodologies designed to assess them; (2) the roles of distress tolerance in the onset and maintenance of psychopathology; (3) the possible impact of psychological symptoms and psychopathology on distress tolerance; and (4) the most effective means of translating this knowledge to inform prevention and treatment approaches. In an effort to fill this gap, the present book attempts to systematically distill information on the nature of distress tolerance and its associations with related variables as well as psychological symptoms and disorders. In the present chapter, we provide a relatively brief overview of the distress tolerance literature by clarifying its historical underpinnings, theoretical bases, and various measurement tools and techniques. Initially, we highlight distinctions between distress tolerance and theoretically related constructs. Thereafter, we describe key distress tolerance constructs, measures of distress tolerance constructs, and their postulated theoretical bases and summarize how they have been used in empirical research. Our broad intention is to provide a contextual framework for distress tolerance research as an introduction to the following chapters in this volume.

## DISTINGUISHING DISTRESS TOLERANCE FROM OTHER CONSTRUCTS

Perspectives on distress tolerance constructs generally pertain to tolerance of various types of experiential distress. For example, some models are theoretically oriented with respect to tolerance for aversive physical sensations (Schmidt & Cook, 1999), whereas others are focused more generally on noxious emotional states (Simons & Gaher, 2005), or the possibility of personal threat as a result of ambiguous (Furnham & Ribchester, 1995) and uncertain (Dugas, Gagnon, Ladouceur, & Freeston, 1998) life circumstances. Although there are indeed important distinctions between these specific models of distress tolerance, these perspectives are all broadly related to "experiential states" that tend to be subjectively aversive or personally threatening in some way (e.g., negative emotions, bodily perturbations). The degree to which they are experienced as aversive reflects individual differences related presumably to individual differences in tolerance of such states. Such a viewpoint is consistent with basic models of affective processing positing that aversive experiential states (e.g., negative affect) are directly linked to emotional reactivity and to biobehavioral adaptation more generally (Lang, 1994). It should be noted that this focus on experiential distress does not intend to suggest that explanatory or clinical merit cannot ultimately be found for tolerance of appetitive experiential states (e.g., positive affect); rather, it simply reflects the current state of behavioral science focused on the distress tolerance construct.

There also is variability in the conceptual and operational definition of the term *tolerance* in the existing literature. Most perspectives on tolerance of distress denote an individual difference in the extent to which a person withstands a certain form and degree of personal discomfort or threat (experiential distress; Otto et al., 2005; Simons & Gaher, 2005). It is, therefore, a construct that encompasses cognitive, affective, and behavioral features.

Inspection of the existing distress tolerance literature indicates that this construct is generally theorized to be related to other affect regulation and sensitivity factors and processes (e.g., Brown et al., 2005; Frenkel-Brunswik, 1948; Hajek, 1991; Schmidt & Cook, 1999; Simons & Gaher, 2005). Although related within a broader nomological network of risk and protective processes, distress tolerance is posited to be distinct conceptually from these other variables, as we describe later (Simons &

Gaher, 2005). Distress tolerance has most typically been linked to the following constructs: experiential avoidance (Hayes et al., 1999); emotional suppression (Richards & Gross, 2000); avoidant (Folkman & Lazarus, 1986) or disengagement coping (Compas, Connor-Smith, Saltzman, Thomsen, & Wadsworth, 2001); emotional dysregulation (Kashdan & Steger, 2006; Linehan, 1993; Rottenberg & Gross, 2003); anxiety sensitivity (McNally, 2002); personality-based perspectives on persistence (Barkley, 1997; Cloninger, Przybeck, & Švrakic, 1991); and perseveration (Ames, Cummings, Wirshing, Quinn, & Mahler, 1994).

Although specific conceptualizations of distress tolerance vary in their degree of overlap with putatively related constructs, in general, this construct is primarily focused on the perceived or actual behavioral capacity to withstand exposure to aversive or threatening stimuli (Brown et al., 2005; Simons & Gaher, 2005). At a global level, distress tolerance may be a function of automatic (e.g., unconscious) and effortful (e.g., voluntary) actions. In contrast, *experiential avoidance* theoretically subsumes a larger constellation of responses functionally aimed at altering the form or frequency of aversive internal experiences (e.g., negative thoughts, bodily sensations) and the contexts that occasion them (Hayes, Wilson, Gifford, Follette, & Strosahl, 1996). It is possible that distress tolerance is a specific type of experiential avoidant process (Hayes et al., 1999), although direct empirical work examining this question is currently lacking. Likewise, *emotional suppression* is generally defined as purposively inhibiting ongoing emotional experiences (Gross, 1998), whereas distress tolerance may or may not actually involve the suppression of an elicited affective state. Thus, distress tolerance and emotional suppression are not conceptually identical constructs. Similarly, *avoidant coping and disengagement coping*, although defined in different ways (Compas et al., 2001; Eisenberg, Fabes, & Guthrie, 1997; Skinner, 1995), from a contemporary perspective, generally reflect conscious, voluntary attempts to manage internal or external stressors that an individual perceives as exceeding psychological-based resources (Folkman & Lazarus, 1986). Furthermore, avoidant coping and disengagement coping are not individual-difference variables characterized by behavioral or perceived capacity to tolerate or persist in the experience of distress. Thus, unlike distress tolerance, such coping is a behavioral strategy and cognitive skill set that influences how one responds to unwanted stimuli, including distress. Distress tolerance may theoretically drive a variety of forms of avoidance, such as avoidant or disengagement coping or experiential avoidance such as suppression, but it is not conceptually one in the same as these (related) processes.

*Emotional dysregulation* involves multiple difficulties in emotional functioning and regulation (Cole, Michel, & Teti, 1994; Mennin, 2004;

Mennin, Heimberg, Turk, & Fresco, 2005; Salovey, Mayer, Goldman, Turvey, & Palfai, 1995). The Contemporary perspectives denote that emotional dysregulation reflects (1) difficulties in the self-regulation of affective states and (2) difficulties in self-control over affect-driven behaviors (Carver, Lawrence, & Scheier, 1996; Gross, 1998). From this perspective, tolerance of distress is a much narrower construct relative to emotional dysregulation. For example, distress tolerance could theoretically be conceptualized as a lower-order component of a higher order emotional dysregulation construct but not isomorphic with it. To the best of our knowledge, no research has been conducted that empirically documents that distress tolerance is, in fact, an aspect (component) of emotional dysregulation, although certain models of psychopathology implicitly allude to such an intriguing possibility (e.g., Linehan, 1993).

Distress tolerance also has been related to *anxiety sensitivity* (Bernstein, Zvolensky, Vujanovic, & Moos, 2009; Zvolensky & Otto, 2007). Anxiety sensitivity is the fear of anxiety and arousal-related sensations and their consequences (Reiss, Peterson, Gursky, & McNally, 1986). Although possibly related but distinct lower-order factors of a putative higher order affect tolerance and sensitivity factor (Bernstein et al., 2009), distress tolerance is not empirically or conceptually equivalent to anxiety sensitivity for a number of reasons. For example, distress tolerance is not related principally to the expectation of negative consequences of anxiety and other interoceptive sensations central to the anxiety sensitivity construct. As another example, although correlated, individual differences in anxiety sensitivity do not reflect cognitive or behavioral capacity to behaviorally tolerate and persist in the experience of unwanted distressing states (Bernstein et al., 2009).

The construct of *persistence* has been operationalized as an individual trait-like dimension of temperament related to propensity to maintain a behavior related to reward contingencies (Barkley, 1997; Cloninger et al., 1991). Models of personality, particularly those of Cloninger and colleagues (1991; Cloninger, Švrakic, & Przybeck, 1993), often suggest that persistence is a subtrait of higher order reward dependence construct. Similar perspectives have been offered in the context of learned industriousness theory (Eisenberger, Kuhlman, & Cotterell, 1992). Individuals at the higher end of variability on this trait tend to persist on tasks despite frustration and fatigue and to increase their task-specific responding when a reward is anticipated (Kose, 2003). From this perspective, persistence would be expected to be related to distress tolerance in the sense that persistence could involve features of distress tolerance (e.g., a propensity to be persistent may involve a willingness to tolerate negative subjective states such as frustration). However, these constructs also are distinct in that persistence typically focuses on reward achievement (Cloninger et al., 1991), whereas distress tolerance is not necessarily reward dependent.

Finally, distress tolerance can be distinguished from *perseveration*. Perseveration involves the tendency to persist in a behavioral pattern beyond a point where the activity is adaptive or rewarding (Ames et al., 1994). Perseveration is closely linked to certain safety-oriented behaviors that attempt to prevent a threat from being realized (e.g., agoraphobic avoidance aimed at preventing panic attacks in public situations; Salkovskis, 1996).

## DISTRESS TOLERANCE PERSPECTIVES: THEORY AND MEASUREMENT

Numerous distress tolerance constructs have been operationalized and studied in the psychopathology literature. As such, there is no single overarching theory that informs all of the work on this topic. As we discussed in the foregoing sections, most distress tolerance perspectives are informed to varying degrees by personality, self-regulation, coping, and, more recently, experiential avoidance literatures. Yet, given the diversity of distress tolerance research, it is important for reasons of clarity and specificity to narrow the focus and define the specific variables and how they are assessed. In this context, the theoretical basis of particular conceptualizations of distress tolerance can be better understood and, ultimately, competing perspectives compared, contrasted, and potentially integrated. Thus, we highlight (1) various perspectives on distress tolerance in the empirical literature and (2) how the constructs have been conceptualized and measured.

### Tolerance of Ambiguity

Perhaps the earliest conceptualization of a distress tolerance construct is *tolerance of ambiguity* (TOA; Frenkel-Brunswik, 1948, 1951, 1959; Hoffeditz & Guilford, 1935). TOA is operationalized as the way people perceive or process information about a situation or stimulus when faced with a set of complicated, foreign, and vague stimuli (Furnham & Ribchester, 1995). At a basic level, TOA is theorized to help "orient" individuals to social and other life situations, influencing affective (e.g., emotional reactivity), cognitive (e.g., how one perceives specific stimuli), and behavioral (e.g., how one copes with specific life events) processes. Informed largely by traditional personality theory, TOA is conceptualized as a stable (trait-like) individual-difference characteristic varying by degree across a single dimension (Budner, 1962). To the extent that individuals have relatively lower levels of TOA, they are expected to react with greater degrees of emotional distress (e.g., anxiety) and in a more impulsive or dysregulated manner (e.g., reactive cognitions and impulsive behaviors) when faced with an ambiguous situation. Furthermore, it is theorized that these individuals may be more apt to avoid such ambiguous stimuli in the future (Furnham & Ribchester, 1995). In contrast, individuals with relatively higher levels of TOA are theorized to perceive ambiguous stimuli as relatively nonthreatening and more personally challenging (Furnham & Ribchester, 1995).

A number of self-report instruments have been developed to assess TOA from a personality-oriented perspective (Budner, 1962; O'Connor, 1952; Rydell & Rosen, 1966). The assessment of TOA, therefore, has presumed a large volitional and self-awareness component. Available TOA measures are listed in Table 1.1. These instruments include the Walk's A Scale (O'Connor, 1952), the Scale of Tolerance–Intolerance of Ambiguity (Budner, 1962), the Rydell–Rosen Tolerance of Ambiguity Scale (Rydell & Rosen, 1966), the Measure of Ambiguity Tolerance Scale—20-item (MAT-20: MacDonald, 1970), the MAT-50 (Norton, 1975), a revision to the Rydell–Rosen scale and the MAT-20 by Kirton (1981), and the Situational Test of Intolerance of Ambiguity (Bhushan & Amal, 1986).

Historically, researchers have attempted to improve TOA scales listed in Table 1.1 by building on from one scale to the next in order to enhance the psychometric properties of such tools and refine the TOA construct (see Furnham & Ribchester, 1995, for a review). Thus, the TOA literature has had a relatively high degree of conceptual interconnection as it developed over time (Furnham & Ribchester, 1995). Despite this historical interconnection, TOA scales have been consistently criticized for lacking a clear operational definition and maintaining relatively poor psychometric properties (see Table 1.1; Ehrlich, 1965).

## Intolerance of Uncertainty

*Intolerance of uncertainty* (IU) has been studied most systematically and extensively in regard to generalized anxiety disorder (GAD), worry more generally, and to a lesser extent obsessive–compulsive and panic psychopathology (Dugas et al., 1998; Dugas, Buhr, & Ladouceur, 2004; Hedayati, Dugas, Buhr, & Francis, 2003; Tolin, Abramowitz, Brigidi, & Foa, 2003). IU is operationalized as individual differences in the tendency to react with limited tolerance (emotionally, cognitively, or behaviorally) to uncertain situations and events (Buhr & Dugas, 2002; Dugas, Schwartz, & Francis, 2004). IU has historically been theorized to be relatively stable and, therefore, akin to a trait-like factor (Dugas et al., 1998).

**TABLE 1.1. Self-Report Measures of Distress Tolerance**

| Distress tolerance construct | Format | Items | Internal consistency |
|---|---|---|---|
| Tolerance of ambiguity (TOA) | | | |
| Walk's A Scale (O'Connor, 1952) | 6-point Likert-type scale ranging from *agree* to *disagree* | 8 | $\alpha$ = .08–.10 (Ehrlich, 1965) |
| Scale of Tolerance–Intolerance of Ambiguity (Budner, 1962) | Forced choice: true–false *or* 6-point Likert-type scale ranging from *strongly agree* to *strongly disagree* | 16 | $\alpha$ = .49–.59 |
| Rydell–Rosen Tolerance of Ambiguity Scale (AT-16; Rydell & Rosen, 1966) from the Self–Other Test, Form C | Forced choice: true–false | 16 | No evidence of internal reliability (Furnham & Ribchester, 1995) |
| Measure of Ambiguity Tolerance Scale (MAT-20; MacDonald, 1970) | Forced choice: true–false | 20 | $\alpha$ = .63–.73 |
| MAT-50 (Norton, 1975) | 7-point Likert-type scale or forced choice yes–no | 55 | $\alpha$ = .75 |
| Tolerance of Ambiguity Scale—Revision to Budner, Rydell & Rosen, and MacDonald measures (Kirton, 1981) | Forced choice: true–false | 18 | $\alpha$ = .71 |
| Situational Test of Intolerance of Ambiguity (STIA; Bhushan & Amal, 1986), based on sample from India | 4-point Likert-type scale ranging from *always* to *never* | 40 | Not reported |
| Intolerance of uncertainty (IU) | | | |
| Intolerance of Uncertainty Scale (IUS—French Version; Freeston et al., 1994) | 5-point Likert scale ranging from *not at all* to *entirely* characteristic | 27 | $\alpha$ = .91 |
| IUS—English Version (Buhr & Dugas, 2002) | 5-point Likert scale ranging from *not at all* to *entirely* characteristic | 27 | $\alpha$ = 0.94 |
| IUS—short version (IUS-12; Carleton et al., 2007) | 5-point Likert scale ranging from *not at all* to *entirely* characteristic | 12 | $\alpha$ = .91 |

**TABLE 1.1.** (*continued*)

| Distress tolerance construct | Format | Items | Internal consistency |
| --- | --- | --- | --- |
| Discomfort intolerance | | | |
| Discomfort Intolerance (Schmidt et al., 2006) | 6-point Likert-type scale ranging from *not at all* to *extremely much like me* | 5 | α = .70 |
| Distress tolerance | | | |
| Distress Tolerance Scale (Simons & Gaher, 2005) | 5-point Likert scale ranging from *strongly agree* to *strongly disagree* | 15 | α = .82 |
| Frustration–Discomfort Scale (Harrington, 2005) | 5-point Likert scale ranging from *absent* to *very strong* | 28 | α = .94 |

The IU construct has been largely informed by cognitive-behavioral perspectives of GAD (Borkovec & Roemer, 1995; Craske 1999; Davey & Tallis, 1994). This GAD work has indicated both theoretically and empirically that worry often involves the prediction of potential future negative outcomes, and that such a prediction may permit a greater sense of perceived control or predictability over these outcomes (Borkovec & Roemer, 1995); such a process, for example, may conceivably foster greater preparatory time to problem solve or avoid the expected outcome (Stöber, 1998). Because day-to-day life experiences often involve uncertain events and outcomes, individual variation in the ability to tolerate uncertainty may be a central construct in understanding the degree to which persons may worry about and experience emotional distress (e.g., elevated state anxiety) in response to such stimuli (Dugas, Buhr, & Ladouceur, 2004). Although the IU construct may share some similarity to TOA, it is distinct from it in the sense that IU is expressly focused on tolerance for uncertain, future-oriented, rather than ambiguous, "here-and-now" life events (Greco & Roger, 2001; Grenier, Barrette, & Ladouceur, 2005). A basic distinction here is that uncertain life events are not necessarily ambiguous (e.g., the relative success of a relationship could involve unexpected outcomes, but the relationship itself is not ambiguous; Greco & Roger, 2001).

Historically, IU has been studied through self-report inventories primarily among adult populations. Freeston, Rhéaume, Letarte, Dugas, and Ladouceur (1994) developed the Intolerance for Uncertainty Scale to measure the construct; both French and English versions of the scale have been successfully developed and tested (Buhr & Dugas, 2002). There have been a variety of factor solutions reported for the IU scales, with most indicating a four- to five-factor solution (see Table 1.1) (Buhr & Dugas, 2002; Freeston et al., 1994; Norton, 2005). It is likely that some of this variability in factor structure may be due to differing sample selection techniques used across studies and factor analytic approaches utilized to explore latent structure (Norton, 2005). Nonetheless, because of the varied factor structures reported in past work, in conjunction with the high interitem correlations, researchers have argued for a more refined IU scale (Carleton, Norton, & Asmundson, 2007). In one such pursuit, Carleton and colleagues (2007) developed an empirically promising 12-item IU scale. Their Intolerance of Uncertainty Scale (IUS-12) includes two factors: prospective anxiety (e.g., "Uncertainty keeps me from having a full life") and inhibitory anxiety (e.g., "Unforeseen events upset me greatly"). Initial work on the IUS-12 indicated it maintained acceptable degrees of internal consistency, and the two observed factors are moderately correlated with one another (Carleton et al., 2007).

## Discomfort Intolerance

Discomfort intolerance is operationalized as individual differences relating to the capacity to withstand uncomfortable physical sensations (Schmidt & Lerew, 1998; Schmidt, Richey, Cromer, & Buckner, 2007; Schmidt, Richey, & Fitzpatrick, 2006). In contrast to constructs that are delimited to specific internal stimuli such as pain (Feldner et al., 2006; Geisser, Robinson, & Pickren, 1992), discomfort intolerance has been conceptualized as relating to interoceptive (bodily) sensations that are uncomfortable, though not necessarily painful, to the individual more generally. Discomfort intolerance is theorized to be a relatively stable (trait-like) construct (Schmidt et al., 2006).

The core idea driving the study of discomfort intolerance is that persons less able to tolerate aversive physical sensations may be motivated to escape or avoid stimuli (e.g., public settings) or activities (e.g., exercise) that may trigger them (Schmidt & Lerew, 1998). If individuals high in discomfort intolerance consistently were unable to withstand physical stress and discomfort associated with fear and anxiety and, by extension, escaped or avoided it, they may place themselves at greater risk for maladaptive anxiety-relevant learning. For example, greater ability to tolerate physical stress (e.g., bodily sensations) may theoretically permit certain people to experience unwanted and feared sensations and/or develop a perceived sense of self-efficacy in experiencing and managing these otherwise unwanted states. This type of perspective is consistent with integrative theoretical models and intervention strategies that attempt to modify anxiety and other problematic emotional states by changing one's maladaptive (typically avoidant or change-oriented) responses to aversive interoceptive (e.g., bodily sensations) and exteroceptive (e.g., stressful life occurrences) events (Hayes & Shenk, 2004; Orsillo et al., 2003; Ramel et al., 2004).

To measure this construct, Schmidt and colleagues (2006) developed the Discomfort Intolerance Scale (DIS), a five-item self-report instrument that examines how much one can tolerate uncomfortable physical sensations. Factor analytic study, using principal-axis factoring, has indicated that the DIS is composed of a global higher order discomfort intolerance factor and two subfactors: intolerance of discomfort or pain (e.g., *"I can tolerate a great deal of physical discomfort" [reverse scored]*) and avoidance of physical discomfort (e.g., *"I take extreme measures to avoid feeling physically uncomfortable"*; Schmidt et al., 2006). Although limited in overall scope, the DIS has thus far demonstrated high levels of internal consistency (see Table 1.1).

## Distress Tolerance (for Negative Emotional States)

Simons and Gaher (2005) conceptualize distress tolerance as an individual's ability to withstand negative psychological states.[1] Whereas other distress tolerance concepts focus on how information is processed (TOA), worry as a consequent of uncertainty (IU), and unpleasant physical discomfort (discomfort intolerance), this perspective focuses on the capacity to withstand negative emotional states (Simons & Gaher, 2005). Simons and Gaher suggested that this distress tolerance construct is multidimensional in nature, involving an individual's anticipation of and experience with negative emotions, including (1) ability to tolerate the negative emotion, (2) assessment of the emotional situation as acceptable, (3) the individual's regulation of the emotion, and (4) the amount of attention absorbed by the negative emotion.

To measure distress tolerance from this perspective, Simons and Gaher (2005) developed the Distress Tolerance Scale (DTS), a 15-item self-report measure that examines one's perceived ability to tolerate emo-

---

[1]Distress tolerance is the general label most frequently given to the body of work reviewed in the current chapter (Zvolensky & Otto, 2007). It is important to recognize that Simons and Gaher (2005) use this same term to reflect a specific type of distress tolerance, as described in this review. Thus, distress tolerance has been used to represent (1) a global area of work and (2) a specific type of tolerance construct. In this section, we use the term *distress tolerance* to refer to the Simons and Gaher (2005) conceptualization. From this point forward in this chapter, however, we clarify whether we are referring to the Simons and Gaher (2005) perspective of the specific construct. In all other instances, it should be presumed we are referring to the putative higher order distress tolerance concept.

tional distress, with questions related to tolerance, appraisal, absorption, and regulation. Factor analytic work based on a relatively healthy college sample indicates a single higher order distress tolerance factor as well as four additional first-order factors: tolerance, appraisal, absorption, and regulation. Although independent psychometric evaluations of the DTS are currently lacking, the measure has thus far demonstrated promising initial psychometric properties (see Table 1.1). Consistent with the trait-like perspective of distress tolerance, the DTS appears to be relatively stable over a 6-month time period (Simons & Gaher, 2005).

## Frustration Tolerance

Harrington (2005) created a self-report measure of frustration tolerance, the Frustration-Discomfort Scale (FDS), the development of which was informed by rational-emotive behavior therapy and the associated conceptualization of intolerance of frustration and discomfort. The scale consists of 28 items and was developed and evaluated on a sample of 254 clinical and 79 nonclinical individuals. Initial work suggests the FDS is multidimensional, consisting of four seven-item subscales, each with good internal consistency: Discomfort Intolerance ($\alpha$ = .88)—demands that life should be easy, comfortable, and free of hassle; Entitlement ($\alpha$ = .85 )—demands for immediate gratification; Emotional Intolerance ($\alpha$ = .87)—beliefs regarding uncertainty, controllability, and aversiveness of emotion; and Achievement Frustration ($\alpha$ = .84)—experiencing difficulties when seeking a specified goal. It is noteworthy that psychometric analysis did not indicate a higher order FDS factor or a global variable of frustration tolerance; however, the full-scale mean interitem correlations for the four-factor model demonstrate strong internal consistency (Table 1.1; $\alpha$ = .94; Harrington, 2005).

## Physical Tolerance Tasks

In addition to self-report measures, there have been a number of approaches used to measure the duration of time an individual can withstand exposure to a specific type of aversive stimulus or task. These assessment procedures, namely thermal stress tolerance and biological challenge (reviewed later), have been used to reflect a behavioral or biologically informed perspective of distress tolerance. *These tasks have been developed without specific reference to a particular conceptual model or theory of distress tolerance.*

One line of work focused on tolerance for physical distress is *thermal stress tolerance.* Research within this area has addressed how individuals tolerate stressful thermal conditions (Hancock, Ross, & Szalma, 2007);

this work is, therefore, oriented on acute physical distress tolerance to specific (thermal) stimuli. There has been little described about the relative stability of this type of thermal stress tolerance over time. However, this body of work implicitly operates from the perspective that variation in thermal stress tolerance is relatively stable for an individual over time, although it could be impacted (e.g., increased or decreased) through exposure-based learning (e.g., repeated exposure to thermal stress exposure may increase the ability to withstand thermal stress) and other contextual factors (e.g., current stress level; Hancock et al., 2007).

Thermal tolerance has primarily been induced through partial body exposures or water immersion (e.g., cold pressor) (Hines & Brown, 1932). The cold-pressor task, for example, involves continual application of an aversive, but safe (i.e., no permanent tissue damage), cold stimulus. Most procedures involve the immersion of an individual's hand, at least up to the wrist, in ice water, typically 1°C (33°F), with instructions to keep the hand still (e.g., Burns, Bruehl, & Caceres, 2004; Hines & Brown, 1932; Neufeld & Thomas, 1977; Willoughby, Hailey, Mulkana, & Rowe, 2002). Pain *threshold* is determined by measuring the time it takes for the individual to indicate to the experimenter that he or she feels "pain" (e.g., Burns et al., 2004; Hines & Brown, 1932; Willoughby et al., 2002) or "discomfort" (Neufeld & Thomas, 1977). *Tolerance* is defined as the time it takes for an individual to report that the pain or discomfort is no longer tolerable and/or to terminate the procedure by removing his or her hand (e.g., Burns et al., 2004; Hines & Brown, 1932; Neufeld & Thomas, 1977). *Endurance* is measured as tolerance minus threshold (Neufeld & Thomas, 1977). It should be noted that, for the purposes of the present review, the tolerance variable and perhaps the endurance variable are most relevant to distress tolerance processes. If the participant has not demonstrated intolerance within 5 minutes, the procedure is generally terminated in order to prevent possible harm (Hackett & Horan, 1980; Neufeld & Thomas, 1977; Willoughby et al., 2002). Some procedures prompt participants to assess their level of discomfort periodically throughout the procedure using a rating scale (e.g., Hackett & Horan, 1980; Willoughby et al., 2002).

Thermal stress has additionally been induced experimentally through whole-body air temperature exposures (see Hancock et al., 2007; Pilcher, Nadler, & Busch, 2002, for reviews). Whole-body methods of examining cold thermal stress (temperatures typically less than 65°F [18.33°C]) (e.g., Sharma & Panwar, 1987; Thomas, Ahlers, House, & Schrot, 1989; van Orden, Benoit, & Osga, 1996) are less common than methodologies used to induce heat thermal stress (temperatures of at least 70°F) (e.g., Hocking, Silberstein, Lau, Stough, & Roberts, 2001; Hygge & Knez, 2001; Razmjou, 1996; Razmjou & Kjellberg, 1992). These procedures typically include exposure to cold (less than 65°F) or hot (greater than 70°F) stimuli over an extended period of time. Temperatures of 90°F or above or 50°F and below are most reliably and strongly related to detrimental cognitive-related task performance (Pilcher et al., 2002).

Radiant heat stimulation also has been used in various procedures to induce cutaneous (skin surface) pain and to measure related tolerance and threshold ratings. Most methods include the application of lightbulb heat to a darkened area of the forehead (Kane, Nutter, & Weckowicz, 1971; Wolff & Jarvik, 1963), wrist (Orbach et al., 1996; Procacci, 1979), or finger of the dominant hand (Rhudy & Meagher, 2003). Participants are asked to indicate when a feeling of warmth changes to a feeling of pain or induces notable bodily sensations (Kane et al., 1971; Rudy & Meagher, 2003); this measurement has been typically referred to as a measure of thermal heat tolerance (Wolff & Jarvik, 1963). To the extent that the measurement is focused expressly on the detection of body temperature changes, however, it may possibly be more akin to an index of sensitivity to thermal heat.

Furthermore, distress tolerance has been examined with respect to behavioral responding to several other procedures, collectively described as *biological challenge tasks*. These are procedures used to manipulate individual oxygen and carbon dioxide ($CO_2$) levels in order to induce physiological activity associated with anxious arousal (Zvolensky & Eifert, 2000). For example, breath holding, voluntary hyperventilation, and inhalation of normal room air with higher concentrations of $CO_2$ have all been used as paradigms to measure tolerance to anxious arousal and related distress or discomfort (Zvolensky & Eifert, 2000).

Breath holding is typically measured with the functional residual capacity estimate of breath-holding duration, whereby participants breathe normally for 30 seconds, completely exhale on the experimenter's instruction, and then inhale and hold their breath for as long as possible; this procedure is then repeated after a 60-second rest period. The longer duration for the two trials is used as the index of maximum breath-holding duration (Hajek, 1991; Hajek et al., 1987; Zvolensky, Feldner, Eifert, & Brown, 2001).

The $CO_2$ challenge task developed by Brown and colleagues (2005) to specifically assess distress tolerance lasts 15 minutes and includes two 20% $CO_2$ presentations set to occur at 7 minutes and 12 minutes. The first presentation lasts 25 seconds, while participants determine the length of the final presentation. That is, once the final presentation has begun, participants may opt to terminate the presentation by pressing a button on the provided computer keyboard. The duration of time to the button press is the behavioral measure of distress tolerance. Unbeknownst to participants, if a button press is not made within 60 seconds, the task self-terminates (i.e., at maximum duration, the presentation automatically terminates). This same type of distress tolerance format also has been adapted for voluntary hyperventilation (Marshall et al., 2008).

## Cognitive Tolerance Tasks

Like physical tolerance tasks, a number of approaches have been used to measure the duration of time an individual can withstand exposure to specific types of difficult or frustrating tasks designed to tax cognitive or related psychological resources. The paced auditory serial addition task (PASAT), mirror-tracing task, and anagram persistence task (APT) have been applied as measures of tolerance for psychological or cognitive frustration. The PASAT is a visual and auditory serial addition task originally developed by Gronwall and Sampson (1974) as an index of information processing. Subsequent work suggested that it is better described as an index that taps multiple cognitive functions such as attention, working memory, and ability to perform under time constraints (e.g., Madigan, DeLuca, Diamond, Tramontano, & Averill, 2000). Although the PASAT has been used primarily as an index of sustained attention and concentration, researchers have noted the difficulty associated with its use and its tendency to elicit perceived stress and negative affect as well as unwillingness to engage in—or propensity to terminate—the task early among participants (Tombaugh, 2006). For example, Holdwick and Wingenfeld (1999) found that self-reported negative affect, as measured by the Multiple Affect Adjective Checklist (Zuckerman, Lubin, & Rinck, 1983), increased as a result of PASAT administration.

With the original PASAT, participants are presented, either visually or orally, with a series of single-digit numbers and are instructed to continually sum the two most recently presented digits (Tombaugh, 2006). They must correctly respond prior to the presentation of the next digit in order to receive a correct response score. Each set typically consists of 60 trials, or opportunities to correctly respond, and each trial consists of a set interstimulus interval (ISI), which is the amount of time between digit presentations. Many researchers use several ISIs across several trials and may choose certain trial lengths based on the population being investigated and the potential of ISIs to detect group differences (Tombaugh, 2006).

Lejuez, Kahler, and Brown (2003) proposed a modified, computerized version of the PASAT, or PASAI-C, consisting of three corresponding levels: Level 1—low difficulty (3 minutes); Level 2—medium difficulty (5 minutes); and Level 3—high difficulty (10 minutes). Two formats have been used: in one participants select their response using the computer mouse, and in the other participants provide their response verbally (e.g.,

Daughters, Lejuez, Kahler, Strong, & Brown, 2005). During administration of the PASAT-C, Level 1 transitions immediately into Level 2. Level 2 is followed by a 2-minute rest period before participants are prompted to complete Level 3. Participants are told that at some point during Level 3 they will be given the option to terminate the procedure, but that their reward is contingent on their level of performance. Psychological distress tolerance using the PASAT-C is indexed as time in seconds until task termination of Level 3 (Lejuez et al., 2003). Participants are told they will be awarded one point for each correct response, and incorrect scores or failure to respond will not impact their score. Unbeknownst to the participant, the task self-terminates within 7 to 10 minutes (Daughters et al., 2005; Lejuez et al., 2003). Prior to the task as well as after Level 2, measurement of dysphoria, including self-reported anxiety, difficulty concentrating, bodily discomfort, and irritability, can be obtained to ensure that levels of psychological stress are adequate (demonstration of significant difference between baseline and post–Level 2 dysphoria ratings) (Brown, Lejuez, Kahler, & Strong, 2002). This dysphoria scale has demonstrated acceptable internal reliability ($\alpha = .69$) (Daughters et al., 2005). In addition, Lejuez and colleagues (2003) have found evidence for the PASAT-C in increasing physiological arousal, most strongly evidenced in skin conductance changes but also in heart rate response.

Mirror tracing is another task used to index tolerance to cognitive or psychological frustration or distress. This methodology requires participants to trace the outline of a geometric figure, often a star, while viewing it through a mirror—or as though they are viewing the object through a mirror—thereby demanding a high degree of motor control (Matthews & Stoney, 1988; Quinn, Brandon, & Copeland, 1996). Because of the mirror viewpoint, participants must move the tracer in the exact opposite direction of where they intend for it to go while tracing the star. Each time the tracer falls off the outline of the star, an irritating auditory tone is emitted (Matthews & Stoney, 1988). Performance on this task is determined as the percentage of time during the trial that the tracer is off the figure (Matthews & Stoney, 1988). Research indicates that engagement in this task results in a substantial increase in blood pressure, heart rate, and self-reported stress as well as frustration (Krantz, Manuck, & Wing, 1986; Matthews & Stoney, 1988; Tutoo, 1971).

In research utilizing mirror tracing as a measure of distress tolerance, participants are typically given two practice trials consisting of simple line images that help orient them to the task (Daughters et al., 2005; Quinn et al., 1996). These lines are followed by one or more complex drawings that are extremely difficult, or practically impossible, to trace with accuracy (Daughters et al., 2005; Quinn et al., 1996). Participants are encouraged to try their best and, in some cases, told that their level of performance will impact their monetary compensation (Daughters et al., 2005; Strong et al., 2003). When faced with the complex figures, participants are given the option of discontinuing at any time or moving on once they have completed the figure (Daughters et al., 2005; Quinn et al., 1996). Similar to the PASAT task, after 5 minutes, presentation of the object terminates. When using the task as a measure of distress tolerance, tolerance is measured as the average time spent on tasks that the individual was unable to complete (Daughters et al., 2005; Quinn et al., 1996). Brandon and colleagues (2003) found that the mirror tracing demonstrated good internal consistency when used among a sample of daily smokers ($\alpha = .92$).

A final cognitive task used to induce distress is the APT (Eisenberger & Leonard, 1980). Participants are presented with anagrams, which may range in level of difficulty (Mayzner & Tresselt, 1966), and are told by the experimenter that each presentation contains letters that can be rearranged to form a word. Participants are then asked to either indicate to the experimenter (e.g., by raising hand or verbally; Postman & Solomon, 1950) that they have reached a solution in order to receive a point or to move on to the next presentation stimulus if they cannot solve the word (Eisenberger & Leonard, 1980). It is noteworthy here that the points were simply given as an indication of the number of anagrams accurately solved and not as a reward. Participants are typically given a distinct amount of time in order to solve the anagram (e.g., 3 minutes; Brandon et al., 2003) and are directed to move on to the next card if they do not respond within the time allotted (Eisenberger & Leonard, 1980). For procedures in which the APT is used as a measure of persistence or tolerance, the average time spent on difficult or not-completed anagrams before giving up and proceeding to the next is used as the individual's score (e.g. Quinn et al., 1996). Brandon and colleagues (2003) found that the APT demonstrated good reliability ratings across six trials each when used with a sample of smokers ($\alpha = .85$).

## SUMMARY

Distress tolerance has increasingly been viewed as a potentially important construct in developing new insights about the onset and maintenance of adult psychopathology as well as its prevention and treatment (Zvolensky & Otto, 2007). In the current chapter, we discuss conceptual distinctions between distress tolerance and theoretically related variables, provide an overview of the historical development of distress tolerance research, and highlight a variety of conceptual models and multimethod measures of the constructs. Given the diversity in conceptual models and indices of distress tolerance in the extant literature, our intention for the present chapter was to specifically define the constructs and their measurement because doing so may be imperative to advancing the empirical and theoretical literature on this topic. The remaining chapters in this volume help elucidate the ways in which distress tolerance may relate to specific psychopathological processes and disorders. In the final chapter, we return to the key issues raised within this volume in an effort to synthesize knowledge gained to date and to inform possible future directions in the study of distress tolerance.

## REFERENCES

Ames, D., Cummings, J. L., Wirshing, W. C., Quinn, B., & Mahler, M. (1994). Repetitive and compulsive behavior in frontal lobe degenerations. *Journal of Neuropsychiatry and Clinical Neurosciences, 6,* 100–113.

Barkley, R. A. (1997). Attention-deficit/hyperactivity disorder, self-regulation, and time: Toward a more comprehensive theory. *Journal of Developmental and Behavioral Pediatrics, 18,* 271–279.

Barlow, D. H., Allen, L., & Choate, M. (2004). Toward a unified treatment for emotional disorders. *Behavior Therapy, 35,* 205–230.

Bernstein, A., Zvolensky, M. J., Vujanovic, A. A., & Moos, R. (2009). Integrating anxiety sensitivity, distress tolerance, and discomfort intolerance: A hierarchical model of affect sensitivity and tolerance. *Behavior Therapy, 40,* 291–301.

Bhushan, L., & Amal, S. (1986). A situational test of intolerance of ambiguity. *Psychologia, 29,* 254–261.

Borkovec, T., & Roemer, L. (1995). Perceived functions of worry among generalized anxiety disorder subjects: Distraction from more emotionally distressing topics? *Journal of Behavior Therapy and Experimental Psychiatry, 26,* 25–30.

Brandon, T. H., Herzog, T. A., Juliano, L. M., Irvin, J. E., Lazev, A. B., & Nath Simmons, V. (2003). Pretreatment task persistence predicts smoking cessation outcome. *Journal of Abnormal Psychology, 112,* 448–456.

Brown, R. A, Lejuez, C. W., Kahler, C. W., & Strong, D. R. (2002). Distress tolerance and duration of past smoking cessation attempts. *Journal of Abnormal Psychology, 111,* 180–185.

Brown, R. A., Lejuez, C. W., Kahler, C. W., Strong, D. R., & Zvolensky, M. J. (2005). Distress tolerance and early smoking lapse (theory and clinical implications). *Clinical Psychology Review, 25,* 713–733.

Budner, S. (1962). Intolerance of ambiguity as a personality variable. *Journal of Personality, 30,* 29–50.

Buhr, K., & Dugas, M. J. (2002). The Intolerance of Uncertainty Scale: Psychometric properties of the English version. *Behaviour Research and Therapy, 40,* 931–945.

Burns, J., Bruehl, S., & Caceres, C. (2004). Anger management style, blood pressure reactivity, and acute pain sensitivity: Evidence for "trait × situation" models. *Annals of Behavioral Medicine, 27,* 195–204.

Carleton, R. N., Norton, P. J., & Asmundson, G. J. G. (2007). Fearing the unknown: A short version of the Intolerance of Uncertainty Scale. *Journal of Anxiety Disorders, 21,* 105–117.

Carver, C. S, Lawrence, J. W., & Scheier, M. F. (1996). A control-process perspective on the origins of affect. In L. L. Martin & A. Tesser (Eds.), *Striving and feeling: Interactions among goals, affect, and self-regulation* (pp. 11–52). Hillsdale, NJ: Erlbaum.

Chaney, E., Roszell, D., & Cummings, C. (1982). Relapse in opiate addicts: A behavioral analysis. *Addictive Behaviors, 7,* 291–297.

Cloninger, C. R., Przybeck, T. R., & Švrakic, D. M. (1991). The Tridimensional Personality Questionnaire: U.S. normative data. *Psychological Reports, 69,* 1047–1057.

Cloninger, C. R., Švrakic, D. M., & Przybeck, T. R. (1993). A psychobiological model of temperament and character. *Archives of General Psychiatry, 50,* 975–990.

Cole, P., Michel, M., & Teti, L. (1994). The development of emotion regulation and dysregulation: A clinical perspective. *Monographs of the Society for Research in Child Development, 59,* 73–100.

Compas, B., Connor-Smith, J., Saltzman, H., Thomsen, A., & Wadsworth, M. (2001). Coping with stress during childhood and adolescence: Problems, progress, and potential in theory and research. *Psychological Bulletin, 127,* 87–127.

Craske, M. (1999). *Anxiety disorders: Psychological approaches to theory and treatment.* Boulder, CO: Westview Press.

Daughters, S. B., Lejuez, C. W., Kahler, C. W., Strong, D. R., & Brown, R. A. (2005). Psychological distress tolerance and duration of most recent abstinence attempt among residential treatment-seeking substance abusers. *Psychology of Addictive Behaviors, 19,* 208–211.

Davey, G., & Tallis, F. (1994). *Worrying: Perspectives on theory, assessment and treatment.* Oxford, UK: Wiley.

Dugas, M. J., Buhr, K., & Ladouceur, R. (2004). The role of intolerance of uncertainty in etiology and maintenance. In R. G. Heimberg, C. L. Turk, & D. S. Mennin (Eds.), *Generalized anxiety disorder: Advances in research and practice* (pp. 143–163). New York: Guilford Press.

Dugas, M. J., Gagnon, F., Ladouceur, R., & Freeston, H. (1998). Generalized anxiety disorder: A preliminary test of a conceptual model. *Behavior Therapy and Research, 36,* 215–226.

Dugas, M. J., Schwartz, A., & Francis, K. (2004). Intolerance of uncertainty, worry, and depression. *Cognitive Therapy and Research, 28,* 835–842.

Ehrlich, D. (1965). "Intolerance of ambiguity," Walk's A scale: Historical comment. *Psychological Reports, 17,* 591–594.

Eisenberg, N., Fabes, R., & Guthrie, I. (1997). Coping with stress: The roles of regulation and development. In S. Wolchik & I. N. Sandler (Eds.), *Handbook of children's coping: Linking theory and intervention* (pp. 41–70). New York: Plenum Press.

Eisenberger, R., Kuhlman, D., & Cotterell, N. (1992). Effects of social values, effort training, and goal structure on task persistence. *Journal of Research in Personality, 26,* 258–272.

Eisenberger, R., & Leonard, J. M. (1980). Effects of conceptual task difficulty on generalized persistence. *American Journal of Psychology, 93,* 285–298.

Feldner, M., Hekmat, H., Zvolensky, M., Vowles, K., Secrist, Z., & Leen-Feldner, E. (2006). The role of experiential avoidance in acute pain tolerance: A laboratory test. *Journal of Behavior Therapy and Experimental Psychiatry, 37,* 146–158.

Folkman, S., & Lazarus, R. (1986). Stress processes and depressive symptomatology. *Journal of Abnormal Psychology, 95,* 107–113.

Freeston, M. H., Rhéaume, J., Letarte, H., Dugas, M. J., & Ladouceur, R. (1994). Why do people worry? *Personality and Individual Differences, 17,* 791–802.

Frenkel-Brunswik, E. (1948). Review of personality: A biosocial approach to origins and structure. *Psychological Bulletin, 45,* 348–351.

Frenkel-Brunswik, E. (1951). Personality theory and perception. In R. R. Blake & G. V. Ramsey (Eds.), *Perception: An approach to personality* (pp. 356–419). New York: Ronald Press.

Frenkel-Brunswik, E. (1959). Meaning of psychoanalytic concepts and confirmation of psychoanalytic theories. In M. Levitt (Ed.), *Readings in psychoanalytic psychology* (pp. 29–42). East Norwalk, CT: Appleton-Century-Crofts.

Furnham, A., & Ribchester, T. (1995). Tolerance of ambiguity: A review of the concept, its measurement and applications. *Current Psychology, 14,* 179–199.

Geisser, M., Robinson, M., & Pickren, W. (1992). Differences in cognitive coping strategies among pain-sensitive and pain-tolerant individuals on the cold-pressor test. *Behavior Therapy, 23,* 31–41.

Greco, V., & Roger, D. (2001). Coping with uncertainty: The construction and validation of a new measure. *Personality and Individual Differences, 31,* 519–534.

Grenier, S., Barrette, A., & Ladouceur, R. (2005). Intolerance of uncertainty and intolerance of ambiguity: Similarities and differences. *Personality and Individual Differences, 39,* 593–600.

Gronwall, D., & Sampson, H. (1974). *The psychological effects of concussion.* Oxford, UK: Auckland University Press.

Gross, J. (1998). The emerging field of emotion regulation. *Review of General Psychology, 2,* 271–299.

Gross, J., & Muñoz, R. (1995). Emotion regulation and mental health. *Clinical Psychology: Science and Practice, 2,* 151–164.

Hackett, G., & Horan, J. J. (1980). Stress inoculation for pain: What's really going on? *Journal of Counseling Psychology, 27,* 107–116.

Hajek, P. (1991). Individual differences in difficulty quitting smoking. *British Journal of Addiction, 86,* 555–558.

Hajek, P., Belcher, M., & Stapleton, J. (1987). Breath-holding endurance as a predictor of success in smoking cessation. *Addictive Behaviors, 12,* 285–288.

Hancock, P. A., Ross, J. M., & Szalma, J. L. (2007). A meta-analysis of perfor-mance response under thermal stressors. *Human Factors, 49,* 851–877.

Harrington, N. (2005). The Frustration Discomfort Scale: Development and Psychometric Properties. *Clinical Psychology and Psychotherapy, 12,* 374–387.

Hayes, S., & Shenk, C. (2004). Operationalizing mindfulness without unneces-sary attachments. *Clinical Psychology: Science and Practice, 11,* 249–254.

Hayes, S. C., Strosahl, K. D., & Wilson, K. G. (1999). *Acceptance and commit-ment therapy: An experiential approach to behavior change.* New York: Guilford Press.

Hayes, S., Wilson, K., Gifford, E., Follette, V., & Strosahl, K. (1996). Experien-tial avoidance and behavioral disorders: A functional dimensional approach to diagnosis and treatment. *Journal of Consulting and Clinical Psychology, 64,* 1152–1168.

Hedayati, M., Dugas, M. J., Buhr, K., & Francis, K. (2003, November). *The relationship between intolerance of uncertainty and the interpretation of ambiguous and unambiguous information.* Poster presented at the annual conference for the Association for Advancement of Behavior Therapy, Bos-ton.

Hines, E. A., & Brown, G. E. (1932). A standard stimulus for measuring vasomo-tor reactions: Its application in the study of hypertension. *Proceedings of the Staff Meeting of the Mayo Clinic, 7,* 332–335.

Hocking, C., Silberstein, R. B., Lau, W. M., Stough, C., & Roberts, W. (2001). Evaluation of cognitive performance in the heat by functional brain imaging and psychometric testing. *Comparative Biochemistry and Physiology—A Molecular and Integrative Physiology, 128,* 719–734.

Hoffeditz, E. L., & Guilford, J. P. (1935). The factors present in the fluctuations of fifteen ambiguous phenomena. *Psychological Bulletin, 32,* 726–727.

Holdwick, D., & Wingenfeld, S. (1999). The subjective experience of PASAT testing: Does the PASAT induce negative mood? *Archives of Clinical Neu-ropsychology, 14,* 273–284.

Hygge, S., & Knez, I. (2001). Effects of noise, heat and indoor lighting on cogni-tive performance and self-reported affect. *Journal of Environmental Psy-chology, 21,* 291–299.

Kabat-Zinn, J., Lipworth, L., Burney, R., & Sellers, W. (1987). Four-year follow-up of a meditation based program for the self-regulation of chronic pain: Treatment outcomes and compliance. *Clinical Journal of Pain, 2,* 159–173.

Kane, E., Nutter, R., & Weckowicz, T. (1971). Response to cutaneous pain in mental hospital patients. *Journal of Abnormal Psychology, 77,* 52–60.

Kashdan, T., & Steger, M. (2006). Expanding the topography of social anxiety: An experience-sampling assessment of positive emotions, positive events, and emotion suppression. *Psychological Science, 17,* 120–128.

Kirton, M. J. (1981). A reanalysis of two scales of tolerance of ambiguity. *Journal of Personality Assessment, 45,* 407–414.

Kose, S. (2003). A psychobiological model of temperament and character: TCI. *Yeni Symposium: Psikiyatri, Nöroloji ve Davranis Bilimleri Dergisi, 41,* 86–97.

Krantz, D. S., Manuck, S. B., & Wing. R. R. (1986). Psychological stressors and task variables as elicitors of reactivity. In K. A. Matthews, S. M. Weiss, B. Faulkner, T. Dembroski, & T. Detre (Eds.), *Handbook of stress, reactivity, and cardiovascular disease* (pp. 85–107). New York: Wiley.

Lang, P. (1994). The motivational organization of emotion: Affect–reflex connections. In *Emotions: Essays on emotion theory* (pp. 61–93). Hillsdale, NJ: Erlbaum.

Lejeuz, C. W., Kahler, C. W., & Brown, R. A. (2003). A modified computer version of the paced auditory serial addition task (PASAT) as a laboratory-based stressor. *The Behavior Therapist, 26,* 290–293.

Linehan, M. M. (1993a). *Cognitive-behavioral treatment of borderline personality disorder.* New York: Guilford Press.

Linehan, M. M. (1993b). *Skills training manual for treating borderline personality disorder.* New York: Guilford Press.

Lynch, T. R., & Bronner, L. L. (2006). Mindfulness and dialectical behavior therapy (DBT): Application with depressed older adults with personality disorders. In R. A. Baer (Ed.), *Mindfulness-based treatment approaches: Clinician's guide to evidence base and applications* (pp. 217–236). San Diego, CA: Academic Press.

MacDonald, A. (1970). Revised scale for ambiguity tolerance: Reliability and validity. *Psychological Reports, 26,* 791–798.

Madigan, N., DeLuca, J., Diamond, B., Tramontano, G., & Averill, A. (2000). Speed of information processing in traumatic brain injury: Modality-specific factors. *Journal of Head Trauma Rehabilitation, 15,* 943–956.

Marshall, E., Zvolensky, M., Vujanovic, A., Gregor, K., Gibson, L., & Leyro, T. (2008). Panic reactivity to voluntary hyperventilation challenge predicts distress tolerance to bodily sensations among daily cigarette smokers. *Experimental and Clinical Psychopharmacology, 16,* 313–321.

Matthews, K. A., & Stoney, C. M. (1988). Influences of sex and age on cardiovascular responses during stress. *Psychosomatic Medicine, 50,* 46–56.

Mayzner, M. S., & Tresselt, M. E. (1966). Anagram solution times: A function of multiple-solution anagrams. *Journal of Experimental Psychology, 71,* 66–73.

McNally, R. J. (2002). Anxiety sensitivity and panic disorder. *Biological Psychiatry, 52,* 938–946.

Mennin, D. (2004). Emotion regulation therapy for generalized anxiety disorder. *Clinical Psychology and Psychotherapy, 11,* 17–29.

Mennin, D., Heimberg, R., Turk, C., & Fresco, D. (2002). Applying an emotion regulation framework to integrative approaches to generalized anxiety disorder. *Clinical Psychology: Science and Practice, 9,* 85–90.

Mennin, D., Heimberg, R., Turk, C., & Fresco, D. (2005). Preliminary evidence for an emotion dysregulation model of generalized anxiety disorder. *Behaviour Research and Therapy, 43,* 1281–1310.

Neufeld, R. W. J., & Thomas, P. (1977). Effects of perceived efficacy of a prophylactic controlling mechanism on self-control under pain stimulation. *Canadian Journal of Behavioral Science, 9,* 224–232.

Norton, P. J. (2005). A psychometric analysis of the Intolerance of Uncertainty Scale among four racial groups. *Anxiety Disorders, 19,* 699–707.

Norton, R. W. (1975). Measure of ambiguity tolerance. *Journal of Personality Assessment, 39,* 607–619.

O'Connor, P. (1952). Ethnocentrism, "intolerance of ambiguity," and abstract reasoning ability. *Journal of Abnormal and Social Psychology, 47,* 526–530.

Orsillo, S. M., & Roemer, L. (2005). *Acceptance and mindfulness-based approaches to anxiety: Conceptualization and treatment.* New York: Springer Science + Business Media.

Orsillo, S. M., Roemer, L., & Barlow, D. (2003). Integrating acceptance and mindfulness into existing cognitive-behavioral treatment for GAD: A case study. *Cognitive and Behavioral Practice, 10,* 222–230.

Otto, M., Powers, M., & Fischmann, D. (2005). Emotional exposure in the treatment of substance use disorders: Conceptual model, evidence, and future directions. *Clinical Psychology Review, 25,* 824–839.

Pilcher, J. J., Nadler, E., & Busch, C. (2002). Effects of hot and cold temperature exposure on performance: A meta-analytic review. *Ergonomics, 45,* 682–698.

Postman, L., & Solomon, R. (1950). Perceptual sensitivity to completed and incompleted tasks. *Journal of Personality, 18,* 347–357.

Procacci, P. (1979). Methods for the study of pain threshold in man. In J. J. Bonica, J. C. Leibskind, & D. G. Albe-Fessard (Eds.), *Advances in pain research and therapy* (Vol. 3, pp. 781–970). New York: Raven Press.

Quinn, E. P., Brandon, T. H., & Copeland, A. L. (1996). Is task persistence related to smoking and substance abuse: The application of learned industriousness theory to addictive behaviors. *Experimental and Clinical Psychopharmacology, 4,* 186–190.

Ramel, W., Goldin, P., Carmona, P., & McQuaid, J. (2004). The effects of mindfulness meditation on cognitive processes and affect in patients with past depression. *Cognitive Therapy and Research, 28,* 433–455.

Razmjou, S. (1996). Mental workload in heat: Toward a framework for analyses of stress states. *Aviation, Space, and Environmental Medicine, 67,* 530–538.

Razmjou, S., & Kjellberg, A. (1992). Sustained attention and serial responding in heat: Mental effort in the control of performance. *Aviation, Space, and Environmental Medicine, 63,* 594–601.

Reiss, S., Peterson, R. A., Gursky, M., & McNally, R. J. (1986). Anxiety sensitivity, anxiety frequency, and the prediction of fearfulness. *Behaviour Research and Therapy, 24,* 1–8.

Rhudy, J., & Meagher, M. (2003). Negative affect: Effects on an evaluative measure of human pain. *Pain, 104,* 617–626.

Richards, J., & Gross, J. (2000). Emotion regulation and memory: The cognitive costs of keeping one's cool. *Journal of Personality and Social Psychology, 79,* 410–424.

Roemer, L., & Orsillo, S. (2002). Expanding our conceptualization of and treatment for generalized anxiety disorder: Integrating mindfulness/acceptance-based approaches with existing cognitive-behavioral models. *Clinical Psychology: Science and Practice, 9,* 54–68.

Rottenberg, J., & Gross, J. (2003). When emotion goes wrong: Realizing the promise of affective science. *Clinical Psychology: Science and Practice, 10,* 227–232.

Rydell, S., & Rosen, E. (1966). Measurement and some correlates of need-cognition. *Psychological Reports, 19,* 139–165.

Salkovskis, P. M. (1996). The cognitive approach to anxiety: Threat beliefs, safety-seeking behavior, and the special case of health anxiety obsessions. In P. M. Salkovskis (Ed.), *Frontiers of cognitive therapy: The state of the art and beyond* (pp. 48–74). New York: Guilford Press.

Salovey, P., Mayer, J. D., Goldman, S. L., Turvey, C., & Palfai, T. P. (1995). Emotional attention, clarity, and repair: Exploring emotional intelligence using the Trait Meta-Mood Scale. In J. W. Pennebaker (Ed.), *Emotion, disclosure, and health* (pp. 125–154). Washington, DC: American Psychological Association.

Schmidt, N. B., & Cook, J. H. (1999). Effects of anxiety sensitivity on anxiety and pain during a cold pressor challenge in patients with panic disorder. *Behaviour Research and Therapy, 37,* 313–323.

Schmidt, N. B., & Lerew, D. R. (1998). Prospective evaluation of psychological risk factors as predictors of functional impairment during acute stress. *Journal of Occupational Rehabilitation, 8,* 199–212.

Schmidt, N. B., Richey, J. A., Cromer, K. R., & Buckner, J. D. (2007). Discomfort intolerance: Evaluation of a potential risk factor for anxiety psychopathology. *Behavior Therapy, 38,* 247–255.

Schmidt, N. B., Richey, J. A., & Fitzpatrick, K. K. (2006). Discomfort intolerance: Development of a construct and measure relevant to panic disorder. *Journal of Anxiety Disorders, 20,* 263–280.

Sharma, V. M., & Panwar, M. R. (1987). Variations in mental performances under moderate cold stress. *International Journal of Biometeorology, 31,* 85–91.

Simons, J., & Gaher, R. (2005). The Distress Tolerance Scale: Development and validation of a self-report measure. *Motivation and Emotion, 29,* 83–102.

Skinner, E. (1995). *Perceived control, motivation, and coping.* Thousand Oaks, CA: Sage.

Stöber, J. (1998). Worry, problem elaboration and suppression of imagery: The role of concreteness. *Behaviour Research and Therapy, 36,* 751–756.

Strong, D. R., Lejuez, C. W., Daughters, S. B., Marinello, M., Kahler, C. W., & Brown, R. A. (2003). *Computerized mirror tracing task version 1.* Unpublished manual.

Thomas, J. R., Ahlers, S. T., House, J. F., & Schrot, J. (1989). Repeated exposure to moderate cold impairs matching-to-sample performance. *Aviation, Space, and Environmental Medicine, 60,* 1063–1067.

Tolin, D. R., Abramowitz, J. S., Brigidi, B. D., & Foa, E. B. (2003). Intolerance of uncertainty in obsessive-compulsive disorder. *Anxiety Disorders, 17,* 233–242.

Tombaugh, T. (2006). A comprehensive review of the paced auditory serial addition test (PASAT). *Archives of Clinical Neuropsychology, 21,* 53–76.

Tutoo, D. (1971). Psychodiagnostic applications of the mirror-tracing test. *Indian Educational Review, 6,* 293–303.

Van Orden, K., Benoit, S., & Osga, G. (1996). Effects of cold air stress on the performance of a command and control task. *Human Factors, 38,* 130–141.

Williams, J., Teasdale, J., Segal, Z., & Soulsby, J. (2000). Mindfulness-based cognitive therapy reduces overgeneral autobiographical memory in formerly depressed patients. *Journal of Abnormal Psychology, 109,* 150–155.

Willoughby, S., Hailey, B., Mulkana, S., & Rowe, J. (2002). The effect of laboratory-induced depressed mood state on responses to pain. *Behavioral Medicine, 28,* 23–31.

Wolff, B., & Jarvik, M. (1963). Variations in cutaneous and deep somatic pain sensitivity. *Canadian Journal of Psychology, 17,* 37–44.

Zuckerman, M., Lubin, B., & Rinck, C. (1983). Construction of new scales for the Multiple Affect Adjective Checklist. *Journal of Behavioral Assessment, 5,* 119–129.

Zvolensky, M. J., & Eifert, G. H. (2000). A review of psychological factors/processes affecting anxious responding during voluntary hyperventilation and inhalations of carbon dioxide-enriched air. *Clinical Psychology Review, 21,* 375–400.

Zvolensky, M. J., Feldner, M. T., Eifert, G. H., & Brown, R. A. (2001). Affective style among smokers: Understanding anxiety sensitivity, emotional reactivity, and distress tolerance using biological challenge. *Addictive Behaviors, 26,* 901–915.

Zvolensky, M., & Otto, M. (2007). Affective intolerance, sensitivity, and processing: Advances in clinical science introduction. *Behavior Therapy, 38,* 228–233.

# 2

# Anxiety Sensitivity as a Specific Form of Distress Tolerance in Youth

*Developmental Assessment, Origins, and Applications*

Carl F. Weems

This chapter examines anxiety sensitivity as a specific form of distress tolerance in childhood and adolescence. Distress tolerance has been measured in a number of different ways in the literature (e.g., see Corstorphine, Mountford, Tomlinson, Waller, & Meyer, 2007; Daughters et al., 2009; Nock & Mendes, 2008). For example, assessments have included behavioral indicators of resiliency to distress such as computer-assisted (e.g., Daughters et al., 2009) or in-person (Nock & Mendes, 2008) tests designed to assess persistence in the face of increasingly difficult/frustrating tasks or capacity to endure painful experiences (e.g., Tsao et al., 2004) and self-report assessment of avoidance of affective responses/willingness to accept and manage affect (e.g., Corstorphine et al., 2007).

Although there is variability in the exact form of assessment in youth samples, each of the conceptualizations has a consistent underlying theme. Specifically, and as discussed in the chapters throughout this volume, distress tolerance involves individual differences in the capacity to tolerate aversive internal states (e.g., pain, negative emotions, and body sensations). For example, research using an affect regulation conceptualization of distress tolerance suggests that youth who engage in self-injurious behaviors are unable to tolerate intense emotions such as sadness and so use pain-inducing injuries as a way of escaping from the experience of the emotion (Nock & Mendes, 2008). Although a literature search on distress tolerance in youth samples will generate few (yet highly promising) results, the work on anxiety sensitivity in youth has produced a substantial body of research.

Anxiety sensitivity is defined as an individual difference in beliefs about the consequences of anxiety, specifically that anxiety sensations (e.g., jitteriness, racing heartbeat) have severe and negative consequences (Reiss, 1991). For example, children with high anxiety sensitivity might believe that feeling their heart beat fast means something is seriously physically wrong them or that appearing nervous to others will result in social ridicule. Given these defining characteristics, anxiety sensitivity might then be seen as a specific form of distress tolerance where high anxiety sensitivity involves a decreased capacity to tolerate anxiety states and sensations and, conversely, low anxiety sensitivity involves an increased tolerance for anxiety sensations. Similar to the affect regulation conceptualization of distress tolerance, youth with high anxiety sensitivity are unable or (less likely) to tolerate anxiety-related emotional experience.

Elevated anxiety sensitivity is a risk factor for the development of panic attacks, panic disorder, and other anxiety disorders. Research indicates that anxiety sensitivity levels predict the development of panic attacks in youth and young adults (Hayward, Killen, Kraemer, & Taylor, 2000; Schmidt, Lerew, & Jackson, 1997, 1999; Weems, Hayward, Killen, & Taylor, 2002), and that anxiety sensitivity is concurrently and prospectively related to anxiety disorder symptoms and severe fear reactions in child and adolescent samples (Ginsberg & Drake, 2002; Lau, Calamari, & Waraczynski, 1996; Silverman, Fleisig, Rabian, & Peterson, 1991). Although the research on anxiety sensitivity has tended to focus on its relation to the development and maintenance of anxiety and anxiety disorders, the literature also indicates relations to a variety of problems, including traumatic stress disorder, somatic symptoms, and substance abuse. Such connections suggest that anxiety sensitivity may tap emotional avoidance and affect regulation in a similar manner to more broad conceptualizations/assessments of distress tolerance. The extant literature on anxiety sensitivity in youth may, therefore, inform a developmental understanding of distress tolerance. In the remainder of this chapter, the developmental assessment of anxiety sensitivity is discussed and studies on the validity of the construct, including longitudinal studies and cultural variations, are reviewed. The possible developmental origin of anxiety sensitivity in childhood is next examined, and the chapter concludes by noting some of the clinical applications of the construct for youth and pointing out future directions for research on anxiety sensitivity as a specific form of distress tolerance.

## ASSESSMENT OF ANXIETY
## SENSITIVITY IN YOUTH

The most extensively used measure of anxiety sensitivity in adults is the 16-item Anxiety Sensitivity Index (ASI; Peterson & Reiss, 1987; Reiss, Peterson, Gursky, & McNally, 1986). The measure has been the subject of many psychometric studies (Peterson & Reiss, 1993), which have suggested excellent reliability and validity estimates (e.g., internal consistency reliabilities ranging from .82 to .91, predictive validity; see McNally, 1989; Peterson & Heilbronner, 1987; Reiss, Peterson, Taylor, Schmidt, & Weems, 2008; Telch, Shermis, & Lucas, 1989). Although the ASI has been used in both adult and adolescent samples (Hayward, Weems, et al., 2002; Weems, Berman, Silverman, & Rodriguez, 2002), the most commonly used measure of anxiety sensitivity in youth is the Childhood Anxiety Sensitivity Index (CASI), a modification of the ASI developed by Silverman and colleagues (1991) for use with school-age youth ages 6–17 years. The 18-item CASI asks youth to rate their fear of the same types of anxiety-related sensations or experiences as on the adult version. The main differences between the ASI and the CASI are simplicity of the item wording and the rating stems and the inclusion of two additional questions. Example questions are "When I notice that my heart is beating fast, I worry that there might be something wrong with me" and "Unusual feelings in my body scare me." Youth rate each item on the CASI as either *none* (1), *some* (2), or *a lot* (3). Total scores may thus range from 18 to 54 (vs. the ASI, which ranges from 0 to 64). The CASI can be obtained from Dr. Silverman and the ASI from *www. anxietysensitivityindex.com*; a full copy of the CASI was also published in Silverman and Weems (1999).

Weems, Taylor, Marks, and Varela (2010) recently tested a parent-report version of the CASI (CASI-P) in a sample of 202 youth ages 6–17 years and their parents. This 18-item measure was designed to assess parent reports of their children's fear of different symptoms of anxiety. Each item's content is identical to the CASI except that the focus has been changed (e.g., from "I" to "my child"). This strategy has been used in past research on childhood fears and trait anxiety (see, e.g., Piña, Silverman, Saavedra, & Weems, 2001; Weems, Silverman, Saavedra, Piña, & Lumpkin, 1999) and facilitates the development of nonarbitrary metrics (see Blanton & Jaccard, 2006) by utilizing the same metric as the CASI (i.e., levels reported by the child can be directly compared with those reported by the parent). Each item of the CASI-P has identical scoring and score range as the CASI.

## Reliability

The CASI has sound psychometric properties similar to those reported for the adult ASI. The CASI has been shown to have satisfactory internal consistency reliability, with coefficient alphas consistently above .80 (e.g., Silverman et al., 1991). For example, in their study of 280 youth with anxiety disorders, Weems, Hammond-Laurence, Silverman, and Ginsburg (1998) found alphas of .86 for the 6- to 11-year-olds, .89 for the 12- to 17-year-olds, and .87 for the total sample. In a community sample of 145 youth ages 6–17, Weems, Costa, Watts, Taylor, and Cannon (2007) reported internal consistencies of .86 in the full sample, .83 in youth ages 6–11 years, and .88 in youth ages 12–17 years.

Silverman and colleagues (1991) demonstrated good test–retest reliability for CASI scores. Using a 2-week test–retest interval, the correlation was .76 in a clinic-referred sample ($n$ = 33; ages 8–15 years; mean age = 10.6 years) and .79 in a non-clinic-referred sample ($n$ = 72; ages 11–16 years; mean age = 13.3 years). Ginsburg and Drake (2002) showed a 6-month test–retest correlation of .48 in a sample of 66 African American youth (mean age = 15.4 years), and Weems and colleagues (2007) reported a 1-year test–retest correlation for the CASI of $r$ = .48, $p < .01$, in a sample of 52 youth ages 7–17 years. Fullana-Rivas, Servera, Weems, Tortella-Feliu, and Caseras (2003) showed that anxiety sensitivity measured with a Catalan translation of the CASI had retest reliabilities of .66 and .54 over 3-month and 1-year periods, respectively, in 291 Catalan school children (ages 9–17 years; mean age = 13.7 years).

Reliability estimates for the CASI-P suggest similar internal consistency and test–retest associations as those previously reported for the self-report instrument. Weems and colleagues (2010) reported internal consistencies of .89 in the full sample, .88 for parent report on youth ages 6–11 years, and .91 for parent report on youth ages 12–17 years. One-year test–retest correlations on the CASI-P were calculated on a subsample of youth ($n$ = 52) who completed a Time 2 assessment, and the retest correlation was $r$ = .59, $p < .01$.

## Factor and Dimensional Structure

Tests of the factor structure of the ASI and CASI have resulted in a large number of studies. Reiss originally theorized, and concluded, that the ASI had a single-factor structure based on a high alpha coefficient and results of an orthogonal principal-component analysis (see Reiss, Silverman, & Weems, 2001). Subsequent studies, however, have supported a multidimensional model with substantial factor intercorrelations (e.g., Zinbarg, Barlow, & Brown, 1997; Zinbarg, Mohlman, & Hong, 1999). As in adults, anxiety sensitivity in children and adolescents can be understood as a hierarchical construct with several lower order factors (Dehon, Weems, Stickle, Costa, & Berman, 2005; Silverman, Ginsburg, & Goedhart, 1999; Zinbarg et al., 1999). Although findings have varied (Chorpita & Daleiden, 2000; Silverman et al., 1999), factor results have typically centered on physical concerns (e.g., "When my stomach hurts, I worry that I might be really sick"), social concerns (e.g., "Other kids can tell when I feel shaky"), and mental incapacitation (e.g, "When I am afraid, I worry that I might be crazy") concerns.

Silverman and colleagues (1999) evaluated the factor structure of the CASI using both clinic ($n = 258$) and nonclinic ($n = 249$) samples. The results supported a hierarchical, multidimensional model with either three or four first-order factors, with the two most robust factors being physical concerns and mental incapacitation concerns. In a later study of youth from both clinical and nonclinical samples in the United States and Australia, Silverman, Goedhart, Barrett, and Turner (2003) again found that both the three-factor model and the four-factor model, which split the physical scale into disease concerns and unsteady concerns, provided adequate to good fit to the data. They further showed that the factor structure of anxiety sensitivity was invariant across children and adolescents as well as across gender. Evidence for factorial invariance across adults and adolescents has also been demonstrated using the ASI (Dehon et al., 2005). However, anxiety sensitivity in youth appears to have both dimensional and taxonic properties. For example, Bernstein, Zvolensky, Weems, Stickle, and Leen-Feldner (2005) used taxometric analyses to test the latent structure of anxiety sensitivity in a sample of 371 youths ages 7–17 using the CASI. The results indicated that the latent structure of anxiety sensitivity among youth was taxonic, with estimated base rates for the observed childhood anxiety sensitivity taxon between 13.6 and 16.5% (see also Bernstein et al., 2007).

The factor structure of the CASI-P has been examined using exploratory factor analysis procedures (Weems et al., 2010). Velicer's minimum average partials method and modified parallel analysis indicated three factors (Zwick & Velicer, 1986). Use of various extraction and rotation methods (e.g., principal-components analysis with varimax rotation vs. principal-factors extraction with direct oblimin rotation) did not change interpretation of the number of factors (i.e., they produced highly similar results) nor did they appreciably change salient loadings. The three-factor solution was consistent with previous work on the CASI, with the

CASI-P the items loading onto physical concerns, mental concerns, and social concerns.

## Validity Studies

The CASI has been shown to be valid in a number of similar ways as the ASI in adults. Convergent validity between the ASI and the CASI has been reported at $r = .73$, $p < .01$, in a sample of high school youth in grades 9–12 (Weems, Berman, et al., 2002). The factor structure of the ASI appears to be invariant across adults and adolescents (Dehon et al., 2005), and that of the CASI appears to be invariant across children and adolescents (Silverman et al., 2003). This pattern of findings suggests similar validity of measurement across age groups to as young as about 6 or 7.

Moreover, the CASI has been shown to (1) concurrently relate to panic symptoms, fears, and associated constructs consistent with theory and in a manner similar to findings on the ASI; (2) predict anxiety-relevant responding to behavioral-stress challenge tasks and other experimental assessments; (3) be prospectively associated with panic symptoms and anxiety disorder symptoms; and (4) demonstrate incremental validity over other measures (e.g., Calamari et al., 2001; Ginsburg & Drake, 2002; Lau et al., 1996; Rabian, Embry, & MacIntyre, 1999; Rabian, Peterson, Richters, & Jensen, 1993; Silverman et al., 1991; Weems, Berman, Silverman, & Saavedra, 2001; Weems, Silverman, & La Greca, 2000; Weems et al., 2007). Moreover, studies have demonstrated that although CASI scores are related to depression (Weems, Hammond-Laurence, Silverman, & Ferguson, 1997), they are more uniquely associated with anxiety symptoms in youth (Joiner et al., 2002; Weems et al., 2007).

Similar to the ASI findings in adults, on average (across studies) youth who experience panic attacks have the highest CASI scores, followed by children with nonpanic anxiety disorders, children with other emotional problems, and finally youth with no disorder. For example, in Kearney, Albano, Eisen, Allan, and Barlow's (1997) comparison study of children meeting criteria for panic disorder ($n = 20$) and children meeting diagnostic criteria for other anxiety disorders ($n = 20$) using several self-report measures of fear and anxiety and the CASI, only CASI scores differed significantly between the two groups. Furthermore, Lau and colleagues (1996) found a .42 correlation between CASI scores and total number of reported panic symptoms in a community sample of 77 high school adolescents. The CASI was correlated with the number of panic attacks in the past year, with the distress the panic attacks caused, and with the judged seriousness of the attacks. Furthermore, participants were categorized as panickers and nonpanickers, and the 30 panickers scored significantly higher on the CASI than the 47 nonpanickers.

Rabian and colleagues (1993) found CASI scores of 30.6, 28.8, and 26.4, respectively, for 18 children with anxiety disorders, 31 with externalizing disorders, and 62 with no psychiatric diagnosis. The CASI scores were significantly higher for children with anxiety disorders versus those with no disorders. Although the difference between children with anxiety disorders and those with externalizing disorders was not statistically significant, the presence of comorbid conditions, in which some children with anxiety disorder also had extermalizing disorders, may have influenced results. Similarly, Vasey, Daleiden, Williams, and Brown (1995) found significant differences in CASI scores between a group of 12 children with anxiety disorders (mean score = 32.4) and a group of 12 controls matched on age, gender, and intellectual ability who did not meet diagnostic criteria for a psychiatric disorder (mean score = 26).

Incremental validity has been established in a number of studies. Weems and colleagues (1998) investigated whether the CASI could account for variance in fears beyond that explained by trait anxiety and anxiety frequency in both younger and older children. Using similar methodology of demonstrating incremental validity in the prediction of fearfulness as in adult samples (see Reiss et al., 1986), Weems and colleagues showed that the CASI exhibited incremental validity in both children ages 6–11 years and adolescents ages 12–17 years, accounting for 9–16% of unique variance. This finding has been replicated in at least two independent samples (Calamari et al., 2001; van Widenfelt, Siebelink, Goedhart, & Treffers, 2002). Although an initial study questioned the incremental validity in children (a finding suggests that incremental validity may drop off at about age 7 or 8 years, see Chorpita, Albano, & Barlow, 1996), this finding has not been replicated. Indeed, Rabian and colleagues (1999) also performed a behavioral arousal induction validation study of the CASI by using a stair-stepping challenge among 56 elementary school children (ages 8–11 years). The results indicated that the CASI significantly predicted the levels of state anxiety and subjective fear reported in response to the challenge task even after controlling for trait anxiety and pretask levels of state anxiety and fear. The CASI also predicted changes (pre–posttask) in fear experienced in response to the challenge task. Such findings demonstrate that the CASI possesses unique incremental validity relative to measures of trait anxiety and also provided a behavioral validation of the CASI in preadolescent children.

These results are similar to earlier findings by Mattis and Ollendick (1997), who investigated children's cognitive responses to the physical symptoms of panic in a sample of nonreferred third, sixth, and ninth graders. Specifically, children listened to a tape recording describing a panic attack and were told to imagine that they were experiencing the condition described. Mattis and Ollendick found that only the children's CASI scores predicted their tendencies to make internal catastrophic attributions (e.g., thoughts of going crazy, losing control, or dying).

Anxiety sensitivity has also been validated within a broader emotional development perspective. Specifically, anxiety problems are thought to result from deviations in the normative mechanisms of the anxiety fight-or-flight response system (Barlow, 2002). There are a number of important behavioral, social, biological, and cognitive risk factors that have been identified (Vasey & Dadds, 2001). Cognitive models of anxiety disorders focus on the hypothesis that anxiety disorders can result from or be maintained by faulty, biased, or negative ways of thinking. The research on cognitive models of anxiety in youth has focused on biased interpretation, biased judgment, biased memory, and selective attention (see, e.g., Vasey & MacLeod, 2001). These various biases are hypothesized to work together at various stages of information processing to foster and maintain heightened anxiety (Watts & Weems, 2006).

Anxiety-related interpretive biases involve being predisposed toward negative or erroneous interpretations of neutral, ambiguous, or potentially threatening stimuli or situations. For example, catastrophizing involves expecting the worst possible outcome of an event or situation (i.e., interpret the event in the worse possible manner: e.g., "If it rains there will be a flood"). Similar negative interpretations of anxiety-related sensations have been the focus of research on anxiety sensitivity. On the basis of this integrative theorizing, Weems and colleagues (2007) examined the interrelations among CASI scores, negative cognitive errors, and anxiety control beliefs and explored their unique and specific associations with anxiety symptoms in a community sample of 145 youth ages 6–17. The results of this study indicated that although negative cognitive errors, anxiety sensitivity, and anxiety control beliefs were associated with each other, each demonstrated unique concurrent associations with childhood anxiety disorder symptoms (anxiety sensitivity accounted for 8–12% of unique variance). Moreover, anxiety sensitivity showed specificity in its association with anxiety symptoms versus depressive symptoms. Similarly, Hunt, Keogh, and French (2007) demonstrated that CASI scores were associated with an attention bias for threat/emotional words ($r = .40$) using the dot-probe paradigm in a sample of 166 youth ages 8–10 years. Eley, Shirling, Ehlers, Gregory, and Clark (2004) demonstrated that the CASI was associated with heartbeat perception assessed via a mental tracking paradigm and also found that the CASI predicted unique variance in panic symptoms beyond heartbeat perception in a sample of ($n = 79$) 8- to 11-year-olds.

Cross-informant validity has also recently been tested. Weems and colleagues (2010) examined parent reports of children's anxiety sensitivity (CASI-P) and explored the effects of age, sex, and ethnicity on cross-informant associations with child reports (CASI) using complementary statistical models. Parents and children ($n$ = 202; ages 6–17 years) also completed instruments assessing fears and manifest anxiety. Results indicated that the CASI-P demonstrated incremental and concurrent validity estimates similar to those previously reported for the self-report instrument. Moreover, reliability and validity were highly similar across age and child sex. However, age and ethnicity were found to significantly influence cross-informant associations, and the statistical method used to examine cross-informant associations produced differing conclusions. Using a procedure to eliminate extremely discrepant parent–child pairs on a behaviorally salient construct (i.e., report of fears on the Fear Survey Schedule for Children—Revised [FSSC-R] parent and child versions), the correlation between the CASI and CASI-P was $r$ = .30, $p <$ .001 ($n$ = 162, or 80% of the sample). Moreover, hierarchical regression analyses indicated that the CASI-P was a significant incremental predictor of FSSCR-R (child report) scores beyond the CASI (child report) ($\Delta R^2$ = .02, $\beta$ = 0.16, $p < .01$).

## Longitudinal Studies

Most of the longitudinal studies published to date on anxiety sensitivity have used the ASI. Maller and Reiss (1992) reported the first longitudinal data using a 3-year follow-up study on college students who had scored either high ($n$ = 23) or low ($n$ = 25) on the ASI. Students with high anxiety sensitivity were significantly more likely than those with low anxiety sensitivity to have a *Diagnostic and Statistical Manual of Mental Disorders* (third edition, revised [DSM-III-R]; American Psychiatric Association, 1987) anxiety diagnosis 3 years later. Furthermore, three of four students who experienced panic attacks for the first time during the follow-up period were in the high–anxiety sensitivity group. Schmidt and colleagues have conducted (1997) and replicated (1999) a large-scale study of anxiety sensitivity as a risk factor for spontaneous panic attacks among individuals undergoing basic military training. Using the ASI, the authors found that approximately 20% of the cadets with high anxiety sensitivity experienced a panic attack during the 5-week follow-up period compared with only 6% for all other cadets.

In terms of studies in youth, Hayward and colleagues (2000) prospectively evaluated negative affectivity, female sex, anxiety sensitivity, and childhood separation anxiety disorder as predictors of panic. The sample included 2,365 high school students assessed over a 4-year period. Both ASI and negative affectivity predicted the onset of four-symptom panic attacks, but ASI did not predict the onset of depression (risk ratio for high negative affectivity = 3.3 and for high ASI scores = 2.1; hazard ratio for negative affectivity = 2.39 and for ASI scores = 1.04). Weems, Hayward, and colleagues (2002) analyzed Hayward and colleagues' (2000) data, focusing on anxiety sensitivity, and used cluster analyses to identify different developmental pathways in levels of anxiety sensitivity. Groups of adolescents with stable low, stable high, and escalating anxiety sensitivity levels were identified. Adolescents with stable high or escalating anxiety sensitivity were significantly more likely to report experiencing a panic attack than those with stable low anxiety sensitivity.

A few longitudinal studies using the CASI have been reported. In a short-term prospective study, Ginsburg and Drake (2002) assessed anxiety sensitivity and panic symptoms among 66 African American adolescents (ages 14–17 years; mean age = 15.6 years) at the initial evaluation and again after 6 months. The results indicated that anxiety sensitivity was concurrently correlated with panic symptoms at both the initial and follow-up assessments. Moreover, initial anxiety sensitivity was significantly associated with anxiety sensitivity and panic symptoms assessed at follow-up. A subsample of 52 participants in Weems and colleagues (2007) completed follow-up assessments 1 year later. Hierarchical regression analyses were conducted to determine which of the cognitive biases predicted anxiety levels at Time 2. CASI scores and negative cognitive errors were significant predictors of anxiety disorder symptoms, jointly accounting for 27% of the variance in anxiety disorders symptoms. More longitudinal research is needed.

## Cultural Variation

Anxiety sensitivity has been reliably measured across several cultures (Taylor, 1999). In children, the CASI has been translated and assessed in a number of languages in addition to English, including Spanish (e.g., Sandin, 1997; Varela, Weems, Berman, Hensley, & de Bernal, 2007), Catalan (e.g., Fullana-Rivas et al., 2003), and Dutch (van Widenfelt et al., 2002). Results among the different translations have been highly consistent. For example, van Widenfelt and colleagues (2002) found that the Dutch CASI predicted fear beyond a measure of trait anxiety and reported a similar three-factor solution (physical concerns, mental concerns, and social concerns) as found in English language samples.

However, there does appear to be some important cultural variation in scoring and validity estimates. For example, Weems, Hayward, and colleagues (2002) and Pina and Silverman (2004) have found that Latino youth report higher anxiety sensitivity than white youth. Although studies have found Latino youth to report more anxiety sensitivity, Pina and Silverman and Varela and colleagues (2007) have reported evidence suggesting that it may be certain facets of anxiety sensitivity that Latino youth find more distressing relative to white non-Latino youth, although these findings have not been consistent. Moreover, Weems, Hayward, and colleagues found that among ethnic minorities (Asian and Hispanic) high stable anxiety sensitivity and escalating anxiety sensitivity (i.e., increasing over time) were not as strongly related to panic attacks compared with European American youth. One possible explanation for these findings is that anxiety sensitivity may be more normative within certain cultures and thus not amplify anxiety symptoms for those youth as much as it does for white non-Latino youth. Although the evidence to date supports this idea (Varela et al., 2007; Weems, Hayward, et al., 2002; Weems et al., 2010), additional research on cultural variation in the expression of anxiety sensitivity in youth is needed.

## DEVELOPMENTAL ORIGINS

Although panic disorder is relatively rare among very young children, accurate and comprehensive assessment of anxiety sensitivity in children may allow for the identification of an important developmental precursor. Indeed, research points to the preschool years as an important time in the development of risk for anxiety problems (Kagan, Reznick, & Gibbons, 1989; Lonigan & Phillips, 2001; Ollendick, King, & Hamilton, 1991). An understanding of the development of anxiety sensitivity might also inform an understanding of the development of distress tolerance more generally. Figure 2.1 presents a schematic representation of possible theoretical processes involved in the development of anxiety sensitivity. The model is tentative because the existing research literature does not allow exact statements about the interrelations among the various mechanisms (i.e., the interactive processes hypothesized among the mechanisms are in need of empirical tests). The model is heuristic/schematic because it is possible that high anxiety sensitivity may have other specific mediational and interactive processes involved in its development. Moreover, the arrows leading to anxiety sensitivity are not are intended to suggest that these processes invariably lead to elevated anxiety sensitivity. For example, certain other social, cognitive, and learning factors may protect those with a biological risk. It is also important to note that each of the paths may not be important for all individuals, and that for some certain factors (paths) may more important than others. Finally, the relationships may be altered by moderators such as gender, ethnicity, and age (see also Daughters et al., 2009) or a function of other meditational processes not shown.

As pointed out in Figure 2.1, anxiety sensitivity is thought to have a genetic basis, and evidence for its heritability has been found in adult sam-

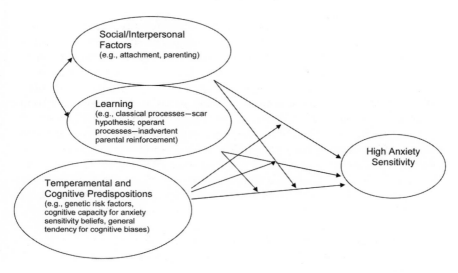

**FIGURE 2.1.** Schematic representation of possible theoretical processes involved in the development of anxiety sensitivity.

ples (e.g., Stein, Jang, & Livesley, 1999). In addition, Reiss and McNally (1985), in their initial theorizing on anxiety sensitivity, reasoned that acquired beliefs (e.g., learning) about the consequences of anxiety can strengthen or weaken individual differences in anxiety sensitivity. Indeed, research has suggested a role for parental anxiety and parental modeling of anxiety (e.g., the social and behavioral factors from Figure 2.1) in the development of anxiety sensitivity (Watt, Stewart, & Cox, 1998).

Theoretically, the cognitive capacities for anxiety sensitivity beliefs begin at about age 4 or 5 (see Muris, Vermeer, & Horselenberg, 2008). Although the full range of metacognitive abilities is still developing at this age (Flavell, Green, & Flavell, 1993, 1995), children as young as 4 or 5 can understand beliefs and the role that beliefs can have in directing action and emotion (Harris, Johnson, Hutton, Andrews, & Cooke, 1989; Muris et al., 2008). Therefore, children approximately 4 to 5 years old could begin to cognitively understand the potential negative implications of anxiety sensations. In studies of anxiety sensitivity, the youngest participants have been in the 6- to 10-year age range, and typically, the CASI items are read to very young children (Calamari et al., 2001; Weems et al., 1997, 1998).

Reiss and Havercamp (1998) put forth an evolutionary genetic argument for the origins of anxiety sensitivity. According to the sensitivity theory of motivation (Reiss & Havercamp. 1998; Reiss & McNally, 1985), genetic variation causes individual differences in sensitivity to anxiety that could be largely independent of experience. Research has begun to explore both predisposition (Jang, Stein, Taylor & Livesley, 1999; Stein et al., 1999) and learning models (Schmidt, Lerew & Joiner, 2000; Watt et al., 1998) of anxiety sensitivity in adult samples. Even given a strong genetic basis, acquired beliefs (e.g., learning) about the consequences of anxiety might strengthen or weaken individual differences in anxiety sensitivity. That is, it is likely that there are gene–environment interactions such that changes in the predisposed level of an individual's anxiety sensitivity may occur through cognitive, operant, or respondent conditioning processes (see, e.g., Reiss & McNally, 1985; Schmidt et al., 2000; Watt et al., 1998; Weems, Hayward, et al., 2002). For example, the experience of panic may affect the vulnerability that anxiety sensitivity imposes, "scarring" the individual to be prone to elevated anxiety sensitivity (Schmidt et al., 2000; see also the classical conditioning model of Goldstein & Chambless, 1978).

Empirical research in a young adult sample has tested this scar hypothesis and suggests that the experience of spontaneous panic may increase anxiety sensitivity levels over relatively short time spans. Specifically, Schmidt and colleagues (2000) reported that the experience of panic attacks as well as general stressors (i.e., symptoms of depression) was associated with increases in the level of anxiety sensitivity, as assessed with the ASI, in a sample of 1,296 young adults (army cadets) followed over a 5-week period (basic training). Although Weems, Hayward, and colleagues (2002) did not find similar strong support for a scar effect in high school–age adolescents, panic attacks predicting change in ASI scores did emerge in one of the three 1-year intervals examined.

In a similar vein, Taylor (2003) suggested that traumatic experiences may also foster the development of anxiety sensitivity. This makes conceptual sense given that reexperiencing arousal and images related to the traumatic event is a core feature of posttraumatic stress disorder (American Psychiatric Association, 1994). Anxiety sensations may be seen as foreboding a recurrence of the trauma, therefore making anxiety symptoms a particularly negative experience for those exposed to trauma. Traumatic stress has been linked to anxiety sensitivity in youth who experienced trauma related to the Hurricane Katrina disaster. For example, Hensley and Varela (2008) reported a correlation of $r = .21$, $p < .05$, with more traumatic experiences related to higher CASI scores (see also Leen-Feldner, Feldner, Reardon, Babson, & Dixon, 2008).

In terms of the development of anxiety sensitivity within the broader developmental literature, research has indicated that insecurely attached children may be at risk for later psychosocial difficulties, including anxiety problems (see Manassis & Bradley, 1994, for a review). Indeed, the original Strange Situation paradigm (Ainsworth, Blehar, Waters, & Wall, 1978) might reasonably be seen as a historically early assessment of distress tolerance (i.e., children are separated from their mothers, and their emotional and behavioral reactions are observed and classified). Weems, Berman, and colleagues (2002) hypothesized that the internal working models (the developmentally later cognitive form of attachment style) of insecurely attached children might also involve distorted and selective encoding of anxiety-related sensations and information regarding the consequences of experiencing anxiety symptoms. For example, the internal working model of insecurely attached individuals is characterized by an increased sensitivity to and fear of rejection (Bartholomew, 1990). This rejection sensitivity is similar to the sensitivity to anxiety-related sensations in individuals with high anxiety sensitivity (Reiss & Havercamp. 1998; see also Reiss, Silverman, & Weems, 2001). Each of these sensitivities may have their origins in the distorted thinking and selective encoding characteristic of insecurely attached individuals.

To test this attachment idea, Weems, Berman, and colleagues (2002) examined the relation between attachment style and anxiety sensitivity in a sample of high school students ($n$ = 203; mean age = 15.7 years) and university students ($n$ = 324; mean age = 21.7 years). It was hypothesized that individuals classified as having insecure attachment styles characterized by a fear of abandonment (i.e., preoccupied and fearful styles) would have elevated anxiety sensitivity scores relative to those with secure or dismissive attachment styles. The Experiences in Close Relationships (Brennan, Clark, & Shaver, 1998) was used to classify participants' characteristic attachment style, and the ASI (Peterson & Reiss, 1987) was used to assess anxiety sensitivity. Results supported the hypothesis in that individuals classified as preoccupied and fearful had significantly higher anxiety sensitivity scores than securely attached individuals in both the high school and college samples. The association between attachment and anxiety sensitivity has been replicated in at least two independent samples (using the CASI, Viana & Rabian, 2008; replicating with the ASI, Watt, McWilliams, & Campbell, 2005), and although Austin, Jamieson, Richards, and Winkelman (2006) reported a failure to replicate, the findings were in the expected direction with a medium-sized effect (i.e., Cohen's $d$ calculated from the information supplied in Austin et al., 2006, was about 0.5, similar to Weems, Berman, et al., 2002, and Watt et al., 2005), and the sample size for insecure individuals was only 14 participants. Moreover, the attachment measure was a modified measure. Thus, the one failure to replicate was likely due to a lack of statistical power given the similarity in effect size.

## CLINICAL APPLICATIONS

The CASI has been used for several clinical applications in youth samples, including as an outcome measure and to help prescribe treatment emphasis. In terms of its use as an outcome variable, Ollendick (1995) used the CASI in a multiple-baseline design study of cognitive-behavioral treatment for panic disorder with agoraphobia in four adolescents ages 13, 14, 16, and 17. The Ollendick investigation examined the effects of progressive muscle relaxation and breathing training, exposure, and cognitive coping procedures. The results suggest that the CASI was sensitive to change in the treatment of the four adolescents. In addition to its use as a treatment outcome measure, the CASI has been used to prescribe type of treatment (Eisen & Silverman, 1993, 1998).

Eisen and Silverman (1993, 1998) showed that children did better when they received a prescribed treatment in accordance with their specific response classes (or symptom patterns) of anxiety. For example, Eisen and Silverman (1998) used a multiple-baseline design across subjects to examine the efficacy of prescriptive versus nonprescriptive cognitive-behavioral intervention for four boys (one 8-year-old, one 11-year-old, and two 12-year-olds) who met DSM-III-R criteria for a primary diagnosis of overanxious disorder as well as DSM-IV criteria for generalized anxiety disorder. Using the CASI and other measures, the children were classified into either a somatic response class (i.e., elevated anxiety sensitivity, high somatic symptoms) or a cognitive response class (i.e., a lot of worry and negative cognitions). The results indicated that participants receiving prescriptive treatment had positive effects, with symptoms falling within normal limits on the response class measures, and gains were maintained at the 6-month follow-up. In contrast, nonprescriptive treatment failed to produce meaningful change, and in one case after nonprescriptive treatment, functioning deteriorated with an increase in levels of distress on the CASI (i.e., an increase from 26 to 34 points).

## FUTURE DIRECTIONS FOR DISTRESS TOLERANCE AND ANXIETY SENSITIVITY IN YOUTH

Anxiety sensitivity in youth may be related to other distress tolerance–related constructs and behavioral problems more broadly. For example, anxiety sensitivity may enhance the fear of pain (Asmundson, 1999). Measures of anxiety sensitivity and pain sensitivities are highly correlated (Asmundson, 1999; Reiss & Havercamp. 1998). Using a classic distress-inducing technique, the cold presser challenge task, in a sample of 22 patients with panic disorder and 22 nonclinical controls, Schmidt and Cook (1999) reported that ASI scores were predictive of both pain and anxiety responses to the task. Several studies have begun to explore these associations in youth. Muris, Vlaeyen, and Meesters (2001) investigated the relationship between anxiety sensitivity and fear of pain in 200 adolescents using a revised, item-expanded version of the CASI (designed to measure four specific domains of anxiety sensitivity: fear of cardiovascular symptoms, fear of respiratory symptoms, fear of loss of control, and fear of publicly observable anxiety symptoms). They found that anxiety sensitivity was positively correlated to fear of pain even when controlling for somatization symptoms, trait anxiety, and panic disorder symptoms.

Lipsitz and colleagues (2004) examined anxiety sensitivity among 65 youth with noncardiac (i.e., medically unexplained) chest pain and 45 comparison youngsters with benign heart murmurs. Results indicated that, compared with the asymptomatic benign-murmur group, youngsters with chest pain had higher levels of anxiety sensitivity. Tsao and colleagues (2004) examined the relationships among anxiety sensitivity, state task-specific anticipatory anxiety, and laboratory pain responses in healthy children and adolescents ($n$ = 118; ages 8–18 years) using thermal, pressure, and cold pain tasks. They found that anticipatory anxiety accounted for a substantial portion of unique variance in pain report across tasks, and a smaller but significant amount of unique variance in thermal tolerance, but that anxiety sensitivity was unrelated to pain responses. Research is needed to clarify these findings. It may be that anxiety sensitivity is related to cognitive aspects of pain in nonclinical youth (Muris et al., 2001) and in clinic-referred youth (Lipsitz et al., 2004), but is not related to actual pain tolerance in nonreferred youth (Tsao et al., 2004). The CASI has also been shown to be related to other health concerns in youth.

Hensley and Varela (2008) found that CASI scores moderated the relationship between trait anxiety and posttraumatic stress symptoms in a sample of sixth- and seventh-grade students ($n$ = 302) exposed to Hurricane Katrina. Specifically, they found that high trait anxiety coupled with high subscale scores on the CASI was associated with the relatively highest posttraumatic stress disorder symptoms and somatic symptoms. Their model suggests that anxiety sensitivity creates a cycle of anxiety amplification, resulting in extremely high levels of net anxiety and rendering children less likely to adequately process and cope with the traumatic experience, which is more than would occur with just high trait anxiety alone.

Comeau, Stewart, and Loba (2001) found that low CASI scores predicted enhancement motives for alcohol use and high anxiety sensitivity predicted conformity motives for alcohol and marijuana use in a sample of 508 adolescents (mean age = 15 years). Moreover, CASI scores moderated the association between trait anxiety and coping motives for alcohol and cigarette use (see also Feldner, Leen-Feldner, Trainor, Blanchard, & Monson, 2008). This research converges with other studies on distress tolerance using broader conceptualizations of the construct. For example, Daughters and colleagues (2009) found that low distress tolerance (measured behaviorally using a computerized increasing-difficulty task paradigm) conferred increased risk for alcohol use (but only among white participants). The research dovetails with the work on anxiety sensitivity in terms of predicting substance use–related variables but also with the work suggesting that ethnicity may moderate predictive relations (Varela et al., 2007; Weems, Hayward, et al., 2002).

An important line of research suggested by this similarity is the examination of the relative predictive ability of anxiety sensitivity versus general measures of distress tolerance, similar to the work couching anxiety sensitivity within broader cognitive models (Weems et al., 2007). For example, two questions arise: Can CASI scores predict anxiety problems (or alcohol and cigarette use) beyond distress tolerance measured more broadly, such as by an increasing-difficulty/frustrating task paradigm? Conversely, do distress tolerance measures predict anxiety problems (or alcohol and cigarette use) beyond CASI scores? Indeed, research in adult samples has suggested that broader measures of distress tolerance may mediate previously reported relationships between anxiety sensitivity and eating disorder symptoms (e.g., see Anestis, Selby, Fink, & Joiner, 2007). Thus, as the negative outcomes that researchers try to predict become more diverse, broader conceptualizations of distress tolerance may be more effective predictors than anxiety sensitivity. It is possible that anxiety sensitivity may only be reasonably thought of as a specific form of distress tolerance related to anxiety problems. In adult samples the association between anxiety sensitivity (ASI) and self-report measures of general distress tolerance is relatively small (e.g., $r = -.28$; Anestis et al., 2007). However, the whole concept of distress tolerance in youth may benefit from testing the incremental validity of assessments/measures of the construct, similar to the work done on anxiety sensitivity. As noted previously, the original Strange Situation paradigm (Ainsworth et al., 1978) might reasonably be seen as a historically and developmentally early assessment of distress tolerance; it will thus be important to ensure that measures of distress tolerance are not simply tapping, for example, general negative affect (similar to the work on anxiety sensitivity vs. trait anxiety and negative affect; Weems et al., 1998, 2007).

# SUMMARY AND CONCLUSIONS

This chapter examined anxiety sensitivity as a specific form of distress tolerance in youth. Anxiety sensitivity, defined as an individual difference in beliefs that anxiety has severe and negative consequences, results in decreased capacity to tolerate anxiety states and sensations (i.e., is associated with anxiety disorders in youth) and also may be associated with pain and other somatic symptoms. Indeed, anxiety sensitivity is a predictive risk factor for the development of panic attacks in youth and young adults (Hayward et al., 2000; Schmidt, Lerew, & Jackson, 1999; Weems, Hayward, et al., 2002). Anxiety sensitivity in youth can be assessed with the ASI for older adolescents and with the CASI for youth as young as 6 years, and may be further facilitated by the use of parent reports (CASI-P).

Examining the development of anxiety sensitivity may help with the identification of an important developmental precursor for panic and anxiety disorders, and the assessment of anxiety sensitivity in clinical settings may help prescribe treatment for youth with anxiety. However, more research on the developmental origins and clinical applications of anxiety sensitivity in youth is needed. Research points to genetic, learning, and social factors as important in the development of anxiety sensitivity. Additional research clarifying the interrelations and incremental predictive ability of anxiety sensitivity and broader measures of distress tolerance are also needed. Research is also needed to clarify the association among anxiety sensitivity, pain, and other somatic responses.

# REFERENCES

Ainsworth, M. D., Blehar, M. C., Waters, E., & Wall, S. (1978). *Patterns of attachment: A psychological study of the strange situation.* Hillsdale, NJ: Erlbaum.

American Psychiatric Association. (1987). *Diagnostic and statistical manual of mental disorders* (3rd ed.). Washington, DC: Author.

American Psychiatric Association. (1994). *Diagnostic and statistical manual of mental disorders* (4th ed.). Washington, DC: Author.

Anestis, M. D., Selby, E. A., Fink, E. L., & Joiner, T. E. (2007). The multifaceted role of distress tolerance in dysregulated eating behaviors. *International Journal of Eating Disorders, 40,* 718–726.

Asmundson, G. (1999). Anxiety sensitivity and chronic pain: Empirical findings, clinical implications, and future directions. In S. Taylor (Ed.), *Anxiety sensitivity: Theory, research, and treatment of the fear of anxiety* (pp. 269–285). Mahwah, NJ: Erlbaum.

Austin, D. W., Jamieson, R. S., Richards, J. C., & Winkelman, J. (2006). The relationship between attachment style, anxiety sensitivity and interpretive bias among adolescent nonclinical panickers. *Behaviour Change, 23,* 31–41.

Barlow, D. H. (2002). *Anxiety and its disorders: The nature and treatment of anxiety and panic* (2nd ed.). New York: Guilford Press.

Bartholomew, K. (1990). Avoidance of intimacy: An attachment perspective. *Journal of Social and Personal Relationships, 7,* 147–178.

Bernstein, A., Zvolensky, M. J., Norton, P. J., Schmidt, N. B., Taylor, S., Forsyth, J. P., et al. (2007). Taxometric and factor analytic models of anxiety sensitivity: Integrating approaches to latent structural research. *Psychological Assessment, 19,* 74–87.

Bernstein, A., Zvolensky, M. J., Weems, C. F., Stickle, T., & Leen-Feldner, E. (2005). Taxonicity of anxiety sensitivity: An empirical test among youth. *Behaviour Research and Therapy, 43,* 1131–1155.

Blanton, H., & Jaccard, J. (2006). Arbitrary metrics in psychology. *American Psychologist, 61,* 27–41.

Brennan, K. A., Clark, C. L., & Shaver, P. R. (1998). Self-report measurement of adult attachment: An integrative overview. In J. A. Simpson & W. S. Rholes (Eds.), *Attachment theory and close relationships* (pp. 46–76). New York: Guilford Press.

Calamari, J. E., Hales, L. R., Heffelfinger, S. K., Janeck, A. S., Lau, J. J., Weerts, M. A., et al. (2001). Relations between anxiety sensitivity and panic symptoms in nonreferred children and adolescents. *Journal of Behavior Therapy and Experimental Psychiatry, 32,* 117–136.

Chorpita, B. F., Albano, A. M., & Barlow, D. H. (1996). Child Anxiety Sensitivity Index: Considerations for children with anxiety disorders. *Journal of Clinical Child Psychology, 25,* 77–82.

Chorpita, B. F., & Daleiden, E. L. (2000). Properties of the Childhood Anxiety Sensitivity Index in children with anxiety disorders: Autonomic and nonautonomic factors. *Behavior Therapy, 31,* 327–349.

Comeau, N., Stewart, S. H., & Loba, P. (2001). The relations of trait anxiety, anxiety sensitivity, and sensation seeking to adolescents' motivations for alcohol, cigarette, and marijuana use. *Addictive Behaviors, 26,* 803–825.

Corstorphine, E., Mountford, V., Tomlinson, S., Waller, G., & Meyer, C. (2007). Distress tolerance in the eating disorders. *Eating Behaviors, 8,* 91–97.

Daughters, S. B., Reynolds, E. K., MacPherson, L., Kahler, C. W., Danielson, C. K., Zvolensky, M., et al. (2009). Distress tolerance and early adolescent externalizing and internalizing symptoms: The moderating role of gender and ethnicity. *Behaviour Research and Therapy, 47,* 198–205.

Dehon, C., Weems, C. F., Stickle, T. R., Costa, N. M., & Berman, S. L. (2005). A cross-sectional evaluation of the factorial invariance of anxiety sensitivity in adolescents and young adults. *Behaviour Research and Therapy, 43,* 799–810.

Eisen, A. R., & Silverman, W. K. (1993). Should I relax or change my thoughts? A preliminary study of the treatment of overanxious disorder in children. *Cognitive Psychotherapy Research, 7,* 265–280.

Eisen, A. R., & Silverman, W. K. (1998). Prescriptive treatment for generalized anxiety disorder in children. *Behavior Therapy, 29,* 105–123.

Eley, T. C., Shirling, L., Ehlers, A., Gregory, A. W., & Clark, D. M. (2004). Heart-beat perception, panic/somatic symptoms and anxiety sensitivity in children. *Behaviour Research and Therapy, 42,* 439–448.

Feldner, M. T., Leen-Feldner, E. W., Trainor, C., Blanchard, L., & Monson, C. M. (2008). Smoking and posttraumatic stress symptoms among adolescents: Does anxiety sensitivity matter? *Addictive Behaviors, 33,* 1470–1476.

Flavell, J. H., Green, F. L., & Flavell, E. R. (1993). Children's understanding of the stream of consciousness. *Child Development, 64,* 387–398.

Flavell, J. H., Green, F. L., & Flavell, E. R. (1995). Young children's knowledge about thinking. *Monographs of the Society for Research in Child Development, 60,* 1–96.

Fullana-Rivas, M. A., Servera, M., Weems, C. F., Tortella-Feliu, M., & Caseras, X. (2003). Reliability and validity of the Catalan version of the Childhood Anxiety Sensitivity Index. *Anxiety, Stress, and Coping, 16,* 99–107.

Ginsburg, G. S., & Drake, K. L. (2002). Anxiety sensitivity and panic attack symptomology among low income African-American adolescents. *Journal of Anxiety Disorders, 16,* 83–96.

Goldstein, A. J., & Chambless, D. L. (1978). A reanalysis of agoraphobia. *Behavior Therapy, 9,* 47–53.

Harris, P. L., Johnson, C. N., Hutton, D., Andrews, G., & Cooke, T. (1989). Young children's theory-of-mind and emotion. *Cognition and Emotion, 3,* 379–400.

Hayward, C., Killen, J. D., Kraemer, H. C., & Taylor, C. (2000). Predictors of panic attacks in adolescents. *Journal of the American Academy of Child and Adolescent Psychiatry, 39,* 207–214.

Hensley, L., & Varela, R. E. (2008). PTSD symptoms and somatic complaints following Hurricane Katrina: The role of trait anxiety and anxiety sensitivity. *Journal of Clinical Child and Adolescent Psychology, 37,* 542–552.

Hunt, C., Keogh, E., & French, C. C. (2007). Anxiety sensitivity, conscious awareness and selective attentional biases in children. *Behaviour Research and Therapy, 45,* 497–509.

Jang, K. L., Stein, M. B., Taylor, S., & Livesley, W. J. (1999). Gender differences in the etiology of anxiety sensitivity: A twin study. *Journal of Gender-Specific Medicine, 2*(2), 39–44.

Joiner, T. E., Jr., Schmidt, N. B., Schmidt, K. L., Laurent, J., Catanzaro, S. J., Perez, M., et al. (2002). Anxiety sensitivity as a specific and unique marker of anxious symptoms in youth psychiatric inpatients. *Journal of Abnormal Child Psychology, 30,* 167–175.

Kagan, J., Reznick, J. S., & Gibbons, J. (1989). Inhibited and uninhibited types of children. *Child Development, 60,* 838–845.

Kearney, C. A., Albano, A. M., Eisen, A. R., Allan, W. D., & Barlow, D. H. (1997). The phenomenology of panic disorder in youngsters: An empirical study of a clinical sample. *Journal of Anxiety Disorders, 11,* 49–62.

Lau, J. J., Calamari, J. E., & Waraczynski, M. (1996). Panic attack symptomology and anxiety sensitivity in adolescents. *Journal of Anxiety Disorders, 10,* 355–364.

Leen-Feldner, E. W., Feldner, M. T., Reardon, L. E., Babson, K. A., & Dixon, L.

(2008). Anxiety sensitivity and posttraumatic stress among traumatic event-exposed youth. *Behaviour Research and Therapy, 46,* 548–556.

Lipsitz, J. D., Masia-Warner, C., Apfel, H., Marans, Z., Hellstern, B., Forand, N., et al. (2004). Anxiety and depressive symptoms and anxiety sensitivity in youngsters with noncardiac chest pain and benign heart murmurs. *Journal of Pediatric Psychology, 29,* 607–612.

Lonigan, C. J., & Phillips, B. M. (2001). Temperamental influences on the development of anxiety disorders. In M. W. Vasey & M. R. Dadds (Eds.), *The developmental psychopathology of anxiety* (pp. 60–91). London: Oxford University Press.

Maller, R. G., & Reiss, S. (1992). Anxiety sensitivity in 1984 and panic attacks in 1987. *Journal of Anxiety Disorders, 6,* 241–247.

Manassis, K., & Bradley, S. J. (1994). The development of childhood anxiety: Toward an integrated model. *Journal of Applied Developmental Psychology, 15,* 345–366.

Mattis, S. G., & Ollendick, T. H. (1997). Children's cognitive responses to the somatic symptoms of panic. *Journal of Abnormal Child Psychology, 25,* 47–57.

McNally, R. J. (1989). Is anxiety sensitivity distinguishable from trait anxiety?: Reply to Lilienfeld, Jacob, and Turner (1989). *Journal of Abnormal Psychology, 98,* 193–194.

Muris, P., Vermeer, E., & Horselenberg, R. (2008). Cognitive development and the interpretation of anxiety-related physical symptoms in 4- to 12-year-old non-clinical children. *Journal of Behavior Therapy and Experimental Psychiatry, 39,* 73–86.

Muris, P., Vlaeyen, J., & Meesters, C. (2001). The relationship between anxiety sensitivity and fear of pain in healthy adolescents. *Behaviour Research and Therapy, 39,* 1357–1368.

Nock, M. K., & Mendes, W. B. (2008). Physiological arousal, distress tolerance, and social problem-solving deficits among adolescent self-injurers. *Journal of Consulting and Clinical Psychology, 76,* 28–38.

Ollendick, T. H. (1995). Cognitive behavioral treatment of panic disorder with agoraphobia in adolescents: A multiple baseline design analysis. *Behavior Therapy, 26,* 517–531.

Ollendick, T. H., King, N. J., & Hamilton, D. I. (1991). Origins of childhood fears: An evaluation of Rachman's theory of fear acquisition. *Behaviour Research and Therapy, 29,* 117–123.

Peterson, R. A., & Heilbronner, R. L. (1987). The Anxiety Sensitivity Index: Construct validity and factor analytic structure. *Journal of Anxiety Disorders, 1,* 117–121.

Peterson, R. A., & Reiss, S. (1987). *Anxiety Sensitivity Index manual.* Orland Park, IL: International Diagnostic Systems.

Peterson, R. A., & Reiss, S. (1993). *Anxiety Sensitivity Index revised test manual.* Worthington, OH: IDS Publishing.

Piña, A. A., & Silverman, W. K. (2004). Clinical phenomenology, somatic symptoms, and distress in Hispanic/Latino and European American youths with anxiety disorders *Journal of Clinical Child and Adolescent Psychology, 33,* 227–236.

Piña, A. A., Silverman, W. K., Saavedra, L. S., & Weems, C. F. (2001). An analysis of the RCMAS lie scale in a clinic sample of anxious children. *Journal of Anxiety Disorders, 15,* 443–457.

Rabian, B., Embry, L., & MacIntyre, D. (1999). Behavioral validation of the Childhood Anxiety Sensitivity Index in children. *Journal of Clinical Child Psychology, 28,* 105–112.

Rabian, B., Peterson, R. A., Richters, J., & Jensen, P. S. (1993). Anxiety sensitivity among anxious children. *Journal of Clinical Child Psychology, 22,* 441–446.

Reiss, S. (1991). Expectancy model of fear, anxiety, and panic. *Clinical Psychology Review, 11,* 141–153.

Reiss, S., & Havercamp, S. M. (1998). Toward a comprehensive assessment of fundamental motivation: Factor structure of the Reiss profiles. *Psychological Assessment, 10,* 97–106.

Reiss, S., & McNally, R. J. (1985). The expectancy model of fear. In S. Reiss & R. R. Bootzin (Eds.), *Theoretical issues in behavior therapy* (pp. 107–121). New York: Academic Press.

Reiss, S., Peterson, R. A., Gursky, D. M., & McNally, R. J. (1986). Anxiety sensitivity, anxiety frequency and the prediction of fearfulness. *Behaviour Research and Therapy, 24,* 1–8.

Reiss, S., Peterson, R., Taylor, S., Schmidt, N. B., & Weems, C. F. (2008). *Anxiety Sensitivity Index consolidated test manual: ASI, ASI-3, and CASI.* Worthington, OH: IDS Publishing. (Available from *www.anxietysensitivityindex.com*)

Reiss, S., Silverman, W. K., & Weems, C. F. (2001). Anxiety sensitivity. In M. W. Vasey & M. R. Dadds (Eds.), *The developmental psychopathology of anxiety* (pp. 92–111). London: Oxford University Press.

Sandin, B. (1997). *Ansidad miedos y fobias en ninos y adolescents* [Anxiety, fears and phobias in children and adolescents]. Madrid: Dykinson.

Schmidt, N. B., & Cook, J. H. (1999). Effects of anxiety sensitivity on anxiety and pain during a cold pressor challenge in patients with panic disorder. *Behaviour Research and Therapy, 37,* 313–323.

Schmidt, N. B., Lerew, D. R., & Jackson, R. J. (1997). The role of anxiety sensitivity in the pathogenesis of panic: Prospective evaluation of spontaneous panic attacks during acute stress. *Journal of Abnormal Psychology, 106,* 355–364.

Schmidt, N. B., Lerew, D. R., & Jackson, R. J. (1999). Prospective evaluation of anxiety sensitivity in the pathogenesis of panic: Replication and extension. *Journal of Abnormal Psychology, 108,* 532–537.

Schmidt, N. B., Lerew, D. R., & Joiner, T. E. (2000). Prospective evaluation of the etiology of anxiety sensitivity: Test of a scar model. *Behaviour Research and Therapy, 38,* 1083–1095.

Silverman, W. K., Fleisig, W., Rabian, B., & Peterson, R. (1991). Childhood Anxiety Sensitivity Index. *Journal of Clinical Child Psychology, 20,* 162–168.

Silverman, W. K., Ginsburg, G. S., & Goedhart, A. W. (1999). Factor structure of the Childhood Anxiety Sensitivity Index. *Behaviour Research and Therapy, 37,* 903–917.

Silverman, W. K., Goedhart, A. W., Barrett, P., & Turner, C. (2003). The facets of anxiety sensitivity represented in the Childhood Anxiety Sensitivity Index: Confirmatory analyses of factor models from past studies. *Journal of Abnormal Psychology, 112,* 364–374.

Silverman, W. K., & Weems, C. F. (1999). Anxiety sensitivity in children. In S. Taylor (Ed.), *Anxiety sensitivity: Theory, research and the treatment of the fear of anxiety* (pp. 239–268). Mahwah, NJ: Erlbaum.

Stein, M. B., Jang, K. L., & Livesley, W. J. (1999). Heritability of anxiety sensitivity: A twin study. *American Journal of Psychiatry, 156,* 246–251.

Taylor, S. (Ed.). (1999). *Anxiety sensitivity: Theory, research and the treatment of the fear of anxiety.* Mahwah, NJ: Erlbaum.

Taylor, S. (2003). Anxiety sensitivity and its implications for understanding and treating PTSD. *Journal of Cognitive Psychotherapy, 17,* 179–186.

Telch, M. J., Shermis, M. D., & Lucas, J. A. (1989). Anxiety sensitivity: Unitary construct or domain specific appraisals. *Journal of Anxiety Disorders, 3,* 25–32.

Tsao, J. C., Myers, C. D., Craske, M. G., Bursch, B., Kim, S. C., & Zeltzer, L. K. (2004). Role of anticipatory anxiety and anxiety sensitivity in children's and adolescents' laboratory pain responses. *Journal of Pediatric Psychology, 29,* 379–388.

Van Widenfelt, B. M., Siebelink, B. M., Goedhart, A. W., & Treffers, P. D. A. (2002). The Dutch Childhood Anxiety Sensitivity Index: Psychometric properties and factor structure. *Journal of Clinical Child and Adolescent Psychology, 31,* 90–100.

Vasey, M. W., & Dadds, M. R. (Eds.). (2001). *The developmental psychopathology of anxiety.* London: Oxford University Press.

Vasey, M. W., Daleiden, E. L., Williams, L. L., & Brown, L. (1995). Biased attention in childhood anxiety disorders: A preliminary study. *Journal of Abnormal Child Psychology, 23,* 267–279.

Vasey, M. W., & MacLeod, C. (2001). Information-processing factors in childhood anxiety: A review and developmental perspective. In M. W. Vasey & M. R. Dadds (Eds.), *The developmental psychopathology of anxiety* (pp. 253–277). London: Oxford University Press.

Varela, R. E., Weems, C. F., Berman, S. L., Hensley, L., & de Bernal, M. C. R. (2007). Internalizing symptoms in Latinos: The role of anxiety sensitivity. *Journal of Youth and Adolescence, 36,* 429–440.

Viana, A. G., & Rabian, B. (2008). Perceived attachment: Relations to anxiety sensitivity, worry, and GAD symptoms. *Behaviour Research and Therapy, 46,* 737–747.

Watt, M. C., McWilliams, L. A., & Campbell, A. G. (2005). Relations between anxiety sensitivity and attachment style dimensions. *Journal of Psychopathology and Behavioral Assessment, 27,* 191–200.

Watt, M. C., Stewart, S. H., & Cox, B. J. (1998). A retrospective study of the learning history origins of anxiety sensitivity. *Behaviour Research and Therapy, 36,* 505–525.

Watts, S. E., & Weems, C. F. (2006). Associations among selective attention, memory bias, cognitive errors and symptoms of anxiety in youth. *Journal of Abnormal Child Psychology, 34,* 838–849.

Weems, C. F., Berman, S. L., Silverman, W. K., & Saavedra, L. M. (2001). Cognitive errors in youth with anxiety disorders: The linkages between negative cognitive errors and anxious symptoms. *Cognitive Therapy and Research*, 25, 559–575.

Weems, C. F., Berman, S. L., Silverman W. K., & Rodriguez, E. (2002). The relation between anxiety sensitivity and attachment style in adolescence and early adulthood. *Journal of Psychopathology and Behavioral Assessment*, 24, 159–168.

Weems, C. F., Costa, N. M., Watts, S. E., Taylor, L. K., & Cannon, M. F. (2007). Cognitive errors, anxiety sensitivity and anxiety control beliefs: Their unique and specific associations with childhood anxiety symptoms. *Behavior Modification*, 31, 174–201.

Weems, C. F., Hammond-Laurence, K., Silverman, W. K., & Ferguson, C. (1997). The relation between anxiety sensitivity and depression in children referred for anxiety. *Behaviour Research and Therapy*, 35, 961–966.

Weems, C. F., Hammond-Laurence, K., Silverman, W. K., & Ginsburg, G. S. (1998). Testing the utility of the anxiety sensitivity construct in children and adolescents referred for anxiety disorders. *Journal of Clinical Child Psychology*, 27, 69–77.

Weems, C. F., Hayward, C., Killen, J. D., & Taylor, C. B. (2002). A longitudinal investigation of anxiety sensitivity in adolescence. *Journal of Abnormal Psychology*, 111, 471–477.

Weems, C. F., Silverman, W. K., & La Greca, A. M. (2000). What do youth referred for anxiety problems worry about?: Worry and its relation to anxiety and anxiety disorders in children and adolescents. *Journal of Abnormal and Child Psychology*, 28, 63–72.

Weems, C. F., Silverman, W. K., Saavedra, L. S., Piña, A. A., & Lumpkin, P. W. (1999). The discrimination of children's phobias using the revised Fear Survey Schedule for Children. *Journal of Child Psychology and Psychiatry and Allied Disciplines*, 40, 941–952.

Weems, C. F., Taylor, L. K., Marks, A., & Varela, R. E. (2010). Anxiety sensitivity in childhood and adolescence: Parent reports and factors that influence associations with child reports. *Cognitive Therapy and Research*, 34, 303–315.

Zinbarg, R. E., Barlow, D. H., & Brown, T. A. (1997). Hierarchical structure and general factor saturation of the Anxiety Sensitivity Index: Evidence and implications. *Psychological Assessment*, 9, 277–284.

Zinbarg, R. E., Mohlman, J., & Hong, N. N. (1999). Dimensions of anxiety sensitivity. In S. Taylor (Ed.), *Anxiety sensitivity: Theory, research and the treatment of the fear of anxiety* (pp. 83–114). Mahwah, NJ: Erlbaum.

Zwick, W. R., & Velicer, W. F. (1986). A comparison of five rules for determining the number of components to retain. *Psychological Bulletin*, 99, 432–442.

# 3

## Distress Overtolerance
## and Distress Intolerance
### *A Behavioral Perspective*

Thomas R. Lynch *and* Guy A. Mizon

In this chapter we examine distress tolerance from a modern behavioral perspective, and introduce the concept of "distress overtolerance." First, we briefly define what we mean by modern behaviorism. Second, we outline our theoretical perspective, defining distress intolerance and distress overtolerance as maladaptive patterns of behavior resulting from an interaction between *distress tolerance capacity* and *distress awareness and judgment* and involving habitual avoidance or overtolerance of aversive tension. Third, we review domains that we consider important when conducting a functional analysis of distress intolerance and distress overtolerance, including (1) biological predispositions, (2) sociobiographic factors, (3) contextual factors, (4) cue factors and discriminant stimuli that signify the availability of reinforcement, and (5) reinforcing factors. Fourth, we discuss how habitual avoidance of aversive tension or distress can exacerbate problems experienced in dealing with everyday life. Finally, we define healthy distress tolerance in the context of acceptance-based therapy approaches and review the theory and practice behind a mindfulness-based approach hypothesized to maximize nonavoidance.

### MODERN BEHAVIORISM
### AND ITS ANTECEDENTS

Behavioral theory and methods are not restricted to the observation of overt behavior, although this assumption is quite common. Currently, three distinct developmental periods have been identified in behavior therapy, with concomitant increases in the empirical basis and conceptual sophistication at each stage (Hayes, Masuda, Bissett, Luoma, & Guerrero, 2004). The first wave focused primarily on the techniques associated with operant and classical conditioning principles. Influenced heavily by Watson (1924), the first wave essentially made the metaphysical claim that the "mind" did not exist (thus reducing the percept of "thinking" to mere subvocal speech); consequently, the only relevant unit of analysis was overt behavior. In addition, Watson argued, even were the mind to exist, it was impossible to study, given that there was no scientifically appropriate method to study it (Hayes, Follette, & Follette, 1995). Thus, the first wave would analyze distress-intolerant behavior as either respondent (i.e., behavior controlled by antecedent external stimuli) and/or operant (i.e., behavior controlled by the external reinforcing or punishing contingencies) and considered mediators such as cognition to be irrelevant.

As a reaction to the lack of recognition given by first-wave thinkers to the possibility of cognitions having any effect on overt behavior, the second wave attempted to use empirical methods to study the functioning of the mind (Hayes et al., 1995) and favored the idea that behavior could be caused by private mental events such as cognitions or appraisals. Although second-wave behavioral therapies still aimed for behavioral change, cognitions were now added to the list of potential clinical targets to be addressed during treatment (Bandura, 1969; Beck, Rush, Shaw, & Emery, 1979). Thus, the second wave of behavioral therapy would not only have examined distress-intolerant behavior from a respondent–operant perspective but also would have accounted for the influence of modeling, cognition, beliefs, and/or schemas.

The third wave began in part as the result of a reevaluation of the extent to which the newer second-wave cognitive techniques were supported by the type of experimental and empirical methods that had formed the scientific basis of behavioral approaches from the outset (Corrigan, 2001). Third-wave proponents argued that explanations that give causal priority to one form of behavior over another were incomplete (Hayes et al., 1995). From this perspective, *cognitions are behaviors* and, as such, are not qualitatively different from overt behavior. The reasoning is that assigning cognitions a special causal or mediational status erroneously prioritizes one type of behavior over another, placing undue emphasis on changing private experience. In addition, third-wave approaches attempt to understand behavior not in terms of its topography but rather in terms of its function. Thus, two acts of distress-intolerant behavior may appear similar but functionally be quite different. For example, a particular behavior such as substance abuse might function to elicit nurturance for one person and to reduce aversive emotions in another. As such, the third wave challenged the fundamental first- and second-wave principles that focused primarily on changing the form or frequency of problematic behavior (e.g., changing dysfunctional schemas, behavior, sensations, or emotions) by empirically testing therapeutic methods that altered the *function* of a behavior *without* altering its form (Hayes, 2004). This resulted in the development of a number of new treatments emphasizing acceptance of and contact with the present moment. Examples of these treatments include dialectical behavior therapy (DBT; Linehan, 1993), acceptance and commitment therapy (Hayes, Strosahl, & Wilson, 1999), functional analytic psychotherapy (Kohlenberg & Tsai, 1994), integrative behavioral couple therapy (Christensen, Jacobson, & Babcock, 1995), and mindfulness-based cognitive therapy (Segal, Williams, & Teasdale, 2002). In acceptance-based strategies, the patients' aim of controlling their private experience (e.g., thoughts, feelings, and sensations) is itself targeted for change rather than the private experience (Hayes, Wilson, Gifford, Follette, & Strosahl, 1996). From an acceptance perspective, trying to willfully change, suppress, or inhibit unwanted physical pain, thoughts, or emotions may actually exacerbate the problem (e.g., Cukrowicz, Ekblad, Cheavens, Rosenthal, & Lynch, 2008; Lynch, Cheavens, Morse, & Rosenthal, 2004; Lynch, Robins, Morse, & Krause, 2001; Lynch, Schneider, Rosenthal, & Cheavens, 2007). It is from this third-wave behavioral perspective that we address the functions of and influences on distress-intolerant and distress-overtolerant behavior in this chapter.

## DEFINING DISTRESS
## OVERTOLERANCE AND INTOLERANCE

A widely used definition of *distress tolerance* (DT) is "the perceived ability to experience and endure negative emotional states" (Simons & Gaher, 2005). The term also has an acknowledged physical dimension, as noted in the definition "the ability to tolerate negative affect or aversive psychological or physical states" (Bernstein, Trafton, Ilgen, & Zvolensky, 2008). However, DT can be used to refer both to the *capacity* to withstand negative emotional states (i.e., a trait) and to *acts* of withstanding negative emotional states (i.e., behaviors). As such, the term distress *in*tolerance (DI) could be used to refer to a *lack of capacity* to withstand distress and to *acts or behaviors* whose function is to avoid distress. To preempt any possible ambiguity, in this chapter we refer to distress-tolerance capacity (*DT capacity*), distress-tolerant behavior (*DT behavior*), and distress-intolerant behavior (*DI behavior*) as separate labels for the trait and the associated behaviors. In talking about a capacity to withstand distress, we refer to a capacity to not impulsively or habitually attempt to change or escape an aversive emotional or physical experience. As such, we view DT capacity as related to, and DI behaviors as a subset of, the broader concept of "experiential avoidance," which refers to "the phenomenon that occurs when a person is unwilling to remain in contact with particular private experiences (e.g., bodily sensations, emotions, thoughts, memories, behavioral predispositions) and takes steps to alter the form or frequency of these events and the contexts that occasion them" (Hayes et al., 1996). Experiential avoidance is a broader concept because it can also encompass avoidance of experiences that are not necessarily distressing, and even positive (e.g., Kashdan, Barrios, Forsyth, & Steger, 2006). In contrast, we use DI behavior to refer specifically to behaviors whose function is to avoid the experience of distress. Moreover, to emphasize the physical as well as psychological aspects of distress, we at times use the terms "distress" and "aversive tension" interchangeably because "aversive tension" is a concept that reflects the experience of aversive physical sensations of unknown physical or psychological origin (Stiglmayr, Shapiro, Stieglitz, Limberger, & Bohus, 2001).

As other chapters in this volume amply demonstrate, DT is growing as a research focus in the empirical literature. However, empirical attention to the maladaptive side of DT has been primarily focused on people with *low* levels of DT behavior, in fields such as smoking cessation (Brown, Lejuez, Kahler, Strong, & Zvolensky, 2005), substance abuse (Daughters et al., 2005), and self-injury (Nock & Mendes, 2008). In this chapter, we seek to draw attention also to the members of the population with tendencies for *overly high* levels of DT behavior because we view this as an important concept that has been relatively understudied. We use the terms *distress overtolerance* (DO) and *DO behavior* to refer to situations in which an individual tolerates a high amount of distress, in a manner that does not fit with his or her long-term values or interests, resulting in adverse long-term consequences. An everyday example of DO behavior would be if an individual were to tolerate an extended period of inadvertent mistreatment by a co-worker for fear of the consequences of objecting to that treatment. In the following sections, we outline our view of the functions of, and relationship between, DI and DO behaviors.

## THE PROBLEM OF DISTRESS OVERTOLERANCE AND INTOLERANCE

Our view is that the relationship between the amount of distress people tolerate in their lives and the level of adaptive behavior they demonstrate (as well as the level of well-being they experience) is best described by an inverse-U-shaped function (quadratic function; see Figure 3.1), such that in general the people at the extremes of the curve—those tolerating the most and least distress—are the ones who exhibit the most maladaptive behaviors and who experience the lowest levels of well-being.

It is important to emphasize that our prediction of a quadratic relationship with adaptive behavior/well-being applies to a person's DT behavior rather than DT capacity. This distinction is important because we predict a different relationship between adaptive behavior/well-being and DT capacity. Specifically, we predict that these factors will be related but that this relationship will be strongly mediated by other factors, such as judgment and distress awareness. We predict that people high in those traits will be placed in the midsection of the curve according to their DT capacity, and that people low in those traits will be placed at the low extreme if they have low DT capacity and at the high extreme if they have high DT capacity.

*Judgment and distress awareness* are, in our view, crucial to healthy DT because they allow an individual to determine the boundaries within which tolerating distress is appropriate for them. Distress awareness entails conscious awareness of internal states, such as physical sensations, emotions, and action urges. There is evidence that a lack of awareness of internal states is associated with psychopathology and maladap-

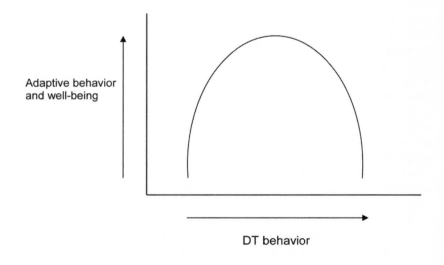

Adaptive behavior and well-being

DT behavior

**FIGURE 3.1.** Proposed "inverse-U" relationship between distress tolerance (DT) and adaptive behavior/well-being.

tive behavior; for instance, there is evidence that difficulty identifying feelings (alexithymia) is highly predictive of a broad range of levels of psychopathology (Conrad, Wegener, Imbierowicz, Liedtke, & Geiser, 2009; Grabe, Spitzer & Freyberger, 2004), whereas an unusually low awareness of pain has also been associated with various forms of psychopathology (Bohus et al., 2000; Claes, Vandereycken, & Vertommen, 2006; Dworkin, Crawford Clark, & Lipsitz, 1995). Awareness of internal states is a prerequisite for decision making regarding those states, but this decision-making process also requires adequate judgments to be made about how DT in a given situation relates to one's goals and how adaptive it would be to continue to tolerate the distress. For example, a successful marathon runner must discriminate between situations in which physical pain should be tolerated and those in which it should be attended to as a sign of potential injury. In later sections, we discuss the factors we view as important determinants of an individual's DT capacity, distress awareness, and judgment, which together contribute to coping style.

Our view of the relationship between DT and well-being/adaptive behavior is similar to predictions of quadratic relationships between behavior regulation and social functioning (Eisenberg & Fabes, 1992; Eisenberg, Fabes, Guthrie, & Reiser, 2000). Eisenberg and colleagues (2000) propose that both very low and very high levels of behavior regulation are maladaptive and related to poor social functioning outcomes. Not only do we predict a similar relationship between our constructs of interest, but we also suggest more broadly that Eisenberg and colleagues' concept of behavioral regulation fits into a set of temperaments that are associated with DO/DI, including the concepts of behavioral inhibition/activation (Gray, 1982, 1991), and impulsivity/risk aversion. Eisenberg and colleagues discuss three styles of behavioral regulation: highly inhibited, undercontrolled, and optimally controlled. Importantly, they distinguish between voluntary behavioral inhibition, or the purposeful exertion of control over behavior in a goal-directed manner, and involuntary behavioral inhibition, which is an overlearned tendency to be closed to new experiences and behavior. They propose that highly inhibited individuals are "high in involuntary behavioral inhibition ..., low to average in voluntary inhibitory control, low in activation control (the ability to get oneself to do things that one might not be motivated to do, e.g., do a difficult task), low to moderate in attentional regulation, and low in problem-focused coping strategies," while undercontrolled individuals are "low in emotion and behavior regulation, including inhibitory, attentional, and activational control, and low in adaptive problem-focused and proactive coping behavior" (p. 139). We propose that individuals with an undercontrolled temperament would also be prone to DI behavior, whereas those with a highly inhibited temperament would be prone to DO behavior. Also, in the same vein as Eisenberg and colleagues' (2000) proposal that emotionality and behavioral control are separate capacities interacting to produce a pattern of behavior, we propose that distress awareness and DT are separate capacities, with an interaction that is mediated by the capacity for judicious application of DT.

The constructs of undercontrol and overcontrol can be mapped onto two broad categories of maladaptive coping: dramatic-erratic tendencies toward behavioral undercontrol and constricted-controlled tendencies toward behavioral overcontrol. Clinically, the former category includes emotionally dysregulated, impulsive, and dramatic–erratic disorders such as borderline personality disorder (BPD), bulimia nervosa, binge-eating disorder, substance abuse disorders, histrionic personality disorder, and antisocial personality disorder and populations such as adolescents engaging in intentional self-injury. In contrast, the latter category encompasses disorders that are characterized by being overcontrolled, emotionally constricted, closed to new experience, perfectionistic, cognitively/behaviorally rigid, and highly risk averse, such as paranoid personality disorder (PPD), obsessive–compulsive personality disorder (OCPD), avoidant personality disorder (APD), and anorexia nervosa (AN) and populations such as older adults with chronic depression (see Lynch & Cheavens, 2008, for more discussion of this contrast).

## ARE DISTRESS INTOLERANCE AND DISTRESS OVERTOLERANCE INDEPENDENT CONSTRUCTS?

An important issue to address is the precise nature of the relationship between the constructs of DI and DO. With respect to this issue, our theoretical perspective is that although these constructs do lie on a single continuum of "distress tolerated" (the $x$-axis of Figure 3.1), thus making sense to characterize someone's general response style as either DI or DO (or somewhere in between), this constraint only applies when aggregating behavior over time. When examining individual behavioral responses to individual situations, we suggest that it is perfectly possible for someone to exhibit a DO response to one situation and a DI response to the next. However, in general, we argue that each of us tends to acquire a particular style of managing distress that is the result of a transaction between our unique biological predispositions and sociobiographic histories that is reinforced such that it becomes an overlearned behavioral response (i.e., likely to be exhibited independent of context).

## INDIVIDUAL-DIFFERENCE FACTORS
## PREDICTING DISTRESS OVERTOLERANCE:
## LEARNED INDUSTRIOUSNESS
## AND EMOTIONAL REACTIVITY

In thinking about individual difference factors that may be systematically related to the expression of these two constructs, we propose that the concept of *learned industriousness* (Eisenberger, 1992) will show an important relationship to DO/DI. Learned industriousness theory holds that people's level of industriousness will be determined by their learning history, such that if they have had to exert a high degree of effort in order to gain rewards in the past, they will be more likely to do so again. If, on the other hand, rewards have tended to come with relatively little effort expended and/or if attempts to escape the task itself have been intermittently reinforced, they will be less likely to persist with high effort in a given endeavor. This notion is supported by experimental evidence demonstrating that the level of effort required in a training task determines the degree of effort expended in a later task (e.g., Boyagian & Nation, 1981; Eisenberger, Heerdt, Hamdi, Zimet, & Bruckmeir, 1979; Eisenberger, Kuhlman, & Cotterell, 1992). We propose that individuals with high levels of learned industriousness, if they are to develop one or other type of maladaptive response to distress, are much more likely to develop DO tendencies than DI tendencies because their learning history will push them toward persistence in the face of adversity. However, it is important to make a clear theoretical distinction between general task persistence, seen as a standard result of learned industriousness, and DO, which involves continued persistence in an activity that elicits high levels of distress despite evidence that the desired goal may not be achieved and/or that the effort of persistence itself may result in damaging effects. It is interesting to note that some otherwise excellent research has treated DT and task persistence as essentially equivalent, referring to "measures of distress tolerance, or task persistence" (Brandon et al., 2003, p. 449). The relevance of this distinction is made clear when considering individuals who are able to persist longer than most with tasks that are normally experienced as aversive but for whom those tasks are not particularly aversive. For example, an individual who *enjoys* spending lengthy and intense periods engaged in solving mathematical problems—a task experienced as aversive by many—should not be seen as exhibiting DO behavior. However, another individual who persists at length with highly stressful attempts to solve these problems, despite experiencing a high degree of distress as a result and for whom persistence has no apparent benefit (e.g., he or she is not cramming for a math exam the next day) might well be characterized as engaging in DO behavior.

Thus, we see the degree of distress experienced by the individual *combined* with the utility of behaving persistently at any given moment to be important determinants of whether a persistent behavior should be classed as DO or simply as persistence. Similarly, it is important to distinguish DO behavior, which does require a degree of task persistence, from behavioral patterns in which an individual maintains a distressed state for long periods of time but is constantly engaged in attempts to escape that distress. Such behavior overlaps with DO behavior in that it falls under the general rubric of experiential avoidance, but it does not constitute DO behavior because it does not involve maladaptive overtolerance of the distress experienced

Another individual-difference factor that we view as likely to be systematically related to DO/DI behavior is *emotional reactivity*. A link between DI and emotional reactivity has been suggested by other authors, citing evidence that individuals who scored highly on measures of affective reactivity also showed reduced persistence in aversive tasks (e.g., Brown, Lejuez, Kahler, & Strong, 2002). We suggest that a degree of emotional reactivity is an important precursor for either strong patterns of DI *or* DO behavior because it will determine the degree of distress experienced in daily life and will, therefore, accentuate any tendencies toward maladaptive coping. However, we predict that emotional reactivity alone is not sufficient to determine whether an individual adopts a DI or a DO coping style. Rather, the combination of emotional reactivity and learned industriousness will lead to a DO pattern, whereas a low level of learned industriousness will combine with emotional reactivity to produce a DI pattern. Thus, we view both task persistence and subjective distress as key components of DO behavior, and we predict that individual differences in learned industriousness (which will affect task persistence) and emotional reactivity (which will affect subjective distress) will be key determinants of the emergence of DO behavior.

## MEASUREMENT OF
## DISTRESS OVERTOLERANCE

Because DO is essentially a new construct, there are no tools dedicated to its measurement as yet. However, we now examine the extent to which existing measures of DT may capture the relevant information for assessing DO.

The best known self-report measure of DT is the Distress Tolerance Scale (Simons & Gaher, 2005). This 15-item questionnaire has four subscales: Tolerance, Appraisal, Absorption, and Regulation. Of these, the items relating to the Tolerance, Appraisal, and Absorption subscales can all be seen to pertain to the intensity and nature of the experience of distress, whereas only the Regulation subscale contains items that pertain to behavioral tendencies relating to dealing with distress. The Regulation subscale items all assess the tendency to act with urgency to avoid feeling upset. As such, they are suited to measurement of tendencies toward DI behavior but not DO behavior. The other three subscales might have some utility in measuring the emotional reactivity that we view as being an important precursor to DO behavior, but this would need to be done in conjunction with further measures to capture DO patterns accurately.

Behavioral measures of DT have tended to involve measurement of persistence in a task either assumed or assessed as aversive to the participants, for example, breath-holding endurance (e.g., Hajek, Belcher, & Stapleton, 1987), inhalation of carbon dioxide–enriched air (e.g., Brown et al., 2002), a time-pressured mathematical task that increases in difficulty (e.g., the paced auditory serial addition task; Holdwick & Wingenfeld, 1999), an anagram task that increases to extreme difficulty (Eisenberger et al., 1992), and hand tracing of difficult geometric figures while observing one's own hand movements in a mirror (Quinn, Brandon, & Copeland, 1996). Such measures would seem to lend themselves well to measurement of DO behavior because they are likely to be sensitive to extremes of high DT. However, we offer two caveats. First, as discussed, it is essential that any measure of DO behavior actually measures real distress. It is possible that some individuals show high levels of task tolerance simply because they find it less aversive. Therefore, it is important to accompany any task assumed to be aversive with some kind of manipulation check to be sure that each individual in question found it to be so and, ideally, to obtain a separate measure of distress that could be used as a covariate in analyses. In addition, as mentioned, DO behavior is considered problematic precisely because continued task persistence is damaging for individuals; to our knowledge, this has yet to be accounted for in measures of DT and doing so may present ethical and practical challenges to researchers. Second, as already discussed, we distinguish between DT *capacity* and actual tendencies to tolerate distress in everyday life. As such, laboratory measures can only be a proxy for the issue at hand, which is the extent to which excessive DT causes problems in a person's life. With this in mind, it may be that self-report measures are best suited to this purpose, and perhaps the next step in investigating the concept of DO would be to design a self-report measure that assesses the extent to which a tendency to tolerate high levels of distress causes problems in an individual's life.

## DISTRESS-INTOLERANT AND DISTRESS-OVERTOLERANT BEHAVIOR AS AN OPERANT RESPONSE

Our theoretical perspective conceptualizes DI behavior as a set of operant responses, reinforced by the short-term benefits of relief from aversive tension, despite potential long-term negative consequences. We consider urges to engage in DI behavior and the aversive tension that precede DI behavior to generally be classically conditioned, whereas actual DI behaviors (e.g., impulsive overspending, self-injury) are operantly reinforced via reductions in aversive tension and/or other short-term rewards. In contrast, we propose that DO behavior (e.g., inhibiting the expression of distress and/or avoiding labeling pain) is maintained by reinforcing contingencies that are expressed in a different pattern and over a longer period than those pertaining to the impulsive responding more typical of DI behaviors. We believe that DO behavior is less likely to be reinforced via reductions in arousal because, by its very nature, DO behavior does not immediately eliminate the distress experienced. Although we propose that immediate contingencies and properties of the current situation do exert some influence on DO behavior, we suggest that far more important is a learned coping style, acquired over an extended period of time, that involves inhibiting engagement with new stimuli and situations and tolerating any discomfort that arises. This constricted style of coping inherently reduces the salience of current stimuli and their potential to influence behavior.

We expand this position in the following sections, in which we address and discuss the relative importance of, the different factors that influence DO/DI behavior: (1) *biological predispositions* for DO/DI behavior or traits that may lead to it; (2) *sociobiographic feedback* that may set up conditions for DO/DI behavior to emerge and be reinforced; and (3) *overtolerant or intolerant* maladaptive coping that is overlearned and characteristic of DO/DI behavior. These are examined via a behavioral analysis of the situations in which a maladaptive DO or DI coping style is learned, including establishing operations, cue factors (stimulus–response–consequence relations), and discriminant stimuli that signify the availability of reinforcement and reinforcing factors that make DO/DI habitual. Our three-factor model of DO/DI behavior is transactional in nature, in that each factor is hypothesized to reciprocally influence the others (see Figure 3.2).

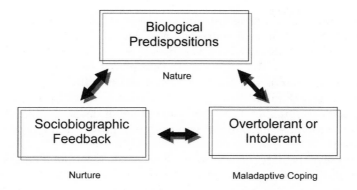

**FIGURE 3.2.** Proposed relationship among biological, social, and regulation (coping) factors in the development of distress overtolerance/distress intolerance behavior.

## BIOLOGICAL PREDISPOSITIONS INFLUENCING DISTRESS–INTOLERANT AND DISTRESS–OVERTOLERANT BEHAVIOR

*Biological vulnerabilities* in this context are the innate predispositions of some individuals to experience atypical physiological reactivity to emotional or pain stimuli (Boyce & Ellis, 2005). Although it is important to acknowledge that "genes represent risk factors and not fated outcomes" (McGuffin & Southwick, 2003), there is nonetheless substantial evidence that such vulnerabilities contribute to explaining why two individuals who have grown up in very similar environments may develop very different patterns of responding to aversive stimuli. For individuals with a dramatic-erratic presentation such as BPD, this vulnerability is hypothesized to consist of greater emotional sensitivity (low threshold for recognition of emotional stimuli), greater emotional reactivity (high amplitude of emotional responses), and a slower return to baseline arousal (long duration of emotional responses), all of which exacerbate difficulties in regulating emotion, making impulsive DO/DI behavior such as self-harm more likely (Linehan, 1993). Although this proposal has yet to be convincingly borne out in the psychophysiological literature, studies using self-report methods consistently find that individuals with BPD report being more emotionally intense and reactive to emotional stimuli relative to controls (see Rosenthal et al., 2008, for a review). A more recent proposal is that some individuals have an innate predisposition toward impulsivity, independent of emotional sensitivity (Crowell, Beauchaine,

& Linehan, 2009), a proposal supported by evidence from family studies of BPD (see White, Gunderson, Zanarini, & Hudson, 2003, for a
review). There is also evidence that people with BPD may have reduced
perception of physical pain, both in relation to self-harm and otherwise
(Bohus et al., 2000). The potential combination in BPD of a heightened
sensitivity to emotional pain and a lowered sensitivity to physical pain
is a potent example of how biological vulnerabilities can increase the
likelihood that a given stimulus will lead to impulsive and dangerous DI
behavior.

At the other end of the spectrum, biological vulnerabilities in individuals with an emotionally constricted presentation such as APD, OCPD,
or AN are hypothesized to include a heightened sensitivity for punishment or threat stimuli relative to reward stimuli (Lynch & Cheavens,
2008). Support for a link between sensitivity for threat stimuli and emotional suppression includes evidence that people with a repressive coping
style demonstrate greater vigilance for threat stimuli (Bonanno, Davis,
Singer, & Schwartz, 1991) or, tellingly, early vigilance and late avoidance
of threat stimuli compared with low-anxious controls (Caldwell & Newman, 2005; Calvo & Eysenck, 2000; see Derakshan, Eysenck, & Myers,
2007, for a review). Tendencies toward overcontrol and emotional repres-
sion are also thought to be related to biological predispositions: There is
evidence suggesting that perfectionism is partially genetically determined
(Lilenfeld et al., 2000), and twin studies have found evidence suggesting
a genetic component to alexithymia (Jørgensen, Zachariae, Skytthe, &
Kyvik, 2007; Valera & Berenbaum, 2001).

More broadly, there is evidence that personality dimensions such
as novelty seeking, harm avoidance, reward dependence, and persistence (Cloninger, 1986, 1987; Gusnard et al., 2003) are heritable, stable
across time, and dependent on genetic and neurobiological factors. We
would expect novelty seeking—defined as a tendency toward exploratory
activity in response to novelty, impulsive decision making, extravagant
approach to reward cues, and quick loss of temper—to be positively correlated with DI behavior and negatively correlated with DO behavior. On
the other hand, we would expect harm avoidance—defined as a tendency
toward inhibition, caution, and apprehension—to be positively correlated with both DI and DO behavior. Although it might seem counterin-
tuitive to predict high harm avoidance tendencies in people showing DI
behavior, especially examples such as self-harm, there is evidence that
self-harm is very frequently used as a means of reducing, rather than
producing, aversive arousal (Haines, Williams, Brain, & Wilson, 1995).
Indeed, people with BPD have been found to have higher than average
levels of harm avoidance (Joyce et al., 2003; Korner, Gerull, Stevenson,
& Meares, 2007). We predict that reward dependence—defined as a

tendency toward sentimentality, social attachment, and dependence on the approval of others—will be relatively low in both people prone to DI behavior and those prone to DO behavior. Individual differences in novelty seeking have been found to be related to variation in the level of activity in the dopaminergic system, whereas differences in harm avoidance have been linked to variability in the serotonergic system. Harm avoidance and reward dependence have been found to be related to polymorphisms of serotonin- and dopamine-related genes (Kim, Kim, Lee, Kim, & Kim, 2006). Furthermore, a recent study using voxel-based morphometry has provided evidence that these personality dimensions are related to structural variation in specific brain regions (Gardini, Cloninger, & Venneri, 2009).

## SOCIOBIOGRAPHIC FEEDBACK INFLUENCING DISTRESS-INTOLERANT AND DISTRESS-OVERTOLERANT BEHAVIOR

Another important factor in the development of DO/DI behavior is sociobiographic influences, referring to a person's learning history from social interactions and the behavioral patterns that result from it. For example, we believe that the most extreme DI behaviors are very likely to have been shaped in part by a pattern of sociobiographic feedback that involves persistent and pervasive invalidation. Such feedback, from caregivers or other important figures in an individual's development, serves to create a learning environment in which the individual's internal experiences and overt behavior are invalidated, and it (1) communicates to the individual that his or her experiences and perceptions (e.g., emotions, beliefs) are wrong and (2) attributes the individual's experiences to socially unacceptable characteristics (e.g., oversensitivity, manipulation) (Linehan, 1993). Should the individual in question be a child who also has a biological predisposition toward intense emotionality, invalidating feedback that involved ignoring, punishing, or contradicting their frequent and intense emotional reactions would be especially confusing and painful. Such invalidation is known to be pervasive among individuals with BPD during childhood, with evidence of high rates of recollected parental denial of the children's feelings (Zanarini et al., 1997) and high rates of physical, sexual, and emotional abuse as well as emotional neglect and separation from significant caretakers (Herman, Perry, & van der Kolk, 1989; Ogata et al., 1990; Zanarini et al., 1997).

Maladaptive coping strategies relating to DT and emotion regulation are thought to be frequent consequences of persistent and pervasively invalidating sociobiographic feedback (Linehan, 1993). We further suggest that such sociobiographic feedback impairs and distorts the development of both appropriate distress awareness and judgment as to how to respond to perceived distress. In particular, a child may learn to suppress emotional reactions and as a result fail to learn how to label emotions. In addition, if extreme emotional reactions sometimes result in a supportive response from the environment, the child is thereby intermittently reinforced for intense displays of emotion. Such a toxic combination of social contingencies leads to a cycle in which the child oscillates between emotional inhibition and extreme emotional reactivity. Empirical support for these notions includes findings that parental punishment or minimization of emotional expression is correlated with children's propensity for frequent or intense negative emotions (e.g., Eisenberg, Fabes, & Murphy, 1996) as well as low socioemotional competence (e.g., Jones, Eisenberg, Fabes, & MacKinnon, 2002). Associations have also been found between childhood emotional invalidation and chronic emotional inhibition in adulthood, emotional inhibition that, in turn, predicts adult psychological distress (Krause, Mendelson, & Lynch, 2003).

DO behavior, on the other hand, is hypothesized to be influenced by sociobiographic feedback characterized by pervasive verbal and nonverbal communication from parents/caregivers/important others that the child is (1) "never good enough" and "mistakes are intolerable" and (2) special and "should" be better than others (e.g., more intelligent, more compliant, more responsible, more religious, more attractive). It is important to note that we predict that escalations of emotion are intermittently reinforced among high-DI individuals, but that high-DO individuals are reinforced for emotion and distress inhibition, with DI displays consistently punished. Thus, DO children learn that it is imperative to avoid mistakes, become highly sensitive to perceived criticism, and see self-worth in relation to the performance and perception of others (Lynch & Cheavens, 2008). In addition, the overall message is that complaining about distress is not appropriate ("Life is tough, get over it"), and instead they are reinforced for control of emotional displays and keeping a "stiff upper lip." The resulting DO behavior is similar to that of "repressors:" high restricted awareness and expression of emotion that is associated with rigid attempts to reduce negative affect through avoidance and constriction of emotional experiences. Over time the sociobiographic environment teaches DO individuals that if they control themselves, good things will happen (e.g., they will be loved) and that being vulnerable (i.e., showing distress) is dangerous. As a consequence, these individuals are likely to avoid situations that may lead to social intimacy or that may require the expression of emotion or distress, finding isolation or rule-governed situations reinforcing because their sense of self is experienced as more stable and less influenced by the whims of others or unknowable demands for intimacy.

Empirical support exists for this prediction of the effects of socio-biographic feedback on DO behavior. Turkat (1985) found that college students classified as having a paranoid personality were more likely to report childhood experiences that reflected parental concern regarding social evaluation. Furthermore, a longitudinal study of a community-based sample found that mothers' reports of childhood emotional abuse (e.g., "I do not praise my child") was associated with an increased risk of APD and PPD (but not BPD) symptoms in their children, even after controlling for childhood abuse (i.e., physical or sexual trauma), neglect (e.g., physical neglect), and other personality disorder symptoms (Johnson, Smailes, Cohen, Brown, & Bernstein, 2000). The effects of adult retrospective report of childhood emotional maltreatment and negative parental reaction to childhood emotional responses on eating disorder pathology also has been shown to be fully mediated by emotion inhibition (Krause, Robins, & Lynch, 2000), suggesting that the symptoms present in adulthood were related to attempts at emotional constriction as opposed to the childhood experiences.

## A BEHAVIORAL ANALYSIS OF SITUATIONAL FACTORS INFLUENCING DISTRESS-INTOLERANT AND DISTRESS-OVERTOLERANT BEHAVIOR

Having examined biological predispositions and sociobiographic history, we now turn our attention to situational factors that we believe influence DO/DI behavior. *Establishing operations* are immediate-term contextual factors that influence the motivational properties (evocative functions and reinforcement salience) of certain stimuli and thus the probability that behaviors associated with those stimuli may be elicited (Dougher, Perkins, Greenway, Koons, & Chiasson, 2002; Michel, Valach, & Waeber, 1994). In this sense, they can be seen as more transient, state versions of the trait concept of biological vulnerabilities. As a simple example, food deprivation is an establishing operation that temporarily increases the salience of food as a form of reinforcement: A hot dog stand is more likely to catch people's attention and elicit action urges if they are hungry. Establishing operations for DO/DI behavior can include a wide variety of events, including lack of sleep or food, the recent loss of a loved one, a recent argument, physical fatigue, alcohol/drug use, and physical pain. The key commonality is that establishing operations for DO/DI behavior in a given individual will temporarily increase the likelihood of aversive tension being elicited. For example, if people seeking to quit smoking are in a situation where they feel less confident than usual, a distressing stimulus (e.g., an uncomfortable sighting of an ex-partner) may be much more likely to provoke DI behavior (a smoking relapse) than if it occurred in a situation where the people feel more self-efficacy (Gwaltney et al., 2002). As stated earlier, we suggest that aversive tension is a less powerful determinant of DO behavior than learned coping style. However, we nonetheless propose that aversive tension may serve to temporarily increase individuals' resolve to fully engage in their DO coping behaviors. To illustrate the role of establishing operations in this process, consider an example of someone with AN who has recently weighed him- or herself (with an outcome found to be unsatisfactory). In this situation, food-related stimuli may temporarily become especially likely to provoke aversive tension, and the individual's resolve to engage in DO behavior such as food restriction or overexercise will be temporarily strengthened (Ogden & Whyman, 1997; Winstanley & Dives, 2005).

*Cue factors* are the motivational properties of the stimuli themselves. Some stimuli will produce aversive tension in almost everyone; these are *unconditioned* stimuli. For example, an unexpected loud bang will elicit a brief fear response. However, with a history of being repeatedly paired with a particular outcome, any given stimulus (or cue) can produce aversive tension and urges for DO/DI behavior across many different contexts; these are *conditioned* stimuli. In addition to conditioned or unconditioned antecedent stimuli that trigger intense emotional states, urges, or other aversive experiences, cue factors for DO/DI behavior also include ideographic discriminant stimuli that signal reinforcement potential. As respondent behavior, aversive tension can be elicited by either unconditioned antecedent stimuli (e.g., a loud bang) or conditioned antecedent stimuli (e.g., time of day signals hunger pangs independent of the actual availability of food); stimuli may include places, persons, objects, sensations, and verbal and/or temporal events. For example, a neutral stimulus (e.g., a certain radio program) automatically elicits aversive tension because it had repeatedly been associated with a negative stimulus (e.g., sexual abuse that occurred while that radio program was on). It is important to note that classically conditioned urges for DO/DI behavior are not cognitively mediated, and conscious cognition is not necessary for the elicitation of conditioned associations (Ohman & Mineka, 2001). In addition, the acquisition of a classically conditioned relationship between two stimuli (e.g., time of day and urge to compulsively tidy) can occur independent of conscious awareness.

Cue factors also involve the case of stimuli that make it possible for particular actions to have particular consequences (stimulus–response–consequence relations). This is called *instrumental* or *operant conditioning* and is defined as learned behavior under the control of reinforcing or punishing consequences. Discriminant stimuli signify the availability of reinforcement. Thus, episodes of DO/DI behavior are more likely to occur if they are preceded by antecedent stimuli that signal the likelihood of reinforcement. For example, for a child who is developing a tendency for DO behavior, a discriminant stimulus might be a parent's mood upon returning home from work: A negative mood might indicate that expressing emotion is likely to be punished (e.g., the parent may get upset or yell in response); therefore, the negative mood signals the potential for reinforcement of the DO behavior (i.e., the child learns that if he or she does not express emotion he or she is less likely to upset the parent).

*Reinforcing factors* are important in any functional analytic approach, which needs to account not only for relevant antecedents but also for reinforcing consequences. Reinforcement of DO/DI behavior can involve psychological, physiological, and social factors. Reinforcing factors for DI behavior are most often immediate in their effect. Many of these effects are obvious, such as the gratification associated with addictive behavior (e.g., smoking) or the immediate relief that comes when simply stopping an aversive activity (e.g., strenuous physical labor). For many, impulsive DI behavior such as self-injury also provides a means by which one can escape aversive tension, through either the reduction of depersonalization that it induces (Wagner & Linehan, 1997), the loss of consciousness that may result from a drug overdose or blood loss, or the physiological/psychological relief secondary to reductions in aversive arousal. Retrospective self-reports suggest that in more than 60% of cases, nonsuicidal self-injury functions to reduce aversive arousal, and psychophysiological arousal has been shown to be immediately and significantly reduced after self-injury imagery (Haines et al., 1995).

For individuals engaging in constricted DO behaviors such as food restriction, reinforcement tends to emerge over the medium term, such as feeling a sense of control over their lives or receiving positive feedback from others about their appearance during initial stages of weight loss (Wade et al., 2008). However, arguably a more important reinforcer, and one that is crucial during the development of an avoidant DO style of coping, is feedback received in social situations (see prior section on sociobiographic feedback). In particular, disapproval of or overreaction to self-expression or excessive punishment of minor mistakes is hypothesized to be a key determinant of the development of DO coping style. In this way, reinforcement for constricted DO behaviors is hypothesized to lead to more of a long-term strategy of risk aversion and overcontrol of behavior and emotional expression in order to avoid the possibility of negative feedback (Lynch & Cheavens, 2008). For example, individuals with APD might find themselves negatively reinforced by reductions in criticism from others when they suppress personal opinions in social situations (Millon, 1991).

## NEGATIVE CONSEQUENCES ASSOCIATED WITH DISTRESS-INTOLERANT AND DISTRESS-OVERTOLERANT BEHAVIOR

There are many obvious negative consequences associated with DI and DO behavior. For example, chronic DI will make it very difficult to achieve anything that requires sustained effort, whereas DO inherently involves the experience of unnecessary aversive tension. However, there are also more subtle consequences of both DO and DI behavioral tendencies. Experiential avoidance, of which DO/DI behavior constitutes a large part, has been shown empirically to have a variety of adverse consequences in comparison to other coping strategies. It is often remarked that the essential irony of experiential avoidance is that attempts to suppress aversive thoughts, feelings, and bodily sensations only serve to increase their frequency and magnitude (Gross, 1998, 2002; Wegner, 1994). Chronic emotional avoidance impedes the possibility of being fully immersed in any given activity, resulting in less frequent experiencing of positive events and dampened positive emotions (Gross & John, 2003; Kashdan & Steger, 2006). Furthermore, yet another source of distress resulting from experiential avoidance is a sense that one is being inauthentic or disconnected from oneself (John & Gross, 2004). The notion that DO/DI behavior and experiential avoidance in general serve to exacerbate psychological vulnerabilities is supported by observations in both clinical and nonclinical samples that experiential avoidance is strongly correlated with measures of general psychopathology (Hayes et al., 2004) as well as specific measures of anxiety and depression (Forsyth, Parker, & Finlay, 2003; Marx & Sloan, 2005; Roemer, Salters, Raffa, & Orsillo, 2005; Starr & Moulds, 2006; Tull, Gratz, Salters, & Roemer, 2004). Avoiding exposure to feared private events impedes processing of potential disconfirming evidence and increases anticipatory anxiety for situations where these unwanted internal events might arise (Salters-Pedneault, Tull, & Roemer, 2004). Furthermore, overcontrolled DO behavior may have negative interpersonal consequences of which the person who is inhibiting the expression of distress is unaware. For example, there is evidence that in a social context people will be (negatively) physiologically aroused by interactions with someone who is inexpressive when the context calls for emotional expression, and that, furthermore, people choose to interact with those who express their emotions more freely versus those who tend to inhibit them (e.g., Butler et al., 2003; Gross, 2002).

In sum, the many negative consequences associated with DO/DI behavior, coupled with the cyclical patterns of reinforcement of both these types of maladaptive coping, can produce a chronic and pervasive set of difficulties—difficulties that require careful treatment if they are to be addressed therapeutically. In the final section, we outline one therapeutic approach that might prove to have utility for this type of presentation.

## USING MINDFULNESS-BASED STRATEGIES TO TREAT DISTRESS INTOLERANCE AND DISTRESS OVERTOLERANCE

From our perspective, healthy DT requires both conscious awareness of internal states (i.e., sensations, emotion, action urges) and an ability to not automatically and without awareness respond to aversive tension with a change strategy (e.g., avoidance) and/or habitually ignore warning signs of distress. As such, healthy DT requires the ability to discriminate when changing or removing the tension is adaptive versus tolerating or not changing the tension or distress. Thus, from our perspective DI and overly tolerant behaviors are more likely to occur without conscious awareness (i.e., they are automatic and overlearned responses). Both extremes involve avoidance of unwanted contingencies: either the pain of the distress itself when distress intolerant or the pain of expressing distress when overly tolerant. As such, therapeutic strategies that are target avoidance are likely to be useful.

One such strategy with growing empirical and clinical interest is known as mindfulness. Mindful practice has been incorporated into a variety of treatment approaches (Hayes et al., 1999; Kabat-Zinn, 1990; Linehan, 1993, Marlatt & Gordon, 1985; Segal et al., 2002) and has garnered growing empirical support (for a review, see Baer, 2003). Mindfulness-based strategies generally teach what might be considered *healthy nonavoidance* of distress, via the practice of nonjudgmental acknowledgment and observation of distressing situations or experience, including aversive sensations (e.g., pain), associated cognitive appraisals (e.g., "This is intolerable"), and action or response tendencies (e.g., to yell, binge, ignore). Mindfulness also relates to the quality of awareness that an individual brings to the present moment and the use of skillful means in finding a balanced way of living between extremes or polarities (Lynch, Chapman, Rosenthal, Kuo, & Linehan, 2006). In DBT the therapist teaches the patient that one goal of mindfulness skills is to achieve a wise state of mind (i.e., "wise mind"), involving a synthesis of reason or logic (reasonable mind) and emotions and intuition (emotion mind; Linehan, 1993). This "wise" or discriminating state of knowing is likely to be essential when learning to change habitual patterns of distress over- or undertolerance. In this context, the goals of mindful practice relate to (1) increasing conscious awareness of habitual tendencies (thoughts, actions, sensations, urges) associated with DI or DO and (2) achieving a discriminating or wise state of mind that allows for effective judgments as to whether to terminate or tolerate distress at any given moment. As such, enhanced awareness of distress and the ability to judge whether to ignore or to respond to signs of tension or distress make up a likely important first step in maximizing healthy DT.

In contrast to behavioral change strategies, mindfulness also entails acceptance of experience, without attempts to fix, alter, suppress, or otherwise avoid the experience. Given that mindfulness involves acceptance and observation of painful internal experiences, mindfulness may work through nonreinforced exposure to previously avoided emotions, thoughts, and sensations. A practice called "urge surfing," originally developed by Marlatt and Gordon (1985), is an example of how mindfulness could prove helpful for increasing an individual's DT capacity. Essentially, this practice involves the skill of learning that it is not always necessary to respond to every sensation, urge, or emotion. Clients might be instructed to observe their breath, to note when an urge to scratch an itch occurs, then to observe this urge with curiosity and openness without responding to it, and then to notice what happens to the urge when they don't respond as they normally might. By allowing aversive tension to be experienced (exposure) without judgment, new associations are acquired (i.e., aversive tension is "just a sensation," a thought that the aversive tension is intolerable is "just a thought," or an impulse to escape the tension is "just an impulse"). By changing the response tendency from automatic avoidance to conscious awareness, mindfulness may alter the meaning of the event (i.e., from something intolerable to something that can be tolerated). Urge surfing and related response prevention strategies may prove particularly useful for those patients who are distress intolerant.

In conclusion, we hope that the concept of DO, as well as our conceptualization of its relationship to and contrasts with DI, may prove useful in future research. Furthermore, we hope that as a field we can inform therapeutic interventions for this type of presentation, in which so much distress is concealed.

## REFERENCES

Baer, R. A. (2003). Mindfulness training as a clinical intervention: A conceptual and empirical review. *Clinical Psychology: Science and Practice, 10,* 125–143.

Bandura, A. (1969). *Principles of behavior modification.* New York: Holt, Rinehart & Winston.

Beck, A. T., Rush, A. J., Shaw, F. F., & Emery, G. (1979). *Cognitive therapy of depression.* New York: Guilford Press.

Bernstein, A., Trafton, J., Ilgen, M., & Zvolensky, M. J. (2008). An evaluation of the role of smoking context on a biobehavioral index of distress tolerance. *Addictive Behaviors, 33,* 1409–1415.

Bohus, M., Limberger, M., Ebner, U., Glocker, F., Wernz, M., & Lieb, K. (2000). Pain perception during self-reported distress and calmness in patients with borderline personality disorder and self-mutilating behavior. *Psychiatry Research, 95,* 251–260.

Bonanno, G. A., Davis, P. J., Singer, J. L., & Schwartz, G. E. (1991). The repressor personality and avoidant information processing: A dichotic listening study. *Journal of Research in Personality, 25,* 386–401.

Boyagian, L. G., & Nation, J. R. (1981). The effects of force training and reinforcement schedules on human performance. *American Journal of Psychology, 94,* 619–632.

Boyce, W. T., & Ellis, B. J. (2005). Biological sensitivity to context: I. An evolutionary-developmental theory of the origins and functions of stress reactivity. *Development and Psychopathology, 17,* 271–301.

Brandon, T. H., Herzog, T. A., Juliano, L., Irvin, J. E., Lazev, A., & Simmons, V. N. (2003). Pretreatment task-persistence predicts smoking cessation outcome. *Journal of Abnormal Psychology, 112,* 448–456.

Brown, R. A., Lejuez, C. W., Kahler, C. W., & Strong, D. R. (2002). Distress tolerance and duration of past smoking cessation attempts. *Journal of Abnormal Psychology, 111,* 180–185.

Brown, R. A., Lejuez, C. W., Kahler, C. W., Strong, D. R., & Zvolensky, M. J. (2005). Distress tolerance and early smoking lapse. *Clinical Psychology Review, 25,* 713–733.

Butler, E. A., Egloff, B., Wilhelm, F. W., Smith, N. C., Erickson, E. A., & Gross, J. J. (2003). The social consequences of expressive suppression. *Emotion, 3,* 48–67.

Caldwell, T. L., & Newman, L. S. (2005). The timeline of threat processing in repressors: More evidence for early vigilance and late avoidance. *Personality and Individual Differences, 38,* 1957–1967.

Calvo, M. G., & Eysenck, M. W. (2000). Early vigilance and late avoidance of threat processing: Repressive coping versus low/high anxiety. *Cognition and Emotion, 14,* 763–787.

Christenson, A., Jacobson, N. S., & Babcock, J. C. (1995). Integrative behavioral couple therapy. In N. S. Jacobson & A. S. Gurman (Eds.), *Clinical handbook of couple therapy* (pp. 31–64). New York: Guilford Press.

Claes, L., Vandereycken, W., & Vertommen, H. (2006). Pain experience related to self-injury in eating disorder patients. *Eating Behaviors, 7,* 204–213.

Cloninger, C. R. (1986). A unified biosocial theory of personality and its role in the development of anxiety states. *Psychiatric Developments, 4,* 167–226.

Cloninger, C. R. (1987). A systematic method for clinical description and classification of personality variants. A proposal. *Archives of General Psychiatry, 44,* 573–588.

Conrad, R., Wegener, I., Imbierowicz, K., Liedtke, R., & Geiser, F. (2009). Alexithymia, temperament and character as predictors of psychopathology in patients with major depression. *Psychiatry Research, 165,* 137–144.

Corrigan, P. W. (2001). Getting ahead of the data: A threat to some behavior therapies. *The Behavior Therapist, 24,* 189–193.

Crowell, S. E., Beauchaine, T. P., & Linehan, M. (2009). A biosocial developmental model of borderline personality: Elaborating and extending Linehan's theory. *Psychological Bulletin, 135,* 495–510.

Cukrowicz, K. C., Ekblad, A. G., Cheavens, J. S., Rosenthal, M. Z., & Lynch, T. R. (2008). Coping and thought suppression as predictors of suicidal ideation in depressed older adults with personality disorders. *Aging and Mental Health, 12,* 149–157.

Daughters, S. B., Lejuez, C. W., Bornovalova, M. A., Kahler, C. W., Strong, D. R., & Brown, R. A. (2005). Distress tolerance as a predictor of early treatment dropout in a residential substance abuse treatment facility. *Journal of Abnormal Psychology, 114,* 729–734.

Derakshan, N., Eysenck, M. W., & Myers, L. B. (2007). Emotional information processing in repressors: The vigilance-avoidance theory. *Cognition and Emotion, 21,* 1585–1614.

Dougher, M., Perkins, D. R., Greenway, D., Koons, A., & Chiasson, C. (2002). Contextual control of equivalence-based transformation of functions. *Journal of the Experimental Analysis of Behavior, 78,* 78–63.

Dworkin, R. H., Crawford Clark, W., & Lipsitz, J. D. (1995). Pain responsivity in major depression and bipolar disorder. *Psychiatry Research, 56,* 173–181.

Eisenberg, N., & Fabes, R. A. (1992). Emotion, regulation, and the development of social competence. In M. S. Clark (Ed.), *Review of personality and social psychology: Vol. 14. Emotion and social behavior* (pp. 119–150). Newbury Park, CA: Sage.

Eisenberg, N., Fabes, R. A., Guthrie, I. K., & Reiser, M. (2000). Dispositional emotionality and regulation: Their role in predicting quality of social functioning. *Journal of Personality and Social Psychology, 78,* 136–157.

Eisenberg, N., Fabes, R. A., & Murphy, B. C. (1996). Parents' reactions to children's negative emotions: Relations to children's social competence and comforting behavior. *Child Development, 67,* 2227–2247.

Eisenberger, R. (1992). Learned industriousness. *Psychological Review, 99,* 248–267.

Eisenberger, R., Heerdt, W. A., Hamdi, M., Zimet, S., & Bruckmeir, M. (1979). Transfer of persistence across behaviors. *Journal of Experimental Psychology: Human Learning and Memory, 5,* 522–530.

Eisenberger, R., Kuhlman, D. M., & Cotterell, N. (1992). Effects of social values, effort training, and goal structure on task persistence. *Journal of Research in Personality, 26,* 258–272.

Forsyth, J. P., Parker, J., & Finlay, C. G. (2003). Anxiety sensitivity, controllability, and experiential avoidance and their relation to drug of choice and addiction severity in a residential sample of substance abusing veterans. *Addictive Behaviors, 28,* 851–870.

Gardini, S., Cloninger, C. R., & Venneri, A. (2009). Individual differences in personality traits reflect structural variance in specific brain regions. *Brain Research Bulletin, 79,* 265–270.

Grabe, H. J., Spitzer, C., & Freyberger, H. J. (2004). Alexithymia and personality in relation to dimensions of psychopathology. *American Journal of Psychiatry, 161*, 1299–1301.

Gray, J. A. (1982). *The neuropsychology of anxiety: An enquiry into the functions of the septo-hippocampal system.* New York: Oxford University Press.

Gray, J. A. (1991). The neuropsychology of temperament. In J. Strelau & A. Angleitner (Eds.), *Explorations in temperament: International perspectives on theory and measurement. Perspectives on individual differences* (pp. 105–128). New York: Plenum Press.

Gross, J. J. (1998). The emerging field of emotion regulation: An integrative review. *Review of General Psychology, 2*, 271–299.

Gross, J. J. (2002). Emotion regulation: Affective, cognitive, and social consequences. *Psychophysiology, 39*, 281–291.

Gross, J. J., & John, O. P. (2003). Individual differences in two emotion regulation processes: Implications for affect, relationships, and well-being. *Journal of Personality and Social Psychology, 85*, 348–362.

Gusnard, D. A., Ollinger, J. M., Shulman, G. L., Cloninger, C. R., Price, J. L. Van Essen, D. C., et al. (2003). Persistence and brain circuitry. *Proceedings of the National Academy of Sciences, 100*, 3479–3484.

Gwaltney, C. J., Shiffman, S., Paty, J. A., Liu, K. S., Kassel, J. D., Gnys, M., et al. (2002). Using self-efficacy judgments to predict characteristics of lapses to smoking. *Journal of Consulting and Clinical Psychology, 70*, 1140–1149.

Haines, J., Williams, C. L., Brain, K. L., & Wilson, G. V. (1995). The psychophysiology of self-mutilation. *Journal of Abnormal Psychology, 104*, 479–489.

Hajek, P., Belcher, M., & Stapleton, J. (1987). Breath-holding endurance as a predictor of success in smoking cessation. *Addictive Behaviors, 12*, 285–288.

Hayes, S. C. (2004). Acceptance and commitment therapy and the new behavior therapies: Mindfulness, acceptance and relationship. In S. C. Hayes, V. M. Follette, & M. M. Linehan (Eds.), *Mindfulness and acceptance: Expanding the cognitive behavioral tradition* (pp. 1–29). New York: Guilford Press.

Hayes, S. C., Follette, W. C., & Follette, V. M. (1995). Behavior therapy: A contextual approach. In A. S. Gunman & S. B. Messer (Eds.), *Essential psychotherapies: Theory and practice* (pp. 128–181). New York: Guilford Press.

Hayes, S. C., Masuda, A., Bissett, R., Luoma, J., & Guerrero, L. F. (2004). DBT, FAP, and ACT: How empirically oriented are the new behavior therapy technologies? *Behavior Therapy, 35*, 35–54.

Hayes, S. C., Strosahl, K. D., & Wilson, K. G. (1999). *Acceptance and commitment therapy: An experiential approach to behavior change.* New York: Guilford Press.

Hayes, S. C., Wilson, K. G., Gifford, E. V., Follette, V. M., & Strosahl, K. (1996). Experiential avoidance and behavioral disorders: A functional dimensional approach to diagnosis and treatment. *Journal of Consulting and Clinical Psychology, 64*, 1152–1168.

Herman, J. L., Perry, C., & van der Kolk, B. A. (1989). Childhood trauma in borderline personality disorder. *American Journal of Psychiatry, 146*, 490–495.

Holdwick, D. J., & Wingenfeld, S. A. (1999). The subjective experience of PASAT testing: Does the PASAT induce negative mood? *Archives of Clinical Neuropsychology, 14,* 273–284.

John, O. P., & Gross, J. J. (2004). Healthy and unhealthy emotion regulation: Personality processes, individual differences, and life span development. *Journal of Personality, 72,* 1301–1333.

Johnson, J. J., Smailes, E. M., Cohen, P., Brown, J., & Bernstein, D. P. (2000). Associations between four types of childhood neglect and personality disorder symptoms during adolescence and early adulthood: Findings of a community-based longitudinal study. *Journal of Personality Disorders, 14,* 171–187.

Jones, S., Eisenberg, N., Fabes, R. A., & MacKinnon, D. P. (2002). Parents' reactions to elementary school children's negative emotions: Relations to social and emotional functioning at school. *Merrill-Palmer Quarterly, 48,* 133–159.

Jørgensen, M. M., Zachariae, R., Skytthe, A., & Kyvik, K. (2007). Genetic and environmental factors in alexithymia: A population-based study of 8,785 Danish twin pairs. *Psychotherapy and Psychosomatics, 76,* 369–375.

Joyce, P. R., Mulder, R. T., Luty, S. E., McKenzie, J. M., Sullivan, P. F., & Cloninger, R. C. (2003). Borderline personality disorder in major depression: Symptomatology, temperament, character, differential drug response, and 6-month outcome. *Comprehensive Psychiatry, 44,* 35–43.

Kabat-Zinn, J. (1990). *Full catastrophe living: Using the wisdom of your mind to face stress, pain and illness.* New York: Dell.

Kashdan, T. B., Barrios, V., Forsyth, J. P., & Steger, M. F. (2006). Experiential avoidance as a generalized psychological vulnerability: Comparisons with coping and emotion regulation strategies. *Behaviour Research and Therapy, 9,* 1301–1320.

Kashdan, T. B., & Steger, M. F. (2006). Expanding the topography of social anxiety: An experience-sampling assessment of positive emotions, positive events, and emotion suppression. *Psychological Science, 17,* 120–128.

Kim, S. J., Kim, Y. S., Lee, H. S., Kim, S. Y., & Kim, C. H. (2006). An interaction between the serotonin transporter promoter region and dopamine transporter polymorphisms contributes to harm avoidance and reward dependence traits in normal healthy subjects. *Journal of Neural Transmission, 113,* 877–886.

Kohlenberg, R. J., & Tsai, M. (1994). Improving cognitive therapy with functional analytic psychotherapy: Theory and case study. *The Behavior Analyst, 17,* 305–319.

Korner, A., Gerull, F., Stevenson, J., & Meares, R. (2007). Harm avoidance, self-harm, psychic pain, and the borderline personality: Life in a "haunted house." *Comprehensive Psychiatry, 48,* 303–308.

Krause, E. D., Mendelson, T., & Lynch, T. R. (2003). Childhood emotional invalidation and adult psychological distress: The mediating role of emotional inhibition. *Child Abuse and Neglect, 27,* 199–213.

Krause, E. D., Robins, C. J., & Lynch, T. R. (2000). A mediational model relating sociotropy, ambivalence over emotional expression and eating disorder symptoms. *Psychology of Women Quarterly, 24,* 328–335.

Lilenfeld, L. R., Stein, D., Bulik, C. M., Strober, M., Plotnicov, K. H., Pollice, C., et al. (2000). Personality traits among currently eating disordered, recovered, and never ill first-degree female relatives of bulimic and control women. *Psychological Medicine, 30,* 1399–1410.

Linehan, M. M. (1993). *Cognitive-behavioral treatment for borderline personality disorder.* New York: Guilford Press.

Lynch, T. R., Chapman, A. L., Rosenthal, M. Z., Kuo, J. R., & Linehan, M. M. (2006). Mechanisms of change in dialectical behavior therapy: Theoretical and empirical observations. *Journal of Clinical Psychology, 62,* 459–480.

Lynch, T. R., & Cheavens, J. S. (2008). Dialectical behavior therapy for co-morbid personality disorders. *Journal of Clinical Psychology, 64,* 1–14.

Lynch, T. R., Cheavens, J. S., Morse, J. Q., & Rosenthal, M. Z. (2004). A model predicting suicidal ideation and hopelessness in depressed older adults: The impact of emotion inhibition and affect intensity. *Aging and Mental Health, 8,* 1–12.

Lynch, T. R., Robins, C. J., Morse, J. Q., & Krause, E. D. (2001). A mediational model of relating affect intensity, emotion inhibition, and psychological distress. *Behavior Therapy, 32,* 519–536.

Lynch, T. R., Schneider, K. G., Rosenthal, M. Z., & Cheavens, J. S. (2007). A mediational model of trait negative affectivity, dispositional thought suppression, and intrusive thoughts following laboratory stressors. *Behaviour Research and Therapy, 45,* 749–761.

Marlatt, G. A., & Gordon, J. R. (1985). *Relapse prevention: Maintenance strategies in the treatment of addictive behaviors.* New York: Guilford Press.

Marx, B. P., & Sloan, D. M. (2005). Peritraumatic dissociation and experiential avoidance as predictors of posttraumatic stress symptomatology. *Behaviour Research and Therapy, 43,* 569–583.

McGuffin, P., & Southwick, L. (2003). Fifty years of the double helix and its impact on psychiatry. *Australian and New Zealand Journal of Psychiatry, 37,* 657–661.

Michel, K., Valach, L., & Waeber, V. (1994). Understanding deliberate self-harm: The patients' views. *Crisis, 15,* 172–178.

Millon, T. (1991). Avoidant personality disorder: A brief review of issues and data. *Journal of Personality Disorders, 5,* 353–362.

Nock, M. K., & Mendes, W. B. (2008). Physiological arousal, distress tolerance, and social problem-solving deficits among adolescent self-injurers. *Journal of Consulting and Clinical Psychology, 76,* 28–38.

Ogata, S. N., Silk, K. R., Goodrich, S., Lohr, N. E., Westen, D., & Hill, E. M. (1990). Childhood sexual abuse and physical abuse in adult patients with borderline personality disorder. *American Journal of Psychiatry, 147,* 1008–1013.

Ogden, J., & Whyman, C. (1997). The effect of repeated weighing on psychological state. *European Eating Disorders Review, 5,* 121–130.

Ohman, A., & Mineka, S. (2001). Fears, phobias, and preparedness: Toward an evolved module of fear and fear learning. *Psychological Review, 108,* 483–522.

Quinn, E. P., Brandon, T. H., & Copeland, A. L. (1996). Is task persistence related to smoking and substance abuse?: Applying learned industriousness theory to addictive behaviors. *Experimental and Clinical Psychopharmacology, 4,* 186–190.

Roemer, L., Salters, K., Raffa, S., & Orsillo, S. M. (2005). Fear and avoidance of internal experiences in GAD: Preliminary tests of a conceptual model. *Cognitive Therapy and Research, 29,* 71–88.

Rosenthal, M. Z., Gratz, K. L., Kosson, D. S., Cheavens, J. S., Lejuez, C. W., & Lynch, T. R. (2008). Borderline personality disorder and emotional responding: A review of the research literature. *Clinical Psychology Review, 28,* 75–91.

Salters-Pedneault, K., Tull, M. T., & Roemer, L. (2004). The role of avoidance of emotional material in the anxiety disorders. *Applied and Preventive Psychology, 11,* 95–114.

Segal, Z. V., Williams, J. M. G., & Teasdale, J. D. (2002). *Mindfulness-based cognitive therapy for depression: A new approach to preventing relapse.* New York: Guilford Press.

Simons, J. S., & Gaher, R. M. (2005). The Distress Tolerance Scale: Development and validation of a self-report measure. *Motivation and Emotion, 29,* 83–102.

Starr, S., & Moulds, M. L. (2006). The role of negative interpretations of intrusive memories in depression. *Journal of Affective Disorders, 93,* 125–132.

Stiglmayr, C., Shapiro, D. A., Stieglitz, R. D., Limberger, M., & Bohus, M. (2001). Experience of aversive tension and dissociation in female patients with borderline personality disorder—A controlled study. *Journal of Psychiatric Research, 35,* 111–118.

Tull, M. T., Gratz, K. L., Salters, K., & Roemer, L. (2004). The role of experiential avoidance in posttraumatic stress symptoms and symptoms of depression, anxiety, and somatization. *Journal of Nervous and Mental Disease, 192,* 754–761.

Turkat, I. D. (1985). Formulation of paranoid personality disorder. In I. D. Turkat (Ed.), *Behavioral case formulation* (pp. 161–198). New York: Plenum Press.

Valera, E. M., & Berenbaum, H. (2001). A twin study of alexithymia. *Psychotherapy and Psychosomatics, 70,* 239–246.

Wade, T. D., Tiggerman, M., Bulik, C. M., Fairburn, C. G., Wray, N. R., & Martin, N. G. (2008). Shared temperament risk factors for anorexia nervosa: A twin study. *Psychosomatic Medicine, 70,* 239–244.

Wagner, A. W., & Linehan, M. M. (1997). The relationship between childhood sexual abuse and suicidal behaviors in borderline patients. In M. Zanarini (Ed.), *The role of sexual abuse in the etiology of borderline personality disorder* (pp. 203–223). Washington, DC: American Psychiatric Association.

Watson, J. B. (1924). *Behaviorism.* New York: Norton.

Wegner, D. M. (1994). Ironic processes of mental control. *Psychological Review, 101,* 34–52.

White, C. N., Gunderson, J. G., Zanarini, M. C., & Hudson, J. I. (2003). Family studies of borderline personality disorder: A review. *Harvard Review of Psychiatry, 11,* 8–19.

Winstanley, S., & Dives, L. (2005). Effects on mood of a bogus weight gain. *European Eating Disorders Review, 13,* 424–426.

Zanarini, M. C., Williams, A. A., Lewis, R. E., Reich, R. B., Vera, S. C., Marino, M. F., et al. (1997). Reported pathological childhood experiences associated with the development of borderline personality disorder. *American Journal of Psychiatry, 154,* 1101–1106.

# 4

# Biological Bases
# of Distress Tolerance

Jodie A. Trafton *and* Elizabeth V. Gifford

Although distress tolerance has been studied using behavioral and psychometric measures in humans and has been shown to be associated with clinical outcomes, its neurobiological underpinnings are rarely discussed (but see Trafton & Gifford, 2008). Differences in terminology and definitional conceptualizations can limit translation of research findings across disciplines, even closely related disciplines such as psychology and neuroscience. Yet understanding the biological processes underlying distress tolerance may improve our ability to interpret findings and understand processes from the psychological literature.

When we examine the candidate neuronal systems underlying distress-tolerance behaviors, it becomes apparent that what has been conceptualized as a single phenomenon by psychologists is likely controlled and regulated by multiple neurobiological processes, each of which may be targeted and modified uniquely by environmental, biological, and genetic factors. Understanding these biological processes and the factors that regulate them may provide new insights into when distress tolerance is likely to be clinically important and how to modify it to improve patient outcomes.

Here we present three core neurobiological processes that would be expected to contribute to distress tolerance. For each of these candidate neurobiological processes, we examine existing systems neuroscience research that has defined some of the structures, connections, and plasticity that regulate behavior. We then discuss the implications of these systems neuroscience findings for understanding distress tolerance and its clinical manifestations.

## A BEHAVIORAL DEFINITION
## OF DISTRESS TOLERANCE

Neurobiology is systematically modified and studied using behavioral tasks in animal models. To integrate across disciplines, we need a unifying behavioral model. Fortunately, this is a relatively simple task because behavioral measures of distress tolerance have been developed in humans. Distress tolerance describes the tendency to refrain from emitting behaviors that would provide immediate relief from experiencing an unpleasant sensation. It is a measure of one's ability to continue experiencing discomfort when an escape is available. In behavioral terms, distress tolerance involves refraining from responding to a negative reinforcement opportunity (Gifford, 1994, 2002). It is a special example of control over responding for an immediate reward (i.e., relief from distress).

This conceptualization suggests that distress intolerance could be one manifestation of an "impulsive" tendency to respond for immediate reinforcement or reward rather than alternative reinforcers available through self-restraint. It also suggests that neurobiological substrates underlying and modulating reward learning and response (i.e., reward circuits) are likely to mediate distress tolerance.

There is extensive neurobiological research studying the mechanisms and neural modulation of reward-driven learning that has possible implications for clinical studies of distress tolerance. It is beyond the scope of this chapter to review this literature in full. Instead, we discuss some general processes that likely underlie the expression of distress tolerance and provide examples from the neurobiological literature to demonstrate possible mechanisms. These examples inevitably oversimplify the processes, neuroanatomical substrates, cell biology, genetics, and molecular targets involved. However, they illustrate several key points:

1.  Distress tolerance is not determined by a single neurobiological process. Instead, a number of anatomically and functionally distinct neurobiological processes can be identified that should modify the expression of distress tolerance. Breaking the concept of distress tolerance into these biologically separate, functionally distinct components may make it easier to interpret findings in human populations and to design interventions to alter distress tolerance.

2.  Processes that underlie distress tolerance involve assigning value to context-specific opportunities based on experience and cognitions,

learning from experienced behavioral consequences, adaptation to the environment at a rate determined by genetics, and executive functions. Thus, we should expect distress tolerance to be context specific; modified by prior experience, learning, beliefs, and expectations; and influenced by genetic background. These mechanisms suggest that distress tolerance is not a static trait, but should be modifiable with a variety of intervention strategies.

We hope that explicating these examples will provide a novel framework for considering the concept of distress tolerance and suggest additional interpretations of clinical literature and potentially new intervention strategies.

## BASIC SCIENCE MODELS AND PREVIOUS RESEARCH

The field of neurobiology is filled with examples of research with a distress-tolerance component. For example, pain tolerance is evaluated using the tail-flick test, hot-plate test, cold-pressor test, and heat and electrical shock tolerance tests. In tail-flick tests, for example, researchers shine a focused light on a rodent's tail and measure the latency until the rodent pulls its tail away from the noxious stimulus. This test has been used to assess the effects of anesthetics, analgesics, and genetic manipulations on tolerance to heat pain (see Le Bars, Gozariu, & Cadden, 2001, or Bannon & Malmberg, 2007, for a review of the test and its uses). Other tests, such as the elevated plus maze and open-field test, are used to assess anxiety tolerance. All of these measures evaluate reactivity to discomfort; some provide a choice between short-term negative reinforcement and delayed positive reinforcement. Testing whether sexually naïve male rodents are willing to approach sexually available female rodents, for example, has been used to identify genes and related brain circuits associated with rodents' willingness to tolerate novelty anxiety in order to gain access to sexual gratification (Barrot et al., 2005). However, studies investigating these tasks in animal models have most often used them as outcome measures to identify candidate drugs, target genes, or interventions for various therapeutic development projects (e.g., analgesics, antidepressants, or antianxiety medications) rather than studying the mechanisms underlying the task behaviors themselves (e.g., Crawley, 1999; Karl, Pabst, & von Hörsten, 2003).

Neurobiological researchers interested in addiction have focused on identifying and exploring some of the processes underlying reward-driven behavior. More recently, investigators have begun to recognize the overlap between the neurobiology of reward learning and pain, anxiety, and stress-tolerance processes and are encouraging research that considers the role of core computational processes in these varied behaviors (e.g., Borsook et al., 2007; Chen et al., 2009; Hikosaka, Bromberg-Martin, Hong, & Matsumoto, 2008).

## CANDIDATE MECHANISMS OF DISTRESS TOLERANCE

The process underlying reward-driven learning has been studied extensively in animal models. As will come to no surprise to those who study reward circuitry, information encoded by dopamine neurons and the excitability of populations of neurons in the nucleus accumbens–ventral striatum (NAc) are implicated in processes that should modify distress tolerance. We propose a model that assumes that distress tolerance is essentially a reward-driven behavior, and that variation in the core processes underlying reward-driven behavior should contribute to variations in distress tolerance.

There are several factors related to decisions on how quickly and vigorously to respond to opportunities in the environment: (1) the expected value of the reward, (2) the availability of reward opportunities in one's experience, and (3) the ability to inhibit immediate responding. Each of these factors corresponds to specific brain systems.

First, opportunities predicted to produce a greater amount of relief will drive more intense behavioral responses. One will try to escape more quickly and vigorously from a highly distressing situation than from a mildly distressing situation. Thus, systems and processes involved in predicting the value of negative reinforcement opportunities (i.e., systems that determine the amount of relief one will experience from escaping the situation) should be important for regulating distress tolerance.

Functionally, dopamine neurons projecting to the NAc and prefrontal cortex have been shown to learn and encode the expected value of the immediate reward predicted to be obtained by performing the trained response (e.g., Schultz, 1998). Dopamine neurons provide an answer to the question "In this situation, how much will I gain by doing my trained response?" The learned value of the expected benefit of doing an escape behavior should contribute to the decision regarding whether to escape or to persist in an unpleasant situation (or, stated behaviorally, contribute to the strength or probability of the learned response contingent on this reinforcer).

Second, the general availability of opportunities in a person's experience will alter his or her enthusiasm for responding to a given opportunity. If opportunities to escape are rarely available, a person will be much more likely to take advantage of a situation when one presents. If opportunities to resolve or escape a potentially dangerous or unpleasant situation are regularly available, then a person may not feel it necessary to take advantage of every opportunity that presents. Thus, systems involved in modifying the tendency to respond to reward opportunities based on their availability in the environment should also be important for regulating distress tolerance.

A cluster of inhibitory medium spiny neurons (MSN) in the NAc control performance of well-trained reward- or relief-seeking behaviors. Their excitability is modified by dopaminergic inputs that indicate the presence and value of opportunities for reward. Altering the excitability of these neurons changes the relationship between reward value and the likelihood/intensity of reward- or relief-seeking response.

Third, the ability to consciously control or inhibit habitual reward or relief seeking should alter tolerance for distress. Although people learn habitual responses to cues indicating opportunities for reward, they generally have the ability to inhibit these habits to allow an alternate response. However, there is substantial individual and contextual variability in how well people can inhibit habits. Poorer ability to inhibit habits increases the probability of expression of escape behaviors even when contextual or longer term contingencies favor distress tolerance. Circuits involving the prefrontal cortex have long been implicated in this executive function.

## Summary

Distress intolerance can be defined as relief seeking during a negative reinforcement opportunity, and thus is a special case of reward seeking. Reward learning can be conceptualized as a process in which associations among a cue, a response, and a reward are learned and driven via a feedback process, which updates the strength of the associations. The intensity of the response will depend on the expected value of the reward to be gained by the response. It will also depend on the amount of effort the individual is willing to put into obtaining rewards of a given value, based on the relative scarcity of opportunities. Last, responses driven by this reward-learning process may be inhibited by conscious control to allow for alternative responding. In the following section, we describe the neurobiology underlying these processes and their behavioral/clinical implications.

# ESTIMATING THE VALUE
# OF OPPORTUNITIES FOR RELIEF

For both short- and long-term decisions, the brain must compare the expected benefits of one choice versus another. A network of neurons that contain the neuromodulator dopamine encodes information about the value of opportunities to work for a reinforcer. The faster these dopamine neurons fire, the greater the expected value of the reward. This has been observed in neurons that terminate in the NAc, where firing is used to guide decisions about whether to perform habitual behaviors to gain immediate relief or reward (Abler, Walter, Erk, Kammerer, & Spitzer, 2006). It is also observed in the orbital frontal cortex, where reward predictions may be used to make more global and conscious decisions about how to respond using well-trained or more novel behaviors (Roesch & Olson, 2004).

These dopamine neurons fire both tonicly and phasicly (Marinelli, Rudick, Hu, & White, 2006; Schultz, 1998). This means that they fire stably at a relatively slow rate in the absence of opportunities (i.e., tonic firing) and fire faster to indicate the presence of opportunities (i.e., phasic firing). Notably, the fact that these neurons fire slowly when no opportunities are present allows them to report when they overestimated the value of an opportunity. They can slow their firing even further to indicate when opportunities that they predicted don't live up to expectations. This slow, constant firing also allows these neurons to convey two different types of information: one about overall resting state and the other about options that are present right now.

These dopamine neurons use a feedback system, or more specifically an error signal model of learning, to develop and update predictions of the value of opportunities for reward or relief (Tobler, O'Doherty, Dolan, & Schultz, 2006). Specifically, learning is guided by a process of prediction with correction via an error signal at the time the predicted reward is expected to materialize. The rate at which the dopamine neurons fire during the prediction encodes the predicted reward value. The sum of (1) the firing during the prediction and (2) the error signal firing at the time of the predicted reward indicates the actual value of the encountered reward. When errors in the original reward prediction occur, they trigger learning of new cues and contingencies. Scientists have observed this process in action in both monkeys (e.g. Schultz, 1998; Tobler et al., 2006) and humans using functional magnetic resonance imaging (fMRI) during learning exercises (e.g., Rodriguez, Aron, & Poldrack, 2006). See Figure 4.1 for an example.

These dopamine neurons consolidate information from a wide variety of sources to generate predictions about the value of opportuni-

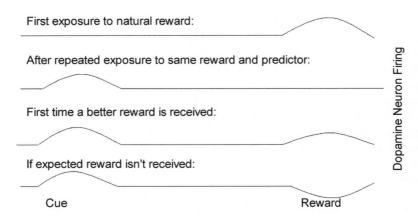

**FIGURE 4.1.** Dopamine neuron firing rates during a process of repeated exposure to a cue and reward. In the first line, the first time a reward is encountered, it is unexpected. Thus, dopamine neurons do not alter their firing rate until the reward is received (i.e., at the first indication that reward opportunities were different than predicted). This dopamine neuron firing provides an error signal, which triggers learning of cues that predict the availability of reward. Thus, after repeated exposure to the same cue and reward (the second line), exposure to the cue will trigger dopamine neuron firing in proportion to the value of the expected reward. If the expected reward is received, dopamine neurons will fire at their basal rate during receipt of the reward. The prediction was perfect; thus, there is no dopamine error signal generated and no new learning occurs. The third line depicts dopamine neuron firing when, in a learned situation, the reward received is better than expected. Dopamine neuron firing increases at the time of the cue in proportion to the expected value of the reward and then again at the time the better reward is received in proportion to the amount that the reward is better than expected. The fourth line depicts dopamine neuron firing when, in a learned situation, the reward is not received or is worse than expected. As before, dopamine neuron firing increases at the time of the cue, in proportion to the expected value of the reward, but at the time a lesser or no reward is received dopamine neuron firing slows below baseline levels in proportion to the value of the reward that was not received. Notably, when dopamine neuron firing indicates an error in prediction, this triggers new learning, updating predictions about reward value and availability in the environment.

ties. Most of these dopamine neurons originate in the ventral tegmental area. Dopamine neuron inputs strongly influence their firing patterns, and thus information from many areas of the brain can modify estimations of the value of an opportunity for reinforcement. For example, the pedunculopontine tegmentum (PPTg) integrates information from auditory, visual, and somatosensory systems with information from the limbic system and prefrontal cortex and can change dopamine neuron firing (Grace, Floresco, Goto, & Lodge, 2007). The PPTg may thereby combine information about what we are seeing, hearing, and feeling with information about our long-term goals and emotional state to alter predictions about relief opportunities. Inputs from the prefrontal cortex can alter the amount these dopamine neurons fire (Del Arco & Mora, 2008), allowing information about longer term goals and intentions to be included in predictions. Hippocampal neurons can increase firing of dopamine neurons by reducing inhibition from the ventral pallidum (Grace et al., 2007), which seems to be important for the effects of novelty on reward value estimates. Through these inputs, these dopamine neurons receive information about what we are currently observing, what we have experienced in the past, and what our goals are for the future. This information shapes the firing patterns of the dopamine neurons to summarize our predictions regarding the value of an opportunity for reward or relief.

## Potential Clinical Implications

This reward value prediction learning process and the varied inputs to the dopamine neurons suggest various strategies for modifying distress tolerance by altering the expected value of an opportunity for relief. First, by altering the outcomes or contingencies associated with an opportunity, one could use the error-learning signal to alter the predicted value of relief opportunities. If the consequences of escaping from a distressing situation were altered, this would change the expected value (and thus the phasic firing rate of dopamine neurons during the distressing situation) of doing escape behaviors. For example, consider the scenario in which someone is asked to continue trying to complete a difficult and annoying task (e.g., a mirror-tracing task paired with a loud buzzing noise) with the promise that he will receive money in proportion to the length of time that he continues to try. Imagine that the first four trials he received 1 cent for every second he persisted in his effort. His dopamine neurons would learn to release dopamine in an amount equivalent to 1 cent/second when he was given the opportunity to attempt the task. If after the fifth trial, he received 5 cents for every second he persisted, we would expect that additional dopamine would be released when the larger-than-expected reward was received. This would trigger learning and increase the predicted value of persisting and the amount of dopamine released when given the opportunity to do the task. Presumably, the increase in the predicted value/dopamine release would lead the person to continue the task longer on the sixth trial.

None of these processes are conscious. Altering conscious expectations about the consequences of the escape response, changing one's long-term goals, or altering longer term contingencies may also alter the predicted reward value via cortical circuits. For example, imagine a pain tolerance test in which a person is asked to tolerate a painful stimulus to the hand until it becomes unbearable. Alone in a room, that person might tolerate the stimulus for 30 seconds. Imagine now that an attractive or highly dominant person comes into the room and clearly indicates that she will be impressed by demonstrations of greater tolerance and disappointed by demonstrations of low tolerance. The value of escaping presumably decreases in this situation because relieving the distress from the painful stimulus will come at the expense of inducing distress by disappointing someone whom this person wished to impress. This will alter the predictions made by dopamine neurons, reducing phasic firing rates in the presence of the pain stimulus, and thereby reducing the drive to do escape behaviors. This presumably would increase the length of time the person would tolerate the painful stimulus, perhaps to 60 seconds. Consistent with these predictions, Magen and Gross (2007) have demonstrated that cognitive manipulations, specifically describing the task as a test of willpower, can increase persistence on unpleasant tasks by reducing the pleasure gained from relief from the task.

## ADAPTING TO RESOURCE AVAILABILITY IN THE ENVIRONMENT

A population of interneurons, specifically a subpopulation of MSN, in the NAc has been shown to gate learned reward-driven behavioral responses (Taha & Fields, 2006). While these neurons fire, reward-driven behaviors are inhibited. When they stop firing, previously learned reward-driven behaviors are released and carried out. For example, a rat is trained that pressing a lever will deliver food when a red light is on. When the light is off, these MSN will fire, inhibiting reward-seeking behaviors like lever pressing. The rat will most likely explore the cage and go about its business. When the light turns on, the dopaminergic projection neurons relay information about this opportunity to the MSN and their activity is inhibited (i.e., they slow their firing). Inhibiting these inhibitory MSN releases trained reward-seeking behaviors, and the rat will be more likely to start pressing the lever.

Making these MSN more difficult to turn off would make it harder to release reward-seeking behaviors. If these neurons were highly excitable, it would take a huge opportunity to slow them down and thus free reward seeking. Thus, the excitability of these neurons determines how much drive is necessary to elicit a reward-driven behavior. If these neurons are rendered more difficult to shut off, by increasing their excitability, the rodent will be less prone to behaviors to gain immediate reward or relief. In other words, making these MSN more difficult to turn off should increase distress tolerance.

A substantial body of research in rodents demonstrates the behavioral effects of altering the excitability of these NAc MSN and supports their importance in regulating distress tolerance. These studies were originally designed to test the effects of modifying the expression and activity of the transcription factor CREB in the NAc. CREB activity is increased within a neuron when various neurotransmitter receptors, such as dopamine receptors, are activated. CREB activity regulates gene expression patterns in the neuron and thereby alters the response characteristics of the neuron. In a series of studies, Nestler and colleagues used viral vectors to either increase expression of CREB or turn off activity of CREB (by increasing expression of a "broken" version of CREB, which would attach to CREB targets but not be active) when they were microinjected into the NAc (see Carlezon et al., 1998, for the initial use of this method, and Nestler, 2004, for a review). Dong and colleagues (2006) showed that increasing the expression of CREB using these viral vectors increased the excitability of MSN. They found that neurons with more CREB fired more times in response to depolarizing currents. More simply put, the neurons showed greater response to the same input and thus would be more difficult to silence. When viral vectors were used to increase CREB expression in the NAc, rats showed decreased responding to positive and negative reinforcers in a variety of behavioral tests (Barrot et al., 2002). On the positive reinforcement side, rats with increased CREB expression drank less sugar water when given free access and showed less preference for environments previously paired with morphine or cocaine injections (Barrot et al., 2002, Pliakas et al., 2001). On the negative reinforcement side, mimicking an increase in distress tolerance, rats with increased CREB expression took longer to pull their tail away when a noxious thermal stimulus was applied, and spent more time in the open arms of an elevated plus maze, demonstrating their reduced response to pain and anxiety stimuli. Rats with increased CREB expression even demonstrated reduced escape from social anxiety, with virgin males being more likely to approach a sexually receptive female (Barrot et al., 2005). Together, these studies suggest that increasing the excitability of MSN in the NAc, in this case by modulating CREB, decreases the tendency to respond for positive and negative reinforcers, making rodents appear more distress tolerant and less reward seeking.

Under normal conditions, the excitability of these neurons is determined by the amount of input received by the dopaminergic neurons, as described earlier. Because these dopamine neurons fire in accordance with expected reward opportunities, the excitability of the MSN should be determined by the amount of exposure to rewards in the environment. Therefore, the more opportunities one encounters, the less likely one will be to aggressively pursue immediate reward or relief. Findings from rodent studies of NAc CREB expression demonstrate this process. For example, Barrot and colleagues (2002, 2005) found that social housing increases and social isolation decreases expression of CREB in the NAc of rats. Social housing provides opportunities for social reward such as being groomed by peers, succeeding in competitions or group endeavors, improving social status, and mating. Altering a rodent's environment by taking away social opportunities decreased CREB expression, and thus presumably decreased the excitability of MSN. This effect should decrease distress tolerance. This was exactly what Barrot and colleagues (2005) observed. Social isolation increased rats' tendency to escape from anxiogenic stimuli. Socially isolated rats spent less time in the open arms of an elevated plus maze (i.e., escaped from the threat of being seen). They were also less likely to approach a receptive female (i.e., escaped the potential threat of engaging a novel social behavior) if, and only if, they were sexually naïve and had not received anxiolytic medications. Moreover, this decreased distress tolerance was reversed by increasing CREB expression in the NAc using viral vectors. Thus, exposure to fewer opportunities led to reduced distress tolerance, with this effect presumably mediated by reductions in the excitability of MSN in the NAc.

## Potential Clinical Implications

Clinically, there are several implications of this process for adapting drive to reward seek based on general availability of reward via modulation of MSN excitability. This process implies that interventions that increase the prevalence of experienced reward opportunities in the environment should increase distress tolerance and thus perhaps facilitate recovery from disorders related to distress intolerance. This is consistent with clinical observations. Virtually every psychosocial treatment involves increasing contact with rewards. These rewards occur both within treatment, where supportive interpersonal interactions provide new social rewards, and outside of treatment, where patients are encouraged to develop skills or engage in activities that are constructive and satisfying and that contribute to their overall well-being. Treatment studies have identified that constructive relationships lead to improvements in acceptance or distress tolerance (e.g., Gifford, Ritsher, McKellar, & Moos, 2006). Therapies that focus explicitly on distress tolerance, such as acceptance and commitment therapy (ACT), also encourage clients to consider their values and explicitly link difficult behaviors (such as quitting smoking) to these rewards (Gifford et al., 2004; Hayes et al., 2004).

A second prediction of this process is that persons who have an impaired ability to increase excitability of their MSN should have relatively poor distress tolerance. Such individuals would be less able to reduce their distress tolerance in resource-rich environments where opportunities are plentiful. Research studies on dopamine deficiency are consistent with this prediction. Because MSN excitability appears to be regulated via signaling from dopamine neurons, persons who release less dopamine or have fewer dopamine receptors might be expected to have difficulty increasing the excitability of their MSN. This might make them more prone to problems associated with low distress tolerance.

A relatively common polymorphism of the D2 dopamine receptor, the A1 allele, is associated with reduced expression of D2 dopamine receptors in the brain (Noble, 2000). Studies of persons with the A1 allele of the D2 dopamine receptor have found that such individuals are more likely to have problems with overuse of addictive substances (i.e., more likely to have tobacco, alcohol, and drug problems or to have greater difficulty quitting) to have gambling problems, and to have posttraumatic stress disorder (PTSD), an anxiety disorder (Comings, Ferry, et al., 1996; Comings, Rosenthal, et al., 1996; Connor, Young, Lawford, Ritchie, & Noble, 2002; Lawford et al., 2000; Lawford, Young, Noble, Kann, & Ritchie, 2006; Noble, 2000; Spitz et al., 1998). Also, in positron emission tomography imaging studies, persons with substance use disorders have been shown to have fewer dopamine receptors or to release less dopamine in reward circuits in response to both drugs of abuse and natural reinforcers (Volkow, Fowler, Wang, Swanson, & Telang, 2004). There is some evidence that these disorders are also associated with low distress tolerance. Smokers, pathological gamblers, and patients entering residential treatment for substance use disorders with low distress tolerance have been shown to be more likely to rapidly relapse during treatment attempts (Brown et al., 2009; Daughters, Lejuez, Bornovalova, 2005; Daughters, Lejuez, Strong, et al., 2005), suggesting that low distress tolerance may contribute to chronicity of these disorders. The relationship between distress tolerance and PTSD is less well studied. However, PTSD patients were found to have less effort tolerance in an ergometric test of work capacity and were more likely to quit the task before reaching 85% capacity, citing palpitations, shortness of breath, chest pain, weakness, and nausea (Shalev, Bleich, & Ursano, 1990). This finding might be reflective of low tolerance for the distressing sensations produced by physical exertion. Although far from conclusive, these observations are consistent with the importance of one's ability to adapt MSN excitability in clinical manifestations of distress tolerance.

## INHIBITING HABITS

When reward-driven behaviors have been learned, practiced, and highly valued, and opportunities to gain these rewards are present, responding for these rewards may become heavily favored or prepotent. In this case, active attempts to inhibit these reward-seeking behaviors may be necessary to prevent their expression. Inhibitory control over prepotent behavior has long been studied as a component of executive functions mediated by circuits, including the prefrontal cortex. Behavioral tasks such as the Stroop color–word task, go/no-go tasks, and stop-signal tasks have been used to examine inhibitory control over prepotent behaviors in human subjects. Neuroimaging and lesion studies using these tasks have investigated brain regions and processes involved in inhibitory control.

Studies of inhibitory control of prepotent behavior have shown that this ability varies over the lifespan and among individuals. On average, performance on the Stroop color–word task improves starting in late childhood and continues to improve until late adolescence, when it stabilizes through adulthood, before declining after about age 65 (Comalli, Wapner, & Werner, 1962). Studies of go/no-go task performance have shown a similar pattern, with children showing increasing efficiency in inhibiting a prepotent motor response (i.e., an ability to inhibit the behavior at an earlier stage of movement) with increasing age and older adults (age > 60) showing more errors in inhibiting a prepotent motor response (Cragg & Nation, 2008; Potter & Grealy, 2008). Imaging studies of response inhibition in persons of various ages have suggested that as children mature, inhibitory control becomes more dependent on the right prefrontal cortex (Chambers, Garavan, & Bellgrove, 2009). With age, inhibition-related activity becomes less lateralized (Nielson, Langenecker, & Garavan, 2002). Impairments in inhibitory control have been observed in patients with a variety of psychiatric disorders. For example, patients with attention-deficit/hyperactivity disorder, obsessive–compulsive disorder, and stimulant addiction have demonstrated deficits in performance on response-inhibition tasks (Chambers et al., 2009).

Imaging studies have demonstrated a cluster of brain regions involved in inhibitory control. In fMRI studies that tested the ability to inhibit a prepotent behavioral response, the ventral prefrontal, right dorsolateral prefrontal, right inferior partial, and anterior cingulate cortex have been found to be particularly important for response inhibition (Chambers et al., 2009; Garavan, Ross, Murphy, Roche, & Stein, 2002).

Performance on tasks that require inhibition of prepotent behaviors may improve with practice, and these improvements may even extrapolate to response inhibition on similar tasks with new stimuli. Kelly, Hester, Foxe, Shpaner, and Garavan (2006) used a go/no-go task with an imbedded working memory challenge to show that regional brain activation associated with task performance changed over 30 minutes of practice. Although performance remained excellent, activation of regions involved in working memory decreased with practice. Simultaneously, there was an increase in the activation of regions (i.e., dorsolateral and inferior prefrontal cortex and inferior parietal cortex) in which greater activation has been associated with greater ability to inhibit prepotent behaviors across individuals. This suggests that practice on response inhibition tasks can alter the cognitive strategies used so that they are more similar to strategies used by individuals who generally perform better on such tasks.

There is weaker evidence that response inhibition may be improved in older adults or that age-related decline in response inhibition may be limited by lifestyle factors or interventions. For example, in cross-sectional, observational studies, Stroop performance declined less in persons with more education (Van der Elst, Van Boxtel, Van Breukelen, & Jolles, 2006) and was positively associated with level of physical activity (Bixby et al., 2007). Also, a 10-month aerobic exercise program was associated with improvements in Stroop performance in adults ages 65–79 (Smiley-Oyen, Lowry, Francois, Kohut, & Ekkekakis, 2008). These studies suggest that practice or lifestyle interventions may be of some benefit in enhancing individual ability to inhibit prepotent behaviors within the range of typical performance.

Behavioral and imaging studies have demonstrated that inhibitory control is highly sensitive to cognitive demands (Chambers et al., 2009). Successful inhibition of behavior requires careful attention and is easily overwhelmed when tasks become more complex, attention is divided, or working memory load is increased. For example, Garvan and colleagues (2002) used a go/no-go task to demonstrate that participants made more errors as the speed of the required response on the task increased. Participants showed greater activation of anterior cingulate cortex and lesser activation of dorsolateral prefrontal cortex on the faster, more difficult inhibition compared with the slower inhibition trials. Notably, activation in dorsolateral prefrontal, inferior parietal, and anterior cingulate cortex was similar regardless of whether the participant successfully inhibited the response; inhibition errors appears to be associated with late activation of these regions rather than a lack of activation of these circuits. This study suggests that the more pressured or automatic the response, the more difficult it becomes to inhibit. In a similar study, Hester and Garavan (2005) showed that increasing working memory load impaired performance on a go/no-go task. Specifically, asking participants to hold five letters versus one letter in working memory impaired performance on a go/no-go task. Activity in dorsolateral prefrontal cortex and anterior cingulate cortex was increased during attempts to inhibit a prepotent button-press response on five-letter trials, indicating the importance of these prefrontal regions for both response inhibition and working memory. Additional studies have suggested that dorsolateral prefrontal cortex activity may be associated with general attentional processes (Fassbender et al., 2006). These studies emphasize that inhibitory control is easily impaired by requirements for concurrent attention or memory, presumably because these processes utilize shared real estate in the prefrontal cortex. Ability to inhibit a habitual response is poor except when one pays full attention to inhibiting the response and nothing else, a state that likely occurs rarely during day-to-day attempts to shape one's lifestyle. Moreover, when habits are stronger and more practiced, inhibitory control systems will be less likely to catch them before they are expressed.

## Potential Clinical Implications

First, clinicians should expect that patient populations with relative deficits in response inhibition, such as children, adolescents, older adults, and patients with certain psychiatric disorders, will have lower tolerance for distress. Distress tolerance should be improved when people actively attend to attempts to persist and should be worsened when distracters are present or cognitive/working memory load is increased. Thus, distress tolerance may be substantially lower during the chaos of day-to-day life than during focused laboratory challenges, particularly in persons who effectively use inhibitory control to mask high expectations or strong drive for immediate gratification.

Interventions to increase distress tolerance that target modifiers others than inhibitory control may be more effective in changing behavior over longer periods, particularly in youth, older adults, and clinical populations. Because inhibitory control requires attention and focus, it may only increase distress tolerance when one is aware of the challenge and is trying to persist. Interventions that increase distress tolerance by modifying reward expectations (i.e., decreasing the value of immediate relief or increasing the value of tolerating distress) or decreasing drive for immediate reinforcement (e.g., by increasing the availability of perceived opportunities in one's life) may be more successful in reducing harmful relief-seeking behaviors over time. Exposure- and acceptance-based therapies (including distress tolerance [Brown et al., 2008], ACT [Hayes, Strosahl, & Wilson, 2003], and cognitive-behavioral treatments for anxiety disorders [Barlow, 2002]) involve experiencing distress while inhibiting the habitual response that would alleviate distress. Clients are encouraged to consciously alter their stance toward their own distress and accept it in the service of greater behavioral control (Gifford et al.,

2004). Directly practicing this response inhibition may improve patients' ability to inhibit this same habit in life.

## DISCUSSION: CAN NEUROBIOLOGY INFORM EFFECTIVE PSYCHOTHERAPY FOR DISTRESS TOLERANCE?

The brain is an organ of adaptation designed to facilitate effective interaction with the environment. Psychotherapy is a method for improving adaptation by providing a structured, enriched environment within which to interact (i.e., the therapeutic encounter). Ideally, what happens in the therapeutic encounter changes how clients perceive, respond to, think about, and interact with their life outside of therapy.

We have discussed a number of candidate neurobiological systems underlying distress tolerance and briefly noted some potential clinical implications. First among these implications is the fact that there are a number of different neurobiological systems involved in distress tolerance. This does not imply that distress tolerance cannot be addressed as a unitary construct; however, considering these different systems may improve our understanding of how to treat distress tolerance.

The biological bases of distress tolerance suggest that shifting the relative emphasis of psychotherapy may improve the efficiency of care. Clinicians need to understand that how clients experience and shape their environment is as important as how they consciously work to control their behavior. Next, we discuss two general strategies for altering distress tolerance: (1) consciously practicing distress tolerance by working to inhibit habitual escape responses and (2) altering distress tolerance by increasing reward availability and perceived reward value.

## INCREASING DISTRESS TOLERANCE BY PRACTICING CONSCIOUS EFFORTFUL CONTROL

Inhibitory control involves executive processes in the prefrontal cortex that address the general issue "If I decide to actively try not to respond, can I stop myself?" Consciously practicing withholding escape behaviors under conditions of distress is likely to increase the efficiency with which restraint is used and applied; however, using such conscious effortful control is apt to provide less consistent increases in distress tolerance than altering experienced rewards and beliefs about rewards. Altering reward value and the gain on reward responding will reduce the inherent drive to escape distress (Trafton & Gifford, 2008). In contrast, the processes involved in conscious inhibition of behavior essentially attempt to break a behavior in process and are naturally limited by capacity constraints. With attention, and under optimal circumstances, people can learn to resist urges to escape distress. However, when they are tired, angry, distracted, or stressed, their capacity to exercise conscious restraint will be compromised, and the preconscious drives of the limbic system are far more likely to dominate. Because it requires attention and uses more complex and thus slower computational logic, the conscious inhibitory system is simply outgunned in complicated circumstances (Saling & Phillips, 2007). Active practice in withholding escape behaviors in contexts that simulate real life (i.e., acceptance and exposure therapies) will likely focus and improve distress tolerance, but relapse under stressful conditions should be anticipated.

## INCREASING DISTRESS TOLERANCE THROUGH ENRICHING EXPERIENCED ENVIRONMENTS

In terms of neurobiological systems, changing reward availability influences how hard individuals are willing to work for immediate relief, and altering the perceived value of rewards influences how highly this immediate relief is valued. Both of these processes involve enriching experienced environments, and there are numerous psychosocial treatment methods that work toward this end. First, to help clients increase contact with rewarding experiences, it is critical to understand how they each experience their environment, both currently and historically. What do they find meaningful and satisfying? To develop this understanding, therapists need to be able to listen empathically and intelligently to their clients and to develop an intimacy that permits their clients to speak honestly and deeply about their experiences and values (cf. Rogers, 1946). This perspective supports the "common factors" and related core clinical skills that are frequently discussed in the psychotherapy literature (Castonguay & Holtforth, 2005). How well one forms a caring relationship with their clients, a relationship that serves as a source of social rewards, matters (Moyers, Miller, & Hendrickson, 2005). Listening and empathizing in ways that permit genuine insight into how clients experience their lives, facilitating values clarification linked to therapeutic goals, and uncovering conscious and unconscious patterns by taking careful histories are not trivial steps before getting to the "real therapy" but rather are processes linked to changes in dopamine signaling with direct potential impact on distress tolerance (Trafton & Gifford, 2008).

Second, it is critical to help clients learn to shape their environment in ways that support their own optimum responding. Adding rewarding experiences, both in the therapeutic relationship and in daily life, should be considered an essential part of treatment (Grawe, 2007). For example, if a client wants to start an exercise program, instead of relying on the intrinsic value of exercise and the long-term benefits of weight loss, it is helpful to engage a supportive social group that highlights and amplifies rewards by adding new social reinforcers to the mix. Rewarding social interactions will add to the inherent benefits of exercise to increase the predicted value of exercising. Contingency management is a treatment that systematically and artificially enhances the reward value for target behaviors using prizes (Petry, Martin, Cooney, & Kranzler, 2000). Far from using "bribery" to "coerce" individuals, it provides a direct means of altering the reward value predictions that drive unconscious habits.

Altering conscious cortical reward value predictions also occurs through common clinical practices. For example, highlighting how specific choices link to long-term values and goals can change how potential rewards are perceived. Helping clients connect with deeply held, meaningful, and rewarding personal values, and directly linking these values to the benefits of quitting drinking or smoking, for example, may increase the perceived value of rewards contingent on quitting (Carrico, Gifford, & Moos, 2007). For example, a smoking client who rewards himself by spending cigarette money instead on dinner out with his grandchildren may experience the benefits of not smoking and also the strong reinforcement of contact with beloved children. Quitting smoking may be consciously linked to these loving relationships through values clarification (e.g, ACT: Gifford et al., 2004; or motivational interviewing: Miller & Rollnick, 2002).

The intensity of treatment needed to alter reward values, experience more opportunities, and practice consciously changing behavior will vary among individuals. A person's genetic profile appears to drive a certain amount of this variability, as does history and experience. Individuals with certain histories and genetic vulnerabilities may require more highly structured intensive environments as well as pharmacological interventions designed to facilitate their ability to respond to these environments more adaptively.

Finally, although we have discussed a variety of brain systems implicated in distress tolerance, the commonality of these systems across disorders points to an integrated approach to psychopathology. Disorders of overavoidance and overconsumption may be understood to have common pathways in the brain (e.g., smoking and obesity) (Gifford & Lillis, 2009). The alcoholic's drink, the obese person's chocolate, the anxious person's escape, and the chronic pain patient's inactivity all trigger the same circuits. It is interesting to note that a neurobiological perspective encourages attention on certain common functional categories (Hayes, Wilson, Gifford, Follette, & Strosahl, 1996), common clinical processes (Barlow, Allen, & Choate, 2004; Salzinger & Serper, 2009), and attendant core clinical competencies in the effort to promote clinical change (Gifford, 2007).

## REFERENCES

Abler, B., Walter, H., Erk, S., Kammerer, H., & Spitzer, M. (2006). Prediction error as a linear function of reward probability is coded in human nucleus accumbens. *NeuroImage, 31,* 790–795.

Bannon, A. W., & Malmberg, A. B. (2007). Models of nociception: Hot-plate, tail-flick, and formalin tests in rodents. *Current Protocols in Neuroscience, 41,* 8.9.1–8.9.15.

Barlow, D. H. (2002). *Anxiety and its disorders: The nature and treatment of anxiety and panic* (2nd ed.). New York: Guilford Press.

Barlow, D. H., Allen, L. B., & Choate, M. L. (2004). Towards a unified treatment for emotional disorders. *Behavior Therapy, 35,* 205–230.

Barrot, M., Olivier, J. D., Perrotti, L. I., DiLeone, R. J., Berton, O., Eisch, A. J., et al. (2002). CREB activity in the nucleus accumbens shell controls gating of behavioral responses to emotional stimuli. *Proceedings of the National Academy of Sciences of the United States of America, 17,* 11435–11440.

Barrot, M., Wallace, D. L., Bolaños, C. A., Grahm, D. L., Perrotti, L. I., Neve, R. L., et al. (2005). Regulation of anxiety and initiation of sexual behavior by CREB in the nucleus accumbens. *Proceedings of the National Academy of Sciences of the United States of America, 102,* 8357–8362.

Bixby, W. R., Spalding, T. W., Haufler, A. J., Deeny, S. P., Mahlow, P. T., & Zimmerman, J. B. (2007). The unique relation of physical activity to executive function in older men and women. *Medicine and Science in Sports and Exercise, 39,* 1408–1416.

Borsook, D., Becerra, L., Carlezon, W., Jr., Shaw, M., Renshaw, P., Elman, I., et al. (2007). Reward-aversion circuitry in analgesia and pain: Implications for psychiatric disorders. *European Journal of Pain, 11,* 7–20.

Brown, R. A., Lejuez, C. W., Strong, D. R., Kahler, C. W., Zvolensky, M. J., Carpenter, L. L., et al. (2009). A prospective examination of distress tolerance and early smoking lapse in adult self-quitters. *Nicotine and Tobacco Research, 11,* 493–502.

Brown, R. A., Palm, K. M., Strong, D. R., Lejuez, C. W., Kahler, C. W., Zvolensky, M. J., et al. (2008). Distress tolerance treatment for early-lapse smokers: rationale, program description, and preliminary findings. *Behavior Modification, 32,* 302–332.

Carlezon, W. A., Jr., Thome, J., Olson, V. G., Lane-Ladd, S. B., Brodkin, E. S., Hiroi, N., et al. (1998). Regulation of cocaine reward by CREB. *Science, 282,* 2272–2275.

Carrico, A., Gifford, E., & Moos, R. H. (2007). Spirituality/religiosity promotes acceptance-based responding and twelve-step involvement. *Drug and Alcohol Dependence, 89,* 66–73.

Castonguay, L., & Holtforth, M. (2005). Change in psychotherapy: A plea for no more "nonspecific" and false dichotomies. *Clinical Psychology: Science and Practice, 12,* 198–200.

Chambers, C. C., Garavan, H., & Bellgrove, M. A. (2009). Insights into the neural basis of response inhibition from cognitive and clinical neuroscience. *Neuroscience and Biobehavioral Reviews, 33,* 631–646.

Chen, A. L., Chen, T. J., Waite, R. L., Reinking, J., Tung, H. L., Rhoades, P., et al. (2009). Hypothesizing that brain reward circuitry genes are genetic antecedents of pain sensitivity and critical diagnostic and pharmacogenomic treatment targets for chronic pain conditions. *Medical Hypotheses, 72,* 14–22.

Comings, D. E., Ferry, L., Bradshaw-Robinson, S., Burchette, R., Chiu, C., & Muhleman, D. (1996). The dopamine D2 receptor (DRD2) gene: A genetic risk factor in smoking. *Pharmacogenetics, 6,* 73–79.

Comalli, P. E., Jr., Wapner, S., & Werner, H. (1962). Interference effects of Stroop color-word test in childhood, adulthood, and aging. *Journal of Genetic Psychology, 100,* 47–53.

Comings, D. E., Rosenthal, R. J., Lesieur, H. R., Rugle, L. J., Muhleman, D., Chiu, C., et al. (1996). A study of the dopamine D2 receptor gene in pathological gambling. *Pharmacogenetics, 6,* 223–234.

Connor, J. P., Young, R. M., Lawford, B. R., Ritchie, T. L., & Noble, E. P. (2002). D(2) dopamine receptor (DRD2) polymorphism is associated with severity of alcohol dependence. *European Psychiatry, 17,* 17–23.

Cragg, L., & Nation, K. (2008). Go or no-go?: Developmental improvements in the efficiency of response inhibition in mid-childhood. *Developmental Science, 11,* 819–827.

Crawley, J. N. (1999). Behavioral phenotyping of transgenic and knockout mice: Experimental design and evaluation of general health, sensory functions, motor abilities, and specific behavioral tests. *Brain Research, 835,* 18–26.

Daughters, S. B., Lejuez, C. W., Bornovalova, M. A., Kahler, C. W., Strong, D. R., & Brown, R. A. (2005). Distress tolerance as a predictor of early treatment dropout in a residential substance abuse treatment facility. *Journal of Abnormal Psychology, 114,* 729–734.

Daughters, S. B., Lejuez, C. W., Strong, D. R, Brown, R. A., Breen, R. B., & Lesieus, H. R. (2005). The relationship among negative affect, distress tolerance, and length of gambling abstinence attempt. *Journal of Gambling Studies, 21,* 363–378.

Del Arco, A., & Mora, F. (2008). Prefrontal cortex-nucleus accumbens interaction: In vivo modulation by dopamine and glutamate in the prefrontal cortex. *Pharmacology, Biochemistry, and Behavior, 90,* 226–235.

Dong, Y., Green, T., Saal, D., Marie, H., Neve, R., Nestler, E. J., et al. (2006). CREB modulates excitability of nucleus accumbens neurons. *Nature Neuroscience, 9,* 475–477.

Fassbender, C., Simoes-Franklin, C., Murphy, K., Hester, R., Meaney, J., Robertson, I. H., et al. (2006). The role of a right fronto-parietal network in cognitive control: Common activations for "cues-to-attend" and response inhibition. *Journal of Psychophysiology, 20,* 286–296.

Garavan, H., Ross, T. J., Murphy, K., Roche, R. A. P., & Stein, E. A. (2002). Dissociable executive functions in the dynamic control of behavior: Inhibition, error detection, and correction. *NeuroImage, 17,* 1820–1829.

Gifford, E. V. (1994). Setting a course for behavior change: The verbal context of acceptance. In S. C. Hayes, N. S. Jacobson, V. M. Follette, & M. J. Dougher (Eds.), *Acceptance and change: Content and context in psychotherapy* (pp. 218–222). Reno, NV: Context Press.

Gifford, E. V. (2002). Socrates and the dodo bird: Clinical behavior analysis and psychotherapy research. *Behavior Analyst Today, 3,* 257–259.

Gifford, E. V. (2007). From the specificity hypothesis to patient-centered process: Advancing the evolution of behavioral treatment research. *Addiction, 102,* 1840.

Gifford, E. V., Kohlenberg, B. S., Hayes, S. C., Antonuccio, D. O., Piasecki, M. M., Rasmussen–Hall, M. L., et al. (2004). Acceptance-based treatment for smoking cessation. *Behavior Therapy, 35,* 689–705.

Gifford, E. V., & Lillis, J. (2009). Avoidance and inflexibility as a common clinical pathway in obesity and smoking treatment. *Journal of Health Psychology,14*(7), 992–996.

Gifford, E. V., Ritsher, J., McKellar, J., & Moos, R. (2006). Acceptance and relationship context: A model of substance use disorder treatment outcome. *Addiction, 101,* 1167–1177.

Grace, A. A., Floresco, S. B., Goto, Y., & Lodge, D. J. (2007). Regulation of firing of dopaminergic neurons and control of goal-directed behaviors. *Trends in Neurosciences, 30,* 220–227.

Grawe, K. (2007). *Neuropsychotherapy: How the neurosciences inform effective psychotherapy.* Mahwah, NJ: Erlbaum.

Hayes, S. C., Strosahl, K. D., & Wilson, K. G. (2003). *Acceptance and commitment therapy: An experiential approach to behavior change.* New York: Guilford Press.

Hayes, S. C., Wilson, K. G., Gifford, E. V., Bissett, R., Piasecki, M., Batten, S. J., et al. (2004). A preliminary trial of twelve-step facilitation and acceptance and commitment therapy with polysubstance-abusing methadone-maintained opiate addicts. *Behavior Therapy, 35,* 667–688.

Hester, R., & Garavan, H. (2005). Working memory and executive function: The influence of content and load on the control of attention. *Memory and Cognition, 3,* 221–233.

Hikosaka, O., Bromberg-Martin, E., Hong, S., & Matsumoto, M. (2008). New insights on the subcortical representation of reward. *Current Opinion in Neurobiology, 18,* 203–208.

Karl, T., Pabst, R., & von Hörsten, S. (2003). Behavioral phenotyping of mice in pharmacological and toxicological research. *Experimental and Toxicologic Pathology, 55,* 69–83.

Kelly, A. M. C., Hester, R., Foxe, J. J., Shpaner, M., & Garavan, H. (2006). Flexible cognitive control: Effects of individual differences and brief practice on a complex cognitive task. *NeuroImage, 31,* 866–886.

Lawford, B. R., Young, R., Noble, E. P., Kann, B., & Ritchie, T. (2006). The D2 dopamine receptor (DRD2) gene is associated with co-morbid depression, anxiety and social dysfunction in untreated veterans with post-traumatic stress disorder. *European Psychiatry, 21,* 180–185.

Lawford, B. R., Young, R. M., Noble, E. P., Sargent, J., Rowell, J., Shadforth, S., et al. (2000). The D(2) dopamine receptor A(1) allele and opioid dependence: Association with heroin use and response to methadone treatment. *American Journal of Medical Genetics, 96,* 592–598.

Le Bars, D., Gozariu, M., & Cadden, S. W. (2001). Animal models of nociception. *Pharmacological Reviews, 53,* 597–652.

Magen, E., & Gross, J. J. (2007). Harnessing the need for immediate gratification: Cognitive reconstrual modulates the reward value of temptations. *Emotion, 7,* 415–428.

Marinelli, M., Rudick, C. N., Hu, X. T., & White, F. J. (2006). Excitability of dopamine neurons: Modulation and physiological consequences. *CNS and Neurological Disorders—Drug Targets, 5,* 79–97.

Miller, W. R., & Rollnick, S. (2002). *Motivational interviewing: Preparing people for change* (2nd ed.). New York: Guilford Press.

Moyers, T., Miller, W., & Hendrickson, S. (2005). How does motivational interviewing work?: Therapist interpersonal skill predicts client involvement within motivational interviewing sessions. *Journal of Consulting and Clinical Psychology, 73,* 590–598.

Nestler, E. J. (2004). Molecular mechanisms of drug addiction. *Neuropharmacology, 47,* 24–32.

Nielson, K. A., Langenecker, S. A., & Garavan, H. (2002). Differences in the functional neuroanatomy of inhibitory control across the adult life span. *Psychology and Aging, 17,* 56–71.

Noble, E. P. (2000). The DRD2 gene in psychiatric and neurological disorders and its phenotypes. *Pharmacogenomics, 1,* 309–333.

Petry, N. M., Martin, B., Cooney, J. L., & Kranzler, H. R. (2000). Give them prizes and they will come: Contingency management for treatment of alcohol dependence. *Journal of Consulting and Clinical Psychology, 68,* 250–257.

Pliakas, A. M., Carlson, R. R., Neve, R. L., Konradi, C., Nestler, E. J., & Carlezon, W. A., Jr. (2001). Altered responsiveness to cocaine and increased immobility in the forced swim test associated with elevated cAMP response element-binding protein expression in nucleus accumbens. *Journal of Neuroscience, 21,* 7397–7403.

Potter, L. M., & Grealy, M. A. (2008). Aging and inhibition of a prepotent motor response during an ongoing action. *Aging, Neuropsychology, and Cognition, 15,* 232–255.

Rodriguez, P. F., Aron, A. R., & Poldrack, R. A. (2006). Ventral-striatal/nucleus-accumbens sensitivity to prediction errors during classification learning. *Human Brain Mapping, 27,* 306–313.

Roesch, M. R., & Olson, C. R. (2004). Neuronal activity related to reward value and motivation in primate frontal cortex. *Science, 304,* 307–310.

Rogers, C. (1946). Significant aspects of client-centered therapy. *American Journal of Psychiatry, 1,* 415–422.

Saling, L. L., & Phillips, J. G. (2007). Automatic behaviour: Efficient not mindless. *Brain Research Bulletin, 73,* 1–20.

Salzinger, K., & Serper, M. R. (2009). *Behavioral mechanisms and psychopathology: Advancing the explanation of its nature, cause, and treatment.* Washington, DC: American Psychological Association.

Schultz, W. (1998). Predictive reward signal of dopamine neurons. *Journal of Neurophysiology, 80,* 1–27.

Shalev, A., Bleich, A., & Ursano, R. J. (1990). Posttraumatic stress disorder: Somatic comorbidity and effort tolerance. *Psychosomatics, 31,* 197–203.

Smiley-Oyen, A. L., Lowry, K. A., Francois, S. J., Kohut, M. L., & Ekkekakis, P. (2008). Exercise, fitness, and neurocognitive function in older adults: The "selective improvement" and "cardiovascular fitness" hypotheses. *Annals of Behavioral Medicine, 36,* 280–291.

Spitz, M. R., Shi, H., Yang, F., Hudmon, K. S., Jiany, H., Chamberlain, R. M., et al. (1998). Case-control study of the D2 dopamine receptor gene and smoking status in lung cancer patients. *Journal of the National Cancer Institute, 90,* 358–363.

Taha, S. A., & Fields, H. L. (2006). Inhibitions of nucleus accumbens neurons encode a gating signal for reward-directed behavior. *Journal of Neuroscience, 26,* 217–222.

Tobler, P. N., O'Doherty, J. P., Dolan, R. J., & Schultz, W. (2006). Human neural learning depends on reward prediction errors in the blocking paradigm. *Journal of Neurophysiology, 95,* 301–310.

Trafton, J. A., & Gifford, E. R. (2008). Behavioral reactivity and addiction: The adaptation of behavioral response to reward opportunities. *Journal of Neuropsychiatry and Clinical Neuroscience, 20,* 23–35.

Van der Elst, W., Van Boxtel, M. P., Van Breukelen, G. J., & Jolles, J. (2006). The Stroop color-word test: Influence of age, sex, and education; and normative data for a large sample across the adult age range. *Assessment, 13,* 62–79.

Volkow, N. D., Fowler, J. S., Wang, G. J., Swanson, J. M., & Telang, F. (2004). Dopamine in drug abuse and addiction: Results from imaging studies and treatment implications. *Molecular Psychiatry, 9,* 557–569.

# PART II

# Distress Tolerance
# and Psychopathology
## Empirical and Clinical Approaches

# 5

## Anxiety and Its Disorders

Norman B. Schmidt, Melissa Mitchell,
Meghan Keough, *and* Christina Riccardi

### STATE OF THE FIELD: THE RELATIONSHIP BETWEEN DISTRESS TOLERANCE AND ANXIETY DISORDERS

In recent years, significant advances have been made in our understanding of anxiety psychopathology (Barlow, 2002). Converging lines of evidence suggest that anxiety disorders in adulthood may represent manifestations of an underlying constitutional vulnerability or diathesis for anxiety that is partly genetic and variably expressed over the life cycle. An individual's overall risk for psychopathology is believed to be a function of personal genetic and nongenetic resiliency and vulnerability factors, environmental risk and protective factors, and an interaction among these factors. This chapter describes a relatively unexplored but promising construct relevant to anxiety psychopathology: distress tolerance (DT). To date, there are very few empirical studies that have evaluated DT and the various anxiety disorders. However, DT appears to coalesce with other factors that have proven their relevance to our understanding of anxiety. Thus, the purpose of this chapter is to review the available literature focused on DT and anxiety. We also integrate the DT literature from other areas of psychopathology in an attempt to describe how this may be relevant to our understanding of anxiety processes. To assist our endeavors, we develop a model that places DT in the context of other, better studied constructs, which will allow us to lay the groundwork for future empirical studies.

There has been increasing interest in the evaluation of emotional sensitivity and affective intolerance in a number of forms of psychopathology (Zvolensky & Otto, 2007). Among the anxiety disorders more specifically, a number of emotion regulation constructs have emerged that attempt to capture processes that appear to be relevant to the onset, exacerbation, and maintenance of these problems. These factors typically involve some type of amplification of a normal anxiety response and include discomfort intolerance (DI) and anxiety sensitivity (AS). DT appears to fit within these sorts of amplifying factors that are believed to play important roles in the pathogenesis of anxiety problems.

To begin, it is important to define these related constructs as well as to develop a conceptual model that attempts to delineate the possible relations among them and their role in anxiety psychopathology. Figure 5.1, consistent with Bernstein, Zvolensky, Vujanovic, and Moos's (2009) investigation of DT, DI, and AS, depicts a possible hierarchical model that describes a number of facets conceivably important in affective intolerance within the anxiety disorders. In this model, we have defined DT as capturing an individual difference in the capacity to effectively manage emotional states. Simons and Gaher (2005) suggest that DT should be broadly defined as the capacity to withstand negative emotional states. Furthermore, they posit that DT is a higher order construct that will affect a variety of processes involved in many aspects of behavior and affect regulation, including deployment of attention, appraisals of distress, and modulation of responses to distress. Thus, DT is believed to affect the evaluation and consequences of experiencing negative emotional states. Those with low DT become overly reactive to stress and distress. Such individuals are also believed to report poor coping abilities with respect to dealing with distress. As a result, people with low DT will attempt to avoid negative emotions and will try to use strategies to quickly remedy negative emotional states.

This model of DT was initially applied to borderline personality disorder and substance use disorders wherein low DT was seen to capture several aspects of these conditions, including perceiving distress to be unbearable and consequent affect dysregulation and poor coping (e.g., substance use) with affect (Linehan, 1993). However, the elements described by Simons and Gaher (2005) can be readily applied to anxiety psychopathology. Most current models of anxiety psychopathology suggest very similar cognitive and behavioral processes relevant to anxiety onset and maintenance. Those with anxiety disorders show information-processing biases that compel them to focus on stimuli relevant to their fears (Bar-Haim, Lamy, Pergamin, Bakermans-Kranenburg, & van IJzen-

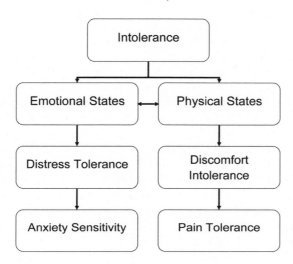

**FIGURE 5.1.** Hierarchical relations among constructs relevant to affective intolerance and sensitivity among the anxiety disorders.

doorn, 2007). In the context of feared stimuli and situations, these individuals show exaggerated threat appraisals along with poor perceived coping. Of course, avoidance of feared situations is a hallmark feature of anxiety disorders along with the use of "quick-fix" remedies, which are often referred to as safety aids (e.g., Parrish, Radomsky, & Dugas, 2008). To make this a bit more concrete, a patient with panic disorder (PD) may be hypervigilant to external (e.g., bridge) or internal (e.g., heart palpitations) cues that have been linked with panic in the past. Upon recognition of the presence of these cues, the patient may have exaggerated threat appraisals (e.g., "I'm going to lose control and drive off the bridge"; "My heart will start racing until I have a heart attack"). This patient may take immediate steps to avoid (e.g., pull off the road) or manage (e.g., take a benzodiazepine) the situation and the impending threat. The considerable similarities between the processes identified by Simons and Gaher (2005) and those noted in contemporary accounts of anxiety clearly suggest that DT may exert some influence in a number of different processes relevant to anxiety.

In turning to the model of affective intolerance and sensitivity described in Figure 5.1, we consider the idea that it may be important to distinguish between tolerance related to emotions and tolerance related to physical cues and sensations. At least among some individuals, tolerance of physical cues, such as pain tolerance, is unrelated to measures of affective states (Geisser, Robinson, & Pickren, 1992), suggesting that the ability to tolerate physical discomfort is not necessarily correlated with the ability to tolerate negative emotions. For example, individuals with borderline personality disorder may become overwhelmed by a variety of strong emotions (i.e., poor DT) but may show higher than average tolerance of painful physical discomfort (e.g., they may engage in nonsuicidal cutting or burning). Therefore, we have paired DT with DI as higher level factors in the model in an attempt to capture the idea that people may have difficulty managing emotions (DT) as well as physical sensations (DI). It is worth noting that the DT literature does not always make a very clear distinction between tolerance of emotions and physical sensations. However, it does seem fairly clear that the DT construct is much more heavily focused on accounting for emotional tolerance and emotion regulation than a tolerance relating to physical sensations. Moreover, measures of DT such as the Distress Tolerance Scale (DTS; Simons & Gaher, 2005) are very focused on emotions (e.g., "Feeling distressed or upset is unbearable"; "I'll do anything to stop feeling distressed or upset").

In contrast, DI is intended to tap individual differences relating to the capacity to withstand uncomfortable physical sensations. Thus, DI is very similar to pain tolerance (or intolerance), but instead of focusing solely on the ability to tolerate painful stimuli, it refers to a much broader array of sensations that are uncomfortable but not necessarily painful. To understand the DI process, consider that an individual is affected by an uncomfortable physical sensation such as shortness of breath, numbness, or chest pressure. In this context, some type of a "sensation detection" filter requires that any stimulus pass above a given threshold in order to be perceived. Finally, a "sensation tolerance" filter will affect the degree to which unpleasant sensations are perceived as manageable. DI, or the trait-like individual-difference variable referring to the capacity to endure physical discomfort, is believed to index the sensation tolerance component of this description.

At the lower level of the model, we have included AS and pain tolerance. In our view, each of these represents a more specific component of the corresponding higher order factor; that is, AS can be viewed as a form of DT and pain tolerance as a form of DI. For our purposes in this chapter, we do not focus much attention on pain tolerance because this is beyond the scope of our discussion. On the other hand, AS is the best researched anxiety-related risk factor, and so it is important to consider AS as it potentially relates to DT.

AS was initially conceptualized as a trait-like cognitive characteristic that predisposes individuals to the development of anxiety problems (Taylor, 1999). Those possessing relatively high levels of AS are theorized to perceive bodily sensations associated with autonomic arousal as a sign of imminent personal harm and, as a result, to potentially react to them with anxiety, panic attacks, or the development of an anxiety disorder. Whereas DT suggests individual differences in tolerance relating to emotions in general, AS can be viewed as tolerance or sensitivity to one specific emotion: fear and fear-related sensations. AS is distinct from trait anxiety (i.e., the tendency to respond with fear to a wide range of stressors) and describes a more specific tendency to respond fearfully to one's own anxiety symptoms. Moreover, AS explains reliable variance unrelated to trait anxiety. In fact, some models indicate that AS and trait anxiety are distinct constructs that appear to be hierarchically organized, with AS operating as a lower order trait that is nested hierarchically within a higher order dimension of trait anxiety (Lilienfeld, Turner, & Jacob, 1993). A more detailed discussion of the trait anxiety–AS hierarchy versus the model proposed here goes a bit beyond the scope of this chapter; however, in our view, both models are compatible if we assume that AS can be subsumed by the more general DT construct.

One additional aspect of Figure 5.1 that should be explained would include the relations among these variables and anxiety psychopathology more specifically. We first consider AS and DI because these constructs have been more clearly linked with anxiety. Unlike many other cognitive conceptualizations of anxiety, AS is believed to be a dispositional characteristic that may precede the development of clinical anxiety symptoms or diagnoses. Empirical studies provide converging evidence that AS does indeed act as a risk factor for anxiety problems. First, laboratory studies indicate that baseline AS predicts fear responses to bodily sensations (Rabian, Embry, & MacIntyre, 1999; Unnewehr, Schneider, Margraf, Jenkins, & Florin, 1996; Zvolensky, McNeil, Porter, & Stewart, 2001). Second, AS levels are elevated among individuals with anxiety disorders compared with those without anxiety disorder (Kearney, Albano, Eisen, Allan, & Barlow, 1997; Taylor, Koch, & McNally, 1992). Perhaps more convincingly, prospective studies with healthy adults (Schmidt, Lerew, & Jackson, 1997, 1999) and adolescents (Hayward, Killen, Kraemer, & Taylor, 2000) indicate that AS predicts the future occurrence of anxiety symptoms and panic attacks. Finally, more recent work has shown that AS increases risk for anxiety disorder diagnoses (Schmidt, Zvolensky, & Maner, 2006).

In regard to DI, models have been proposed to describe the hypothesized role of DI in panicogenesis. When tolerance is high, discomfort is more readily managed. Alternatively, when tolerance is low, noxious stimuli are more likely to be perceived as threatening (i.e., in the sense that they may be perceived to be unmanageable). This, in turn, can lead to fear or panic in the presence of unpleasant somatic sensations, consistent with recent models of PD (Barlow, 2002; Bouton, Mineka, & Barlow, 2001; McNally, 2002). Thus, the DI model is highly consistent with prevailing cognitive and physiological conceptualizations of panic but delineates a pathway focused on the role of uncomfortable somatic perturbations. There has been some empirical work on the DI construct. Consistent with the model specified, Schmidt and Lerew (1998) found that DI prospectively predicted some indices of anxiety-related impairment as well as sick days. In fact, DI, in the context of other risk factors such as AS, has been found to uniquely predict anxiety outcomes (Schmidt & Cook, 1999; Schmidt, Lerew, & Trakowski, 1997). Taken together, these studies provide preliminary evidence that DI may act as a risk factor for anxiety pathology.

Finally, we must consider the role of DT in regard to anxiety. Consistent with the model described in Figure 5.1 and our discussion of AS and DI, we propose that poorer DT could increase the risk for anxiety as well as potentially help maintain problematic anxiety reactions. Individuals with poor DT are believed to be at increased risk for becoming overwhelmed by a wide array of emotions. When their own emotional response is perceived as unpredictable, uncontrollable, and generally unmanageable, we would expect that this would lead to increased negative affect, including anxiety. Extrapolating from cognitive models of anxiety, the detection and interpretation of emotions, including problematic interpretation of arousal sensations (i.e., AS), is believed to be critical in the generation of anxiety (Reiss & McNally, 1985). In the case of PD, for example, these models presume that threatening interpretation of emotions is critical to the onset and maintenance of the condition (Clark, 1986). Thus, when emotions and emotional responses are deemed threatening, the individual should experience fear. Relative to those low in distress tolerance, people with high tolerance of sensations are unlikely to perceive or attend to some sensations. This provides more or less of an opportunity for problematic interpretive processes to take hold. Similarly, DT is likely to influence these interpretive processes. Having a long history of experiencing, tolerating, and recovering from high levels of emotional upheaval may inoculate one against interpreting emotions as threatening. Thus, DT is likely to influence interpretation of sensations, including AS as one key interpretive problem relevant to anxiety psychopathology. Finally, DT may influence coping processes that help maintain anxiety problems. As noted previously, avoidance and the use of other safety behaviors are believed to be common reactions to emotional arousal for those with low DT. The empirical literature clearly shows that avoidance behaviors and other maladaptive safety aids help to maintain fear responses (Powers, Smits, & Telch, 2004; Salkovskis, Clark, Hackmann, Wells, & Gelder, 1999). Although much of this literature focuses on situational avoidance, it is also clear that those with anxiety conditions avoid bodily sensations, and there are some data, consistent with this model, to suggest that patients with anxiety will avoid emotionally arousing situations (Hoffart, Sexton, Hedley, & Martinsen, 2008). Thus, we have reason to believe that DT will affect key perceptual, interpretative, and coping responses relevant to emotions that will increase risk for anxiety problems.

## REVIEW OF RELEVANT EMPIRICAL LITERATURE

Existing DT research has primarily focused on its impact in emotional dysregulation in Axis II disorders (e.g., borderline personality disorder). Yet DT is emerging as a novel construct to assess in Axis I symptoms and syndromes, particularly for substance use as well as anxiety. Unfortunately, very few studies have directly examined DT and anxiety. We review those studies along with others that have assessed DT and anxiety-relevant constructs such as AS.

### Distress Tolerance and Anxiety Psychopathology

There is relatively little research on DT in anxiety psychopathology. Timpano, Buckner, Richey, Murphy, and Schmidt (2009) examined the association between DT and AS in compulsive hoarding in three large samples of nonclinical undergraduates (total $n = 745$) using a cross-sectional design. Each of the three samples was composed of approximately 200–250 individuals about 19 years old, 50–60% of whom were female. Participants completed the DTS (Simons & Gaher, 2005) to index their DT. DT was significantly negatively associated with hoarding in studies of Samples 2 and 3. Furthermore, study of Sample 3 demonstrated that DT and AS interacted such that individuals with high AS and low DT were at greater risk for hoarding symptoms.

Using a longitudinal design, Marshall and colleagues (2008) assessed the number of panic symptoms during an initial hyperventilation challenge to determine whether panic attack status predicted DT in a second hyperventilation challenge (as defined by persistence in an unpleasant task, namely hyperventilation) in 95 adult smokers. The sample was 58% female and were a mean age of 29 years ($SD = 12.2$). Participants smoked a mean of 15.9 cigarettes daily ($SD = 7.31$, range = 4–50) and reported smoking daily for about 12 years ($SD = 10.6$, range = 1–45). Although this was a smoking sample, almost two-thirds met criteria for at least one current Axis I psychopathology, with most of these diagnoses being anxiety disorders. Findings indicated that a panic attack during the first hyperventilation challenge significantly predicted persistence in the second hyperventilation challenge above and beyond AS, NA, DI, and the number of cigarettes smoked per day. This study is one of the most stringent tests to date on DT and anxiety because the authors controlled for multiple third variables that could account for the relationship. On the other hand, it could be argued that persistence during a biological challenge does not tap into some of the core features of DT when it is defined by tolerance of emotions.

Telch, Jacquin, Smits, and Powers (2003) conducted a cross-sectional study examining respiratory distress during panic attacks among individuals with a primary diagnosis of PD with or without agoraphobia (based on *Diagnostic and Statistical Manual of Mental Disorders* [third edition, revised] criteria; American Psychiatric Association, 1987) as well as nonclinical panickers. Of the 149 participants, 59 had PD with agoraphobia, 46 had PD without agoraphobia, and 44 were nonclinical panickers. The sample was primarily female (70.4%). Although not referred to as DT in the article, DT was assessed by the duration of hyperventilation challenge test. In other words, we can adopt the same definition Marshall and colleagues (2008) used for this study. Results indicated that individuals with PD with agoraphobia had significantly shorter hyperventilation duration times, controlling for demographics and clinical measures. Taken together, these two studies provide early evidence for a relationship between panic and decreased DT in relation to unpleasant physical sensations.

Daughters and colleagues (2009) assessed the link between DT and internalizing disorders in 231 community youth (mean age = 10.9 years, $SD$ = 0.9, range = 9–13), 45.5% of whom were female. The Revised Child Anxiety and Depression Scale (Chorpita, Yim, Moffitt, Umemoto, & Francis, 2000) assessed internalizing symptoms, including mood and anxiety diagnoses. Utilizing a cross-sectional design, DT was assessed using the Behavioral Indicator of Resiliency to Distress (BIRD; Lejuez, Daughters, Danielson, & Ruggiero, 2006). In the BIRD, participants click a green dot above one of 10 boxes before it moves to another box on a computer screen. If they are successful, they earn one point; failure earns zero points. The BIRD has three levels of increasing difficulty. DT was measured as the persistence on the final level of the task. Persistence can be assessed based on whether or not participants ended the task. Findings showed that DT interacted with gender such that low DT was associated with greater internalizing symptomatology but only among female youth.

Two other anxiety-related constructs that may influence DT are intolerance of uncertainty (IU; Dugas, Gosselin, & Ladouceur, 2001) and frustration discomfort (FD; Harrington, 2005). IU is the tendency to view the chance of a negative event occurring as unacceptable and threatening regardless of the likelihood of it occurring. Those with relatively high IU may be less able to withstand negative emotion (i.e., low DT). Studies suggest that IU is associated with generalized anxiety disorder, obsessive–compulsive disorder (OCD), and social anxiety disorder (Boelen & Reijntjes, 2009; Dugas et al., 2001). FD is characterized by the refusal to accept the difference between reality and desire. Emotional intolerance, which falls under FD, is similar to Simons and Gaher's (2005) interpretation of DT. Initial results indicated that emotional intolerance was uniquely associated with anxiety, controlling for negative affect and self-worth (Harrington, 2006). More research on IU and FD is needed to further understand their potential relationships with DT and anxiety psychopathology.

Overall, current research on DT suggests that it may function in several ways to influence anxiety psychopathology. First, low DT may be a risk factor for the development of anxiety psychopathology (Daughters et al., 2009). When low DT is combined with other more well-established risk factors for anxiety (i.e., AS), the chance of anxiety symptoms or syndromes developing appears to increase (Timpano et al., 2009). Second, although little research has addressed how DT might maintain anxiety psychopathology, it is likely that for those with clinically significant anxiety an inability or decreased ability to tolerate negative emotions would likely amplify anxiety when it is experienced and maintain the disorder in the future. Third, although there is little research on the role of DT in relapse of anxiety psychopathology, those with low DT have a decreased threshold for withstanding negative emotions. If they encounter noxious stimuli, low DT may play a role in potential relapse of the anxiety symptomatology. Thus, DT may have a bidirectional relationship with anxiety symptoms and syndromes. Specifically, early results suggest that low DT may be associated with greater anxiety symptoms and syndromes (Daughters et al., 2009; Timpano et al., 2009) and anxiety symptoms may be associated with lower DT (Telch et al., 2003).

## Unpublished Research

Although the current literature is beginning to elucidate the role of DT in anxiety, there is a need for a greater research focus in this area to delineate more clearly the role of DT in anxiety and its correlates. To expand upon current knowledge, we have included findings from pilot investigations by our group to address some of the gaps in research regarding the role of DT in anxiety. The following analyses were conducted among a large undergraduate sample ($N = 418$). Participants were recruited from a pool of introductory-level psychology undergraduates at a large public university. Participants were about 19 years old ($SD = 2.40$) and received class credit in exchange for their participation. They completed a battery of self-report measures in groups of approximately 10–30 individuals. The measures assessed anxiety symptomatology and related constructs such as DT and AS.

Despite the theoretical association of DT elevating individuals' risk for the development and maintenance of anxiety problems, only a few investigations have directly examined the link between DT and anxiety symptomatology. The current pilot investigation sought to extend these findings by more broadly examining DT across a wider range of anxiety symptoms. Results of this investigation indicate that DT, as measured by the DTS (Simons & Gaher, 2005), was negatively associated with anxious worry (Penn State Worry Questionnaire; Meyer, Miller, Metzger, & Borkovec, 1990), panic (Panic Disorder Self-Report Scale; Newman, Holmes, Zuellig, Kachin, & Behar, 2006), social anxiety (Social Interaction Anxiety Scale; Mattick & Clarke, 1998), and obsessions and compulsions (Obsessive Compulsive Inventory—Revised; Foa et al., 2002). These results remained significant after controlling for depression (Beck Depression Inventory–II; Beck, Steer, & Brown, 1996). Consistent with Figure 5.1, it appears that DT is generally associated with a broad range of anxiety symptoms, and that this association is not accounted for by depression.

In line with Figure 5.1, initial investigations have demonstrated a link between AS and DT (e.g., Timpano et al., 2009). The same negative association was found among the current sample, such that as DT decreased, AS (as measured by the Anxiety Sensitivity Index [ASI]; Reiss, Peterson, Gursky, & McNally, 1986) increased. Because of the conceptual similarity between DT and AS, it is important to establish whether they are distinct and uniquely predict anxiety symptomatology. To date, no investigations have examined this. Using the same sample as in the prior analyses, we examined whether DT and AS were uniquely associated with anxiety symptomatology. DTS and ASI scores were simultaneously entered into a regression equation for each of the anxiety symptom measures listed previously. We found that AS and DT each uniquely predicted anxiety symptoms for all of the anxiety measures. Similar to findings that AS is distinct from trait anxiety, these findings indicate that DT and AS are distinct constructs.

Additionally, we sought to examine whether DT and AS acted synergistically to predict anxiety symptoms. To examine this effect, we assessed the interaction between the DTS and ASI. Separate regression equations were constructed for each anxiety measure. The centered DTS and ASI scores (Holmbeck, 2002) and their interaction term were entered simultaneously into each multiple regression along with the anxiety symptom measure, which served as the dependent variable. Simultaneously entering the DTS and ASI main effects and the interaction term in the regression equation ensured that observed interactions were not attributable to the main effects of these variables (Cohen & Cohen, 1983). Results indicated that the interaction term did not significantly predict any of the anxiety measures above and beyond the main effects of DTS and ASI. These results indicate that DT and AS uniquely, but not synergistically, predicted panic, obsessive–compulsive, general worry, and social anxiety symptoms.

## Quality/Limitations of Extant Research

The most obvious limitation in this area is the dearth of studies directly evaluating DT and anxiety. Any statements are tentative at this stage of our understanding. The available studies that have directly examined DT and anxiety or anxiety-related constructs are promising because they suggest that DT may play a role in the pathogenesis and maintenance of these conditions.

# THEORETICAL IMPLICATIONS
# AND FUTURE DIRECTIONS

As shown in Table 5.1, current DT research is generally high quality and is also consistent with the theoretical model proposed earlier. Studies have controlled for multiple third variables (e.g., AS, depression) that may better account for the relationship between DT and anxiety. At this time, two types of studies would be most useful to expand upon our knowledge of DT and anxiety. First, we need basic descriptive information regarding the levels of DT as they impact the various anxiety disorders. Currently, extant studies on DT and anxiety as well as our pilot data suggest that DT may be relevant to various anxiety symptoms and indicate that we need to examine all anxiety conditions. Second, we need to include experimental and prospective designs to ascertain whether DT acts as a risk factor in the pathogenesis or maintenance of anxiety problems (e.g., Wilson & Hayward's, 2006, risk factor research on anxiety in youth and adolescents).

**TABLE 5.1. Distress Tolerance and Anxiety: Key Studies**

| Study | Sample size | DT measure | Summary |
|---|---|---|---|
| Timpano et al. (2009) | 745 nonclinical undergraduates | DTS (Simons & Gaher, 2005) | Hoarding was related to low DT. Significant interaction of AS and DT such that those with low DT and high AS may be at greater risk for hoarding symptoms. |
| Marshall et al. (2008) | 95 daily smokers | Time to persist on a second hyperventilation challenge | Panic attacks during the first hyperventilation challenge significantly predicted DT in the second hyperventilation challenge, above and beyond AS, NA, amount of cigarettes per day, and DI. |
| Telch et al. (2003) | 149 individuals diagnosed with panic disorder with or without agoraphobia or nonclinical panickers | Duration of hyperventilation challenge | Individuals with panic disorder with agoraphobia had significantly shorter hyperventilation duration times compared with individuals with panic disorder. The duration of the hyperventilation significantly predicted the presence or absence of agoraphobia in individuals with panic disorder, controlling for demographics and clinical measures. |
| Daughters et al. (2009) | 231 nonclinical youth | BIRD (Lejuez, et al., 2006); DT was measured by the time to persist on the final level of the game | Low DT increased vulnerability for alcohol use in whites, delinquent behavior in African Americans, and internalizing symptomatology in female youth. |

*Note.* DT, distress tolerance; AS, anxiety sensitivity; DTS, Distress Tolerance Scale; BIRD, Behavioral Indicator of Resiliency to Distress; NA, negative affect.

# CLINICAL IMPLICATIONS AND APPLICATIONS

## Clinical Implications

Research has demonstrated that DT plays a role in the development and maintenance of some psychological disorders, but it has only recently been investigated in relation to anxiety pathology. Anxiety is an unpleasant emotion experienced in response to perceived threat. With anxiety disorders, the degree of anxiety is disproportionate to the danger or occurs in the absence of threat. DT affects the ability to withstand and manage emotions, including anxiety. As a result, those with low DT are more susceptible to anxiety-related problems because they perceive anxiety symptoms as overwhelming and unmanageable. Because of the preliminary nature of our understanding, we attempt to build a case for the role of DT in PD and OCD. This section highlights aspects of anxiety that may be influenced by DT and the relevance of those characteristics to particular anxiety disorders.

Several anxiety disorders are related to increased reactivity to emotional stimuli (Lundh, Wikström, Westerlund, & Öst, 1999; Pollatos, Traut-Mattausch, Schroeder, & Schandry, 2007). Anxious individuals show heightened emotionality compared with controls and greater arousal in response to stress (Noteboom, Barnholt, & Enoka, 2001), which is consistent with the idea of poor DT among this group of patients.

The key feature of PD is recurrent panic attacks, which is an acute fear reaction appearing at inappropriate or unexpected times with no apparent trigger. Diagnosing PD requires a consistent and distressing concern about experiencing another panic attack, which may drastically change behavior (e.g., agoraphobia). Low-DT individuals are more likely to attend to somatic sensations and interpret them as dangerous or threatening (high AS), increasing their fear and anxiety. Consequently, low DT leads to greater safety behaviors, including avoidance of emotional sensations associated with anxiety or stress. Avoidance and other safety behaviors play a key role in the maintenance of PD. These behaviors are believed to be common reactions to the emotional arousal accompanying anxiety. Therefore, it stands to reason that low-DT individuals would be more likely to use safety behaviors to cope and, in turn, maintain their anxiety.

Evidence for the role of DT in PD is demonstrated in the onset of panic symptoms. Most individuals with PD report identifiable stressors around the time of their first panic attack (Craske, Miller, Rotunda, & Barlow, 1990), suggesting that the ability to handle stress or DT might influence the development of the disorder. Individuals with PD also actively avoid negative emotions (Hayes, Wilson, Gifford, Follette, & Strosahl, 1996). Compared with controls, individuals with PD use more avoidance-based and less problem-focused coping strategies to handle emotional stress (Vitalinao et al., 1987) and perceive avoidance as the most effective way to deal with stress (Cox, Endler, Swinson, & Norton, 1992). Taken as a whole, these findings are consistent with the idea that individuals with PD have lower DT, and that DT may play a role in the development and maintenance of PD.

DT has also been examined in OCD. The hallmark features of OCD are obsessions or fears accompanied by a ritual, which reduce anxiety associated with the fear. DT may play a role in misinterpretation of the threat that establishes the obsession and its associated safety behaviors (i.e., rituals). For example, an individual with contamination concerns misinterprets the threat posed by germs and experiences anxiety in response to possibly becoming contaminated. Negative emotions such as disgust and fear accompany the worry that he or she will become ill or make someone else ill. To neutralize negative emotions, low DT may increase the desire to ritualize (e.g., hand washing) or avoid situations where contamination may occur.

Research on the relationship between OCD and emotional experiences indicates that DT may influence the development and maintenance of OCD symptoms. The onset of OCD ranges from early adolescence to young adulthood (Rasmussen & Eisen, 1990). Children with OCD and their parents report lower emotional adjustment (i.e., greater reaction to emotional stress) compared with their peers (Sukhodolsky et al., 2005). OCD is also associated with greater sensitivity to negative feedback. Individuals with OCD who overestimate criticism from their families experience more severe OCD symptoms and poorer treatment outcomes (Chambless & Steketee, 1999). Furthermore, individuals with OCD who report being more upset by criticism had greater anxiety symptoms. These results suggest increased emotional reactivity among people with OCD.

Anger and disgust are two emotions of recent interest in OCD research. Studies consistently find that individuals with OCD have greater anger than controls (Radomsky, Ashbaugh, & Gelfand, 2007; Whiteside & Abramowitz, 2005). Increased disgust sensitivity is also associated with OCD (Berle & Phillips, 2006). Increased disgust may increase avoidance and rituals by enhancing the aversiveness of feared stimuli, or it may strengthen contamination beliefs if disgust is misinterpreted as indicating real contamination (Berle et al., 2006). Taken together, there is some support for DT playing a role in OCD.

## Treatment Implications

DT has not been a direct focus of anxiety treatment as it has for other conditions like borderline personality disorder. This is not surprising given that research on DT in the development and maintenance of anxiety pathology is in its infancy. However, current treatment models incorporate some components of DT. Cognitive and behavioral strategies, which are most commonly used to treat anxiety disorders, focus on identifying and changing dysfunctional thoughts, beliefs, and emotions so clients develop skills for changing their beliefs and behaviors, identifying thinking errors, and relating to others in different ways. Distorted beliefs and thinking errors often center around emotional experiences.

As a result, effective strategies to deal with emotional distress are part of many cognitive-behavioral therapy (CBT) protocols. Behavioral strategies, including exposure with or without response prevention, rely upon anxious people confronting their fears to facilitate fear extinction. DT likely plays a key role in the success of the exposure to treat anxiety disorders because it enables patients to better manage fear and other emotions during treatment.

## Clinical Techniques and Therapeutic Tactics

### Assessment

The anxiety literature concerning DT has utilized standard measures of DT, including the DTS (Simons & Gaher, 2005), along with other behavioral indicators such as the paced auditory serial addition task (PASAT; Lejuez, Kahler, & Brown, 2003) and the BIRD (Lejuez et al., 2006). This literature has also included some more unique indicators, including breath holding or biological challenge procedures (inhalation of high concentrations of carbon dioxide), that have been utilized as a result of the unique aspects of the conditions being studied. For example, patients with PD show high sensitivity to bodily cues. Assessments of tolerance to such cues would be highly relevant to these disorders. In summary, there is a very nice variety of procedures across self-report and behavioral domains, including some that tap into domains specific to some of the anxiety conditions.

### Treatment/Prevention

DT is not explicitly addressed in current CBT protocols. However, it may be argued that many, or perhaps all, components of CBT may impact DT. If the goal of treatment is to decrease anxiety and distress though skill building and exposure, we would expect that patients would learn to successfully increase tolerance to anxiety and other distressing emotions. For example, exposure, which is the foundation for most CBT protocols, involves successful tolerance of strong distress so that fear extinction can occur. It can be argued that this process necessarily builds DT over time as patients learn that they can face their anxiety and experience the distress without resorting to maladaptive coping procedures. In terms of prevention as it relates to DT, we know even less. If DT disposes individuals to develop anxiety problems, teaching techniques related to better tolerance of anxiety and distress may become an important preventive intervention.

*Clinical Future Directions*

DT is not currently a direct focus of anxiety treatment, but many components of CBT may impact DT. Should future work clearly implicate DT in anxiety problems, clinicians could consider making DT a central aspect of treatment.

# SUMMARY

## Empirical Literature and Theoretical Implications

Despite theoretical suggestions that DT plays a key role in elevating individuals' risk for the development and maintenance of anxiety problems, research supporting this association is in a nascent stage. To date, there have been several cross-sectional investigations suggesting that anxiety problems are associated with decreased DT. Additionally, DT has been reported to be negatively associated with AS, an important anxiety-related risk factor. Our pilot investigations indicate that both AS and DT uniquely predict panic, obsessive–compulsive, general worry, and social anxiety symptoms. Taken together, these findings provide preliminary evidence that low DT increases risk for anxiety problems. Future investigations are needed to delineate more clearly the link between DT and the development and maintenance of anxiety disorders.

## Clinical Implications and Applications

DT affects one's ability to withstand and manage provocative and emotional experiences (i.e., anxiety). As a result, it is presumed that individuals with low DT are more susceptible to anxiety-related problems because of their perception that anxiety symptoms are overwhelming and uncontrollable. The inability to withstand negative affect is likely to increase individuals' motivation to use maladaptive coping strategies such as avoidance, safety aids, or rituals that have the unintended effect of increasing and potentially maintaining anxiety problems. Although the specific construct of DT is not typically addressed in the treatment of anxiety disorders, it is likely to be an integral aspect of CBT protocols. The key behavioral component of CBT treatment relies on exposing anxious individuals to their feared stimuli. Successful exposure is very likely to hinge on the capacity to tolerate fear and other distressing emotions that occur in the context of these treatment interventions.

## Summary of Future Directions

There are many opportunities for researchers to contribute to our understanding of DT in the anxiety disorders. In addition to basic descriptive research, there are no prospective studies and very few experimental
studies, which will be needed to address questions concerning the causal
status of DT. In terms of measurement issues, one potential strength is
the utilization of a gold standard self-report measure of DT. The development of the DTS (Simons & Gaher, 2005) has helped to create a more
defined conceptualization of DT and subsequently allowed for more consistent research on this construct. On the other hand, other studies have
assessed DT using behavioral assessments (e.g., breath holding, cold-
pressor task, PASAT, computerized mirror-tracing persistence task). Multimodal assessment of a construct is a potential strength, but it would
be helpful for future studies to include both behavioral and self-report
measures. On the theoretical level, we need some additional clarification
of the nature of this construct and how it relates to other anxiety-relevant factors (see Figure 5.1). For example, Simons and Gaher's (2005)
definition of DT emphasizes its psychological dimensions, whereas some
research in this area has focused on behavioral measures of DT such as
breath holding, which may better reflect DI. The model discussed earlier
in the chapter suggests a separation of the capacity to tolerate physical
discomfort (DI) from psychological or emotional discomfort (DT). However, additional work is needed to determine whether a broader view of
DT or the separation of these constructs best captures this construct as it
relates to anxiety.

## REFERENCES

American Psychiatric Association. (1987). *Diagnostic and statistical manual of
mental disorders* (3rd ed., rev.). Washington, DC: Author.

Bar-Haim, Y., Lamy, D., Pergamin, L., Bakermans-Kranenburg, M. J., & van
IJzendoorn, M. H. (2007). Threat-related attentional bias in anxious and
non-anxious individuals: A meta-analytic study. *Psychological Bulletin,
133,* 1–24.

Barlow, D. H. (2002). *Anxiety and its disorders: The nature and treatment of
anxiety and panic* (2nd ed.). New York: Guilford Press.

Beck, A. T., Steer, R. A., & Brown, G. K. (1996). *Manual for Beck Depression
Inventory* (2nd ed.). San Antonio, TX: Psychological Corporation.

Berle, D., & Phillips, E. S. (2006). Disgust and obsessive-compulsive disorder: An
update. *Psychiatry: Interpersonal and Biological Processes, 69,* 228–238.

Bernstein, A., Zvolensky, M. J., Vujanovic, A. A., & Moos, R. (2009). Integrating anxiety sensitivity, distress tolerance, and discomfort intolerance: A hierarchical model of affect sensitivity and tolerance. *Behavior Therapy, 40,* 291–301.

Boelen, P. A., & Reijntjes, A. (2009). Intolerance of uncertainty and social anxiety. *Journal of Anxiety Disorders, 23,* 130–135.

Bouton, M. E., Mineka, S., & Barlow, D. H. (2001). A modern learning theory perspective on the etiology of panic disorder. *Psychological Review, 108,* 4–32.

Chambless, D. L., & Steketee, G. (1999). Expressed emotion and behavior therapy outcome: A prospective study with obsessive compulsive and agoraphobic outpatients. *Journal of Consulting and Clinical Psychology, 67,* 658–665.

Chorpita, B. F., Yim, L. M., Moffitt, C. E., Umemoto, L. A., & Francis, S. E. (2000). Assessment of symptoms of DSM-IV anxiety and depression in children: A revised child anxiety and depression scale. *Behaviour Research and Therapy, 38,* 835–855.

Clark, D. M. (1986). A cognitive approach to panic. *Behaviour Research and Therapy, 24,* 461–470.

Cohen, J., & Cohen, P. (1983). *Applied multiple regression/correlation analysis for the behavioral sciences.* Hillsdale, NJ: Erlbaum.

Cox, B. J., Endler, N. S., Swinson, R. P., & Norton, R. G. (1992). Situations and specific coping strategies associated with clinical and non-clinical panic attacks. *Behaviour Research and Therapy, 30,* 67–69.

Craske, M. G., Miller, P. P., Rotunda, R., & Barlow, D. H. (1990). A descriptive report of features of unexpected panic attacks in minimal and extensive avoiders. *Behaviour Research and Therapy, 28,* 395–400.

Daughters, S. B., Reynolds, E. K., MacPherson, L., Kahler, C. W., Danielson, C. K., Zvolensky, M., et al. (2009). Distress tolerance and early adolescent externalizing and internalizing symptoms: The moderating role of gender and ethnicity. *Behaviour Research and Therapy, 47,* 198–205.

Dugas, M. J., Gosselin, P., & Ladouceur, R. (2001). Intolerance of uncertainty and worry: Investigating specificity in a nonclinical sample. *Cognitive Therapy and Research, 25,* 551–558.

Foa, E. B., Huppert, J. D., Leiberg, S., Langner, R., Kichic, R., Hajcak, G., et al. (2002). The Obsessive–Compulsive Inventory: Development and validation of a short version. *Psychological Assessment, 14,* 485–496.

Geisser, M. E., Robinson, M. E., & Pickren, W. E. (1992). Differences in cognitive coping strategies among pain-sensitive and pain-tolerant individuals on the cold-pressor test. *Behavior Therapy, 23,* 31–41.

Harrington, N. (2005). The Frustration Discomfort Scale: Development and psychometric properties. *Clinical Psychology and Psychotherapy, 12,* 374–387.

Harrington, N. (2006). Frustration intolerance beliefs: Their relationship with depression, anxiety, and anger, in a clinical population. *Cognitive Therapy and Research, 30,* 699–709.

Hayes, S. C., Wilson, K. G., Gifford, E. V., Follette, V. M., & Strosahl, K. (1996). Experiential avoidance and behavioral disorders: A functional dimensional approach to diagnosis and treatment. *Journal of Consulting and Clinical Psychology, 64,* 1152–1168.

Hayward, C., Killen, J. D., Kraemer, H. C., & Taylor, C. B. (2000). Predictors of panic attacks in adolescents. *Journal of the American Academy of Child and Adolescent Psychiatry, 39,* 207–214.

Hoffart, A., Sexton, H., Hedley, L. M., & Martinsen, E. W. (2008). Mechanisms of change in cognitive therapy for panic disorder with agoraphobia. *Journal of Behavior Therapy and Experimental Psychiatry, 39,* 262–275.

Holmbeck, G. N. (2002). Post-hoc probing of significant moderational and mediational effects in studies of pediatric populations. *Journal of Pediatric Psychology, 27,* 87–96.

Kearney, C. A., Albano, A. M., Eisen, A. R., Allan, W. D., & Barlow, D. H. (1997). The phenomenology of panic disorder in youngsters: An empirical study of a clinical sample. *Journal of Anxiety Disorders, 11,* 49–62.

Lejuez, C. W., Daughters, S. B., Danielson, C. W., & Ruggiero, K. (2006). *The behavioral indicator of resiliency to distress (BIRD).* Unpublished manual.

Lejuez, C. W., Kahler, C. W., & Brown, R. A. (2003). A modified computer version of the paced auditory serial addition task (PASAT) as a laboratory-based stressor. *Behavior Therapist, 26,* 290–293.

Lilienfeld, S. O., Turner, S. M., & Jacob, R. G. (1993). Anxiety sensitivity: An examination of theoretical and methodological issues. *Advances in Behavior Research and Therapy, 15,* 147–182.

Linehan, M. M. (1993). *Cognitive-behavioral treatment of borderline personality disorder.* New York: Guilford Press.

Lundh, L. G., Wikström, J., Westerlund, J., & Öst, L. G. (1999). Preattentive bias for emotional information in panic disorder with agoraphobia. *Journal of Abnormal Psychology, 108,* 222–232.

Marshall, E. C., Zvolensky, M. J., Vujanovic, A. A., Gregor, K., Gibson, L. E., & Leyro, T. M. (2008). Panic reactivity to voluntary hyperventilation challenge predicts distress tolerance to bodily sensations among daily cigarette smokers. *Experimental and Clinical Psychopharmacology, 16,* 313–321.

Mattick, R. P., & Clarke, J. C. (1998). Development and validation of measures of social phobia scrutiny fear and social interaction anxiety. *Behaviour Research and Therapy, 36,* 455–470.

McNally, R. J. (2002). Anxiety sensitivity and panic disorder. *Biological Psychiatry, 52,* 938–946.

Meyer, T. J., Miller, M. L., Metzger, R. L., & Borkovec, T. D. (1990). Development and validation of the Penn State Worry Questionnaire. *Behaviour Research and Therapy, 28,* 487–495.

Newman, M. G., Holmes, M., Zuellig, A. R., Kachin, K. E., & Behar, E. (2006). The reliability and validity of the panic disorder self-report: A new diagnostic screening measure of panic disorder. *Psychological Assessment, 18,* 49–61.

Noteboom, J. T., Barnholt, K. R., & Enoka, R. M. (2001). Activation and arousal response and impairment of performance increase with anxiety and stressor intensity. *Journal of Applied Physiology, 91,* 2093–2101.

Parrish, C. L., Radomsky, A. S., & Dugas, M. J. (2008). Anxiety-control strategies: Is there room for neutralization in successful exposure treatment? *Clinical Psychology Review, 28,* 1400–1412.

Pollatos, O., Traut-Mattausch, E., Schroeder, H., & Schandry, R. (2007). Interoceptive awareness mediates the relationship between anxiety and the intensity of unpleasant feelings. *Journal of Anxiety Disorders, 21,* 931–943.

Powers, M. B., Smits, J. A. J., & Telch, M. J. (2004). Disentangling the effects of safety-behavior utilization and safety-behavior availability during exposure-based treatment: A placebo-controlled trial. *Journal of Consulting and Clinical Psychology, 72,* 448–454.

Rabian, B., Embry, L., & MacIntyre, D. (1999). Behavioral validation of the Childhood Anxiety Sensitivity Index in children. *Journal of Clinical Child Psychology, 28,* 105–112.

Radomsky, A. S., Ashbaugh, A. R., & Gelfand, L. A. (2007). Relationship between anger, symptoms, and cognitive factors in OCD checkers. *Behaviour Research and Therapy, 45,* 2712–2715.

Rasmussen, S. A., & Eisen, J. L. (1990). Epidemiology of obsessive-compulsive disorder. *Journal of Clinical Psychiatry, 51,* 10–14.

Reiss, S., & McNally, R. J. (1985). Expectancy model of fear. In S. Reiss & R. R. Bootzin (Eds.), *Theoretical issues in behavior therapy* (pp. 107–121). New York: Academic Press.

Reiss, S., Peterson, R. A., Gursky, D. M., & McNally, R. J. (1986). Anxiety sensitivity, anxiety frequency, and the prediction of fearfulness. *Behaviour Research and Therapy, 24,* 1–8.

Salkovskis, P. M., Clark, D. M., Hackmann, A., Wells, A., & Gelder, M. G. (1999). An experimental investigation of the role of safety-seeking behaviours in the maintenance of panic disorder with agoraphobia. *Behaviour Research and Therapy, 37,* 559–574.

Schmidt, N. B., & Cook, J. H. (1999). Effects of anxiety sensitivity on anxiety and pain during a cold pressor challenge in patients with panic disorder. *Behaviour Research and Therapy, 37,* 313–323.

Schmidt, N. B., & Lerew, D. R. (1998). Prospective evaluation of psychological risk factors as predictors of functional impairment during acute stress. *Journal of Occupational Rehabilitation, 8,* 199–212.

Schmidt, N. B., Lerew, D. R., & Jackson, R. J. (1997). The role of anxiety sensitivity in the pathogenesis of panic: Prospective evaluation of spontaneous panic attacks during acute stress. *Journal of Abnormal Psychology, 106,* 355–364.

Schmidt, N. B., Lerew, D. R., & Jackson, R. J. (1999). Prospective evaluation of anxiety sensitivity in the pathogenesis of panic: Replication and extension. *Journal of Abnormal Psychology, 108,* 532–537.

Schmidt, N. B., Lerew, D., & Trakowski, J. J. (1997). Body vigilance in panic disorder: Evaluation attention to bodily perturbations. *Journal of Consulting and Clinical Psychology, 65,* 214–220.

Schmidt, N. B., Zvolensky, M. J., & Maner, J. K. (2006). Anxiety sensitivity: Prospective prediction of panic attacks and axis I pathology. *Journal of Psychiatric Research, 40,* 691–699.

Simons, J. S., & Gaher, R. M. (2005). The Distress Tolerance Scale: Development and validation of a self-report measure. *Motivation and Emotion, 29,* 83–102.

Sukhodolsky, D. G., do Rosario-Campos, M. C., Scahill, L., Katsocich, L., Pauls, D. L., Peterson, B. S., et al. (2005). Adaptive, emotional, and family functioning of children with obsessive-compulsive disorder and comorbid attention deficit hyperactivity disorder. *American Journal of Psychiatry, 162,* 1125–1132.

Taylor, S. (Ed.). (1999). *Anxiety sensitivity: Theory, research, and treatment of the fear of anxiety.* Mahwah, NJ: Erlbaum.

Taylor, S., Koch, W. J., & McNally, R. J. (1992). How does anxiety sensitivity vary across the anxiety disorders? *Journal of Anxiety Disorders, 6,* 249–259.

Telch, M. J., Jacquin, K., Smits, J. A. J., & Powers, M. B. (2003). Emotional responding to hyperventilation as a predictor of agoraphobia status among individuals suffering from panic disorder. *Journal of Behavior Therapy and Experimental Psychiatry, 34,* 161–170.

Timpano, K. R., Buckner, J. D., Richey, J. A., Murphy, D. L., & Schmidt, N. B. (2009). Exploration of anxiety sensitivity and distress tolerance as vulnerability factors for hoarding behaviors. *Depression and Anxiety, 26,* 343–353.

Unnewehr, S., Schneider, S., Margraf, J., Jenkins, M., & Florin, I. (1996). Exposure to internal and external stimuli: Reactions in children of patients with panic disorder or animal phobia. *Journal of Anxiety Disorders, 10,* 489–508.

Vitalinao, P. P., Katon, W., Russo, J., Maiuro, R. D., Anderson, K., & Jones, M. (1987). Coping as an index of illness behavior in panic disorder. *Journal of Nervous and Mental Disease, 175,* 78–84.

Whiteside, S. P., & Abramowitz, J. S. (2005). The expression of anger and its relationship to symptoms and cognitions in obsessive-compulsive disorder. *Depression and Anxiety, 21,* 106–111.

Wilson, K. A., & Hayward, C. (2006). Unique contributions of anxiety sensitivity to avoidance: A prospective study in adolescents. *Behaviour Research and Therapy, 44,* 601–609.

Zvolensky, M. J., McNeil, D. W., Porter, C. A., & Stewart, S. H. (2001). Assessment of anxiety sensitivity in young American Indians and Alaska natives. *Behaviour Research and Therapy, 39,* 477–493.

Zvolensky, M. J., & Otto, M. W. (2007). Affective intolerance, sensitivity, and processing: Advances in clinical science. *Behavior Therapy, 38,* 228–233.

# 6

# Traumatic Stress

Anka A. Vujanovic, Amit Bernstein,
*and* Brett T. Litz

## THEORETICAL CONSIDERATIONS

Distress tolerance has received only limited empirical attention in the field of traumatic stress (Zvolensky, Leyro, Bernstein, & Vujanovic, Chapter 1, this volume). Distress tolerance is broadly defined as the perceived or actual behavioral capacity to withstand exposure to aversive or threatening stimuli (e.g., negative emotions, uncomfortable physical sensations; Brown, Lejuez, Kahler, Strong, & Zvolensky, 2005; Simons & Gaher, 2005).

Distress tolerance has been studied in relation to a variety of types of clinical syndromes, and it has demonstrated both disorder-specific as well as transdiagnostic relevance (e.g., Zvolensky et al., Chapter 1, this volume). With regard to the anxiety disorders, the majority of research on distress tolerance has evaluated its relations with panic disorder (Marshall et al., 2008; Telch, Jacquin, Smits, & Powers, 2003; Timpano, Buckner, Richey, Murphy, & Schmidt, 2009). Studies have found that lower levels of perceived distress tolerance for emotional distress and physical stress, and a lesser ability to withstand acute episodes of emotional stress, are significantly related to an increased risk of anxiety symptoms and panic attacks (Boelen & Reijntjes, 2009; Bonn-Miller, Zvolensky, & Bernstein, 2009; Daughters et al., 2009; Marshall et al., 2008), fears about the negative consequences of anxiety symptoms (Timpano et al., 2009), and escape behavior in response to somatic arousal (Asmundson & Stein, 1994; Telch et al., 2003). These data have begun to illuminate notable linkages between distress tolerance and anxiety and its disorders. However, limited study or theorizing has been conducted on the potential relations between distress tolerance and posttraumatic stress disorder (PTSD).

Although 50–75% of individuals are exposed to a traumatic life event during the course of their lifetimes, only approximately 7.8–9.8% go on to develop PTSD or other clinical syndromes (Bleich, Koslowsky, Dolev, & Lerer, 1997; Breslau, Davis, Andreski, Federman, & Anthony, 1998; Kessler, Sonnega, Bromet, Hughes, & Nelson, 1995). Although the majority of trauma-exposed individuals experience heightened emotional and physiological responses to trauma-relevant reminders in the immediate aftermath of the event (Rothbaum, Foa, Riggs, Murdock, & Walsh, 1992), a significant minority develop more chronic trauma-related symptoms of reexperiencing, effortful avoidance, emotional numbing, and hyperarousal (King, Leskin, King, & Weathers, 1998). It has been argued that certain individual differences rooted in peoples' attitudes and beliefs about emotion, present before trauma exposure, might predispose some to develop PTSD (e.g., Ansorge, Litz, & Orsillo, 1996). Distress tolerance is one relevant construct within this context.

In the context of adapting to and recovering from trauma, low levels of distress tolerance might predispose an individual to greater levels of emotional dysregulation as a result of insufficient perceived (or actual) capacities to experience without avoiding and to tolerate trauma-related distress. Thus, individuals with lower perceived or actual behavioral capacity to withstand such experiences may demonstrate greater posttraumatic tendencies to use avoidance or to behave impulsively to regulate—perceived or objectively—aversive psychological or physiological states and emotions. Theoretically, these avoidant coping behaviors may be negatively reinforcing for individuals with low distress tolerance and may significantly impair healing and recovery from trauma because they impede opportunities to learn that various forms of trauma-related distress can be tolerated and regulated. Conversely, individuals with higher tolerance of emotional distress may be less likely to perceive or to react with avoidance to posttraumatic stress symptoms following trauma exposure, relative to those lower in distress tolerance; *or* such individuals may perceive their tolerance as greater for coping with trauma-related psychological symptoms. Thus, lower or higher levels of distress tolerance prior to trauma exposure may predispose an individual to a course toward risk or resilience, respectively.

Indeed, several additional theoretical pathways may explain the potential associations between distress tolerance and posttraumatic stress, further underscoring the importance of empirical exploration of this domain. For instance, it is plausible that distress tolerance levels may change (increase *or* decrease) as a function of exposure to traumatic stressors. In addition, posttraumatic stress symptom severity may promote less tolerance of distress over time. Finally, distress tolerance and posttraumatic stress symptom levels may relate bidirectionally or transactionally following trauma exposure.

Interestingly, research to date indicates that distress tolerance skills may be taught (Gratz & Tull, Chapter 9, this volume; Linehan, 1993), and an individual's level of distress tolerance is amenable to change. Interventions that target distress tolerance may serve as a secondary prevention of PTSD or may be useful in tertiary care. The primary therapeutic mechanism of change within this context may involve increased willingness to approach and experience a variety of corrective (posttrauma) experiences without pursuing negative reinforcement or escape–avoidance opportunities. Together, the potential malleability of the distress tolerance construct via intervention underscores its potential significance as a target for empirical study.

## AIMS OF THIS CHAPTER

In this chapter, we review the available literature pertaining to traumatic stress and distress tolerance and related constructs. There is scant empirical research directly addressing distress tolerance and traumatic stress. We, therefore, offer a variety of ideas to stimulate needed future research. We also suggest ideas about intervention strategies applicable to distress tolerance. We opted to devote an entire chapter to the exploration of distress tolerance and traumatic stress, rather than couch the review of research on distress tolerance and trauma within the anxiety disorders chapter, in part, because of ongoing scientific discourse about the possible development of a separate diagnostic classification category for traumatic stress disorders in the revised fifth edition of the *Diagnostic and Statistical Manual of Mental Disorders* (e.g., Resick & Miller, 2009). Moreover, we concluded that a separate chapter on traumatic stress might better (1) underscore the paucity of empirical and theoretical work in this domain; (2) elucidate the potential relevance of this construct to the study of traumatic stress specifically; and (3) build a theoretical argument for the utility of expanding this line of inquiry in terms of potentially enhancing PTSD prevention and treatment efforts.

## LITERATURE REVIEW

There is a relative paucity of studies dedicated specifically to the associations among distress tolerance, traumatic stress, and PTSD. Several relevant constructs have been studied in individuals exposed to trauma: (1) emotion regulation and related facets (i.e., cognitive-emotional processing of threat, emotional numbing, avoidant coping); (2) anxiety sensitivity; and (3) mindfulness and acceptance. In addition to the distress tolerance and traumatic stress literature, these variables are explicated individually, with the understanding that more empirical work is necessary to document their relations with one another and within a greater model of emotion regulation.

## Emotion Regulation

One way to conceptually contextualize our thinking about tolerance of distressing experiential states is within the emotion (dys)regulation literature. Indeed, individuals with low levels of distress tolerance may be at increased risk of developing and maintaining maladaptive beliefs and behaviors related to emotion and vice versa. Conversely, maladaptive beliefs and behaviors related to emotion may theoretically increase the risk of developing and maintaining maladaptive levels of distress tolerance. Furthermore, lower levels of distress tolerance, or conversely excessively high levels of distress tolerance applied rigidly or inflexibly across contexts (see Lynch & Mizon, Chapter 3, this volume), may predispose individuals to the development or maintenance of difficulties regulating emotion. It is also possible that difficulties regulating emotion might lead to lower or inflexible levels of distress tolerance. Notably, the proposed relations between distress tolerance and emotion regulation may be transactional, insofar as emotion dysregulation may promote increasingly maladaptive (in)tolerance of distress or rigid intolerance/overtolerance across contexts (i.e., context inflexibility) and vice versa. Furthermore, it is possible that distress tolerance not only may be related to emotion dysregulation but *distress tolerance* may be an intrinsic aspect of the regulation of emotion such as a core element or dimension of emotional dysregulation. No empirical studies to date have attempted to address or disentangle these conceptual issues. Regardless, it may be theoretically or conceptually useful to consider distress tolerance in the context of emotion (dys)regulation, and we try to do so in the present chapter.

Broadly, emotion regulation has been defined as the implementation of techniques intended to influence the experience and expression of emotions and the context/times at which certain emotions occur (Rottenberg & Gross, 2003). Emotion regulation occurs unconsciously and automatically or strategically and effortfully (see Gross, 1998). Most conceptualizations posit that emotion regulation refers to the ability to tolerate and regulate or cope with the experience of various emotional states (e.g., Briere, 1997). Others have posited that the tolerance *and* acceptance of emotions are central to adaptive emotion regulation (e.g., Amstadter, 2008).

PTSD has been conceptualized as a disorder of emotional and experiential avoidance (Foa & Kozak, 1986), stemming from difficulties managing the enormous emotional demands of trauma. Because they are unprecedented and often unimaginable pretrauma, traumatic experiences are intensely disruptive and disorganizing psychologically, socially, biologically, and emotionally. Consequently, traumatic stress is an important context for the study of emotional dysregulation. For example, individuals suffering from posttraumatic stress frequently experience severe hyperemotionality or negative emotional reactivity to trauma-related cues and, in a reciprocal or phasic fashion, hypoemotionality, in that they might also report emotional numbing and avoidance symptoms. The interplay of these two basic types of emotional experiences has been conceptualized as fundamental to PTSD from numerous intellectual vantage points (Horowitz, 1986; Litz, Orsillo, Kaloupek, & Weathers, 2000; van der Kolk, 1987).

Studies have examined various facets of emotional regulation and processing in individuals with PTSD (e.g., Amdur, Larsen, & Liberzon, 2000; Burriss, Ayers, & Powell, 2007; Litz et al., 2000; Miller & Litz, 2004; Morey, Petty, Cooper, LaBar, & McCarthy, 2008; New et al., 2009; Roemer, Litz, Orsillo, & Wagner, 2001; Tull, Barrett, McMillan, & Roemer, 2007). Cross-sectional, laboratory, and neuroimaging studies have shown that individuals suffering from posttraumatic stress have difficulty regulating emotion (e.g., Lanius et al., 2003; Litz et al., 2000; Luterek, Orsillo, & Marx, 2005; Tull, Barrett, et al., 2007). For example, Tull, Barrett, and colleagues (2007) found that posttraumatic stress symptom severity was significantly associated with a lack of acceptance of emotional experiences, lack of clarity of emotional responses, and limited emotion regulation strategies, as measured by the Difficulties in Emotion Regulation Scale (Gratz & Roemer, 2004).

A comprehensive review of the emotion literature as related to traumatic stress is beyond the scope of the current chapter. Rather, we intend to highlight research of potential relevance to distress tolerance and traumatic stress.

## Cognitive–Emotional Processing of Threat

Cognitive models of PTSD posit that threat perception in the aftermath of trauma is a central risk and maintenance factor for the disorder (Ehlers & Clark, 2000). Symptoms of trauma are thought to persist when survivors process the event such that they continue to perceive imminent threat in its absence (Ehlers & Clark, 2000). Furthermore, several studies have found that individuals' interpretations of emotional experiences are a significant factor in posttraumatic stress symptom severity (e.g., Bryant & Harvey, 1995). For example, the fear of emotions, or interpretation of emotions as threatening, has been linked to more severe posttraumatic stress symptoms among adult survivors of childhood interpersonal violence (Tull, Jakupcak, McFadden, & Roemer, 2007). In a related vein, the fear of the loss of affective control has been associated with posttraumatic stress symptom severity among veterans with military-related PTSD (Price, Monson, Callahan, & Rodriguez, 2006), while alexithymia has been associated with greater PTSD symptoms and poorer physical health outcomes among trauma-exposed veterans (Hyer, Woods, & Boudewyns, 1991; Monson, Price, Rodriguez, Ripley, & Warner, 2004; Polusny, Dickinson, Murdoch, & Thuras, 2008).

Individuals with PTSD tend to prioritize the cognitive processing of threatening or trauma-related information by attending selectively to perceived threat (e.g., Ehlers & Clark, 2000; Engelhard, Macklin, McNally, van den Hout, & Arntz, 2001; McNally, 1998; Milanak & Berenbaum, 2009), particularly to threat related to the type of trauma experienced (e.g., Litz et al., 1997; McNally, English, & Lipke, 1993; Thrasher, Dalgleish, & Yule, 1994). Individuals with PTSD also tend to manifest reduced autobiographical memory specificity and to show discrepancies in the storage and recall of threatening information (e.g., Dalgleish, Rolfe, Golden, Dunn, & Barnard, 2008; Lanius et al., 2003; McNally, Metzger, Lasko, Clancy, & Pitman, 1998). Furthermore, individuals with chronic PTSD tend to utilize emotion- and intrusion-based reasoning (i.e., inferring danger from the presence of anxiety and intrusion-based symptoms, respectively) (Ehlers & Clark, 2000; Engelhard et al., 2001). Individuals with PTSD—by definition, those who are experiencing greater trauma-related distress—may thus have an increased tendency to avoid specific personal or threatening information in efforts to regulate or avoid potentially negative mood states (Dalgleish et al., 2008).

Additionally, the detection and interpretation of emotionally distressing trauma-related symptoms are believed to be critical in the generation of symptom intensity and impairment (Keane & Barlow, 2002). Distress tolerance is directly relevant to the nexus between perception of sensation, interpretation, and, by extension, experience of distressing traumatic symptoms. Relative to those lower in distress tolerance, individuals with higher tolerance of emotional distress may, therefore, be less likely to perceive or attend to some trauma-relevant sensations (e.g., hyperarousal symptoms), or they may perceive greater personal capacity to tolerate and thereby adapt to or cope with trauma-related symptoms.

Thus, individuals with lower levels of distress tolerance may be more apt to perceive such sensations as threatening, experience more intense arousal, and engage in strategic efforts to avoid stimuli that elicited traumatic reactions.

Individual differences in the interpretation of external and internal stimuli (e.g., traumatic events, emotional experiences) may be a mechanism in the development and maintenance of PTSD. Lower levels of distress tolerance may predispose trauma-exposed individuals to being more attuned to perceived threat or to responding to such perceived threat in a behaviorally dysregulated or avoidant manner. Such individuals may judge their capability to regulate trauma-related distress as limited and may thus be hypervigilant and reactive to such threat. This heightened threat perception and processing may, in part, lead trauma-exposed individuals with lower levels of distress tolerance to develop or maintain PTSD.

## Emotional Numbing

Emotional numbing following trauma exposure may be related to the development of PTSD as well as to poor psychosocial functioning outcomes over time (Breslau & Davis, 1992; Kilpatrick & Resnick, 1993; Litz, 1992; Litz et al., 1997). Emotional numbing may have a variety of causes, including (1) chronic avoidance of trauma-related internal and external cues, with such chronically avoidant behavior resulting in the suppression of emotional experiences; (2) depletion of cognitive-affective resources as a result of constant attempts at overregulation of trauma-related reexperiencing and hyperarousal symptoms, which might lead to decreased levels of emotional responsivitiy over time (e.g., Litz, 1992; Litz et al., 1997); and (3) biological factors, such as a decrease in catecholamines resulting from exposure to trauma and the conditioned fear response (e.g., van der Kolk, Greenberg, Boyd, & Krystal, 1985) or conditioned analgesic effects caused by conditioned fear responses, generalized from trauma exposure (e.g., Pitman, van der Kolk, Orr, & Greenberg, 1990).

The role of distress tolerance in the etiology and maintenance of emotional numbing symptoms following trauma exposure has not been explored. Yet individuals who have limited perceived and/or actual levels of distress may be at a higher risk of developing emotional numbing or emotional avoidance symptoms following trauma exposure. Conversely, trauma-exposed individuals' ability to tolerate distress may be affected by their emotion regulatory attempts, such as emotional avoidance and emotional numbing, with greater attempts to avoid resulting in a depleted ability to withstand distress over time.

## Avoidant Coping

Experiential avoidance, defined as the unwillingness to maintain contact with aversive internal experiences (e.g., emotions, cognitions, memories, bodily sensations) and the active as well as automatic nonconscious avoidance of events and contexts related to such internal experiences, may affect posttraumatic adjustment (e.g., Roemer et al., 2001; Tull, Gratz, Salters, & Roemer, 2004; Tull & Roemer, 2003). Not surprisingly, two diagnostic criteria of PTSD refer specifically to the avoidance of internal and external stimuli associated with the trauma (e.g., "efforts to avoid thoughts, feelings, or conversations associated with the trauma"; American Psychiatric Association, 2000, p. 468). Experiential avoidance has been associated with increased posttraumatic stress symptoms (Foa & Kozak, 1986; Marx & Sloan, 2005; Tull et al., 2007). Related studies have suggested that emotional suppression, defined as the conscious inhibition of emotional expression while experiencing emotional arousal, increases physiological reactivity (Gross & Levenson, 1993, 1997). For example, Vietnam War combat veterans with PTSD, compared with those without the disorder, reported frequent and intense intentional, strategic withholding of positive and negative emotional experience (Roemer et al., 2001), even after controlling for co-occurring distress. In addition, the regularity of withholding was related to posttraumatic stress symptom severity in this study. Similarly, externally oriented thinking, defined as the tendency to avert thinking to superficial, external events instead of internal affective experiences, has also been linked to greater PTSD symptoms (Monson et al., 2004). Also, trauma-related experiential avoidance or active suppression of emotional expression may heighten emotional dysregulation, thereby increasing the risk for aggressive behavior among trauma-exposed individuals (Tull, Jakupcak, et al., 2007).

The problematic use of substances to avoid negative mood states has been postulated as a mechanism whereby individuals suffering from posttraumatic stress may attempt to cope with trauma-related symptoms via avoidance. This type of avoidance strategy has been referred to as the self-medication hypothesis or coping model (Khantzian, 1997). With regard to associations between PTSD and substance abuse, emotion-focused coping (Staiger, Melville, Hides, Kambouropoulos, & Lubman, 2009) as well as emotional disconstraint and negative emotionality (Miller, Vogt, Mozley, Kaloupek, & Keane, 2006) have been found to serve mediating roles, suggesting that emotion regulation skills may be key to "self-medication"–related coping. Distress tolerance may similarly be related to avoidant coping. A lower perceived or actual behavioral capacity to tolerate negatively evaluated affective (and related) states may lead to avoidant coping, may be influenced by avoidant coping, or may relate to a higher-order predisposition toward experiential avoidance (e.g., Lynch & Mizon, Chapter 3, this volume). It is thus important for future work to further examine relations among distress tolerance, avoidant coping, including substance use to regulate and reduce negative affective states, and traumatic stress-related psychopathology.

## Anxiety Sensitivity

Anxiety sensitivity (AS) is a cognitive factor defined as the fear of anxiety and anxiety-related sensations (McNally, 2002; Reiss, Peterson, Gursky, & McNally, 1986). It has been conceptualized as a lower-order facet of a higher-order affect tolerance and sensitivity variable (Bernstein, Zvolensky, Vujanovic, & Moos, 2009). Specifically, in a preliminary exploratory factor analytic study, Bernstein and colleagues (2009) found that AS and distress tolerance (Simons & Gaher, 2005) may be distinct but systematically related lower-order facets of a common higher-order affect tolerance and sensitivity factor, whereas discomfort intolerance (i.e., difficulty tolerating uncomfortable physical sensations) (Schmidt, Richey, & Fitzpatrick, 2006) did not appear to demonstrate similar relations with either AS or distress tolerance at the lower-order or higher-order levels. Notably, AS and distress tolerance are not conceptually equivalent, although they are distinct lower-order factors of a higher-order affect tolerance and sensitivity factor (Bernstein et al., 2009). For example, distress tolerance is not related principally to the expectation of negative consequences of anxiety and other interoceptive sensations (Bernstein et al., 2009).

With respect to trauma-related problems, heightened levels of AS have been associated with PTSD (e.g., Bernstein, Zvolensky, Feldner, Lewis, & Leen-Feldner, 2005; Bernstein et al., 2007; Taylor, Koch, & McNally, 1992), and decreases in AS have been associated with PTSD symptom improvement in an intervention trial (Fedoroff, Taylor, Asmundson, & Koch, 2000). Furthermore, higher levels of AS have been found to moderate, or amplify, the association between number of trauma exposure types and posttraumatic stress symptoms among trauma-exposed adults (Feldner, Lewis, Leen-Feldner, Schnurr, & Zvolensky, 2006). More specifically, the psychological concerns facet of the AS construct (e.g., "When I cannot keep my mind on a task, I worry that I might be going crazy") has been differentially associated with posttraumatic stress symptoms (cf. panic symptoms) among trauma-exposed adults (e.g., Vujanovic, Zvolensky, & Bernstein, 2008).

## Mindfulness and Acceptance

Mindfulness and acceptance have been increasingly discussed in relation to PTSD in basic and especially applied clinical contexts (Orsillo &

Roemer, 2005). Although there are a variety of conceptual or theoretical perspectives on mindfulness and related operational definitions and measures (Bishop et al., 2004), most definitions include a reference to present-centered attention and awareness (Brown & Ryan, 2003). Other conceptualizations incorporate an emphasis on regulation of attention and nonjudgmental acceptance of the present moment (e.g., Baer, Smith, & Allen, 2004; Bishop et al., 2004). Emerging acceptance-based approaches to treating PTSD, namely acceptance and commitment therapy (ACT; Walser & Westrup, 2007), emphasize acceptance but also incorporate mindfulness. Mindfulness and acceptance have been conceptualized as skills related to adaptive emotional regulation or emotional functioning processes such that higher levels of each are related to lower levels of emotional dysregulation (Vujanovic, Bonn-Miller, Bernstein, McKee, & Zvolensky, in press). Clinically, ACT (Hayes, Strosahl, & Wilson, 1999) appears to be a potentially promising treatment for PTSD (Walser & Westrup, 2007), although independently replicated clinical trial data are not yet available.

To the best of our knowledge, results of only four cross-sectional and one small-scale intervention trial have focused on the association between mindfulness and/or acceptance and posttraumatic stress. First, among a sample of pain patients and nonpatients in Germany, Michal and colleagues (2007) documented significant (partial) negative correlations among mindful attention and awareness (as indexed by the Mindful Attention and Awareness Scale [MAAS]; Brown & Ryan, 2003) and depersonalization levels, childhood emotional abuse severity, and childhood emotional neglect severity, even after controlling for a variance explained by psychological distress and age. Second, Vujanovic, Youngwirth, Johnson, and Zvolensky (2009) found significant incremental (negative) associations between the Accepting without Judgment subscale (i.e., adopting a nonjudgmental stance about present experience) of the Kentucky Inventory of Mindfulness Skills (KIMS; Baer et al., 2004) and posttraumatic stress symptom severity, and the Acting with Awareness subscale of the KIMS (i.e., focusing fully on present-centered activity) and posttraumatic stress-relevant reexperiencing symptoms, specifically. These effects were observed among a sample of trauma-exposed adults without current Axis I psychopathology, above and beyond the variance accounted for by negative affectivity and number of trauma types reported. Third, in a trauma-exposed sample of undergraduate students, Thompson and Waltz (2010) similarly documented significant, incremental negative relations between the Non-Judgmental Acceptance subscale of the Five Facet Mindfulness Questionnaire (FFMQ; Baer et al., 2008) and posttraumatic stress avoidance symptoms, after controlling for various indices of experiential avoidance. Fourth, in a trauma-exposed adult community sample, Bernstein, Tanay, and Vujanovic (in press) documented significant, incremental negative associations between levels of mindful attention and aware-ness (MAAS; Brown & Ryan, 2003) and posttraumatic stress symptom severity, psychiatric multimorbidity, anxious arousal, and anhedonic depression symptoms, above and beyond the number of traumatic event types. Finally, Kimbrough, Magyari, Langenberg, Chesney, and Berman (2010) conducted an 8-week mindfulness-based stress reduction (MBSR) pilot program (without a randomized control condition) with 27 adult survivors of childhood sexual abuse. This program documented signifi-cant decreases in posttraumatic stress symptoms, particularly symptoms of avoidance/numbing, at the conclusion of the intervention.

Distress tolerance may be a distinct construct related to mindful-ness and acceptance-based processes such that higher levels of mindful-ness and acceptance may be associated with greater perceived or actual abilities to withstand emotional and physical distress (and vice versa). It remains unclear, however, whether distress tolerance may be improved via mindfulness practice.

## Distress Tolerance and Traumatic Stress

### Initial Empirical Findings

The only published work to date directly related to distress tolerance and posttraumatic stress is based on smokers with PTSD. In a theoretical review of factors that might influence smoking relapse among individu-als with PTSD, Cook, McFall, Calhoun, and Beckham (2007) postulated that distress tolerance, defined here as the ability to withstand distress and discomfort, might be a significant factor related to smoking absti-nence among smokers with PTSD. Indeed, lower levels of distress tol-erance might increase the risk of lapse or relapse among smokers with PTSD attempting cessation. Vujanovic, Marshall, Gibson, and Zvolensky (2009) found significantly higher levels of discomfort intolerance, defined as the "capacity to withstand physical perturbations or uncomfortable bodily states" (Schmidt et al., 2006, p. 264), among smokers with PTSD compared with smokers with nonclinical panic attacks only and those without current Axis I psychopathology. This study, albeit cross-sectional and based on a subpopulation of individuals with PTSD, is the first to document levels of discomfort intolerance among individuals with PTSD compared with those without the disorder, underscoring the need for further work in this area focused on the broader distress tolerance con-struct.

In a related domain of study, O'Cleirigh, Ironson, and Smits (2007) examined relations among distress tolerance, assessed using the Dis-tress Tolerance Scale (DTS; Simons & Gaher, 2005), major life events, and mood and substance use outcomes in a sample of 116 HIV-positive patients. In light of the lack of direct distress tolerance and traumatic stress research to date, these preliminary data related to major life events are relevant here. O'Cleirigh and colleagues found that distress tolerance, defined by the DTS as perceived ability to withstand emotional distress, moderated the association among major life events and depressive symptoms, substance use, and medication adherence; lower levels of distress tolerance exacerbated the association.

## Unpublished Studies

We now highlight two unpublished studies, submitted for peer review, that offer a preliminary perspective on the relationship between distress tolerance and posttraumatic stress. First, Vujanovic, Bonn-Miller, Potter, Marshall, and Zvolensky (2009) examined incremental associations between distress tolerance, indexed with the DTS, and posttraumatic stress symptoms, measured with the Posttraumatic Stress Diagnostic Scale (Foa, 1995) among 140 trauma-exposed adults without current Axis I psychopathology. Vujanovic, Bonn-Miller, and colleagues (2009) found significant incremental associations among distress tolerance, posttraumatic stress symptom severity, and severity of the reexperiencing, avoidance, and hyperarousal symptom clusters, examined individually; these effects were significant, even after controlling for the effects of negative affectivity and number of trauma exposure types. As expected, an inverse relationship between distress tolerance and posttraumatic stress symptom severity was established such that lower levels of distress tolerance were related to higher levels of posttraumatic stress symptoms.

Second, Marshall, Vujanovic, Bonn-Miller, Bernstein, and Zvolensky (2010) examined the incremental validity of four indices of distress tolerance in terms of posttraumatic stress symptom severity, indexed with the Clinician Administered PTSD Scale (Blake et al., 1995), among 84 trauma-exposed adults. Marshall and colleagues (2009) concurrently examined two self-report inventories—DTS total score and Discomfort Intolerance Scale (DIS; Schmidt et al., 2006) total score—and two behavioral indices—mirror-tracing task and breath-holding task (see descriptions in Chapter 1)—in terms of the incremental associations of these measures with regard to posttraumatic stress symptom severity. Only DTS total score emerged as significantly predictive of global posttraumatic stress symptom severity and symptom cluster severity, above and beyond variance contributed by number of prior trauma exposures. This study provides preliminary evidence that the perceived ability to withstand emotional distress, indexed by the DTS, as compared with the perceived ability to tolerate physical discomfort (DIS), behavioral frustration tolerance (mirror-tracing task; Strong et al., 2003), and/or behavioral physical discomfort tolerance (breath-holding task; Hajek, Belcher, & Stapleton, 1987), may be of particular concurrent relevance to posttraumatic stress.

## FUTURE RESEARCH DIRECTIONS

In this chapter, we discussed theoretical and empirical models that link distress tolerance to the etiology and maintenance of traumatic stress within the context of several related constructs, including (1) emotion regulation, (2) anxiety sensitivity, and (3) mindfulness and acceptance. Although only limited studies linking distress tolerance to traumatic stress have been conducted to date, a fairly large body of literature linking related variables and traumatic stress symptoms was reviewed. Many of these variables may be contextualized in relation to emotion regulation, broadly, and may be related to distress tolerance in various ways. The extant literature offers an empirical, albeit indirect, basis for considering the role of distress tolerance in relation to these factors and traumatic stress. More extensive study of distress tolerance in the context of its potential nomological network of risk and protective factors may yield a better understanding of the processes underlying the cause and maintenance of traumatic stress. This effort may be of importance to ongoing research efforts focused on identifying malleable risk and protective factors related to posttraumatic stress.

Currently, there are too many methodological limitations in existing studies and too few studies overall to draw conclusions about the directionality of associations between distress tolerance and posttraumatic stress. Not enough is known about the construct to extrapolate its malleability over time or, specifically, the relations between change in distress tolerance and trauma or posttraumatic stress symptoms. It is plausible that distress tolerance levels may change (increase or decrease) as a function of exposure to traumatic stressors. That is, exposure to a traumatic life event might result in an increase in adaptive coping, leading to resilience, posttraumatic growth or related recovery from trauma, and perhaps greater distress tolerance. Conversely, an individual exposed to trauma might have the tendency to respond with affective and experiential avoidance, thereby amplifying posttraumatic stress symptoms over time, potentially leading to lower distress tolerance. Similarly, it is unknown whether levels of distress tolerance prior to trauma exposure may predispose an individual to risk or resilience or whether traumatic stress or posttraumatic stress symptoms may promote greater intolerance of distress. These are important questions for further study.

## CLINICAL IMPLICATIONS AND APPLICATIONS

It may be promising to consider targeting and assessing change in distress tolerance in prevention and treatment programs for traumatic stress psychopathology (e.g., via exposure and related cognitive-behavioral techniques). It may also be fruitful to explicitly study distress tolerance and therapeutic change in distress tolerance in the context of mechanisms of change underlying extant treatments for posttraumatic stress. For example, distress tolerance may be evaluated as a moderating factor underlying treatment effectiveness and/or as a mediator, potentially leading to a greater willingness to engage in approach-oriented coping.

Distress tolerance is targeted directly in dialectical behavior therapy (DBT; Linehan, 1993), unified treatment for emotional disorders (Barlow, Allen, & Choate, 2004), and acceptance-based emotion regulation group therapy (Gratz & Gunderson, 2006). As one example, Iverson, Shenk, and Fruzzetti (2009) pilot-tested a 12-week DBT skills training program, which included emotion regulation, distress tolerance, mindfulness, and interpersonal effectiveness modules, specifically for female victims of domestic abuse. These researchers found preliminary support for this program in reducing depressive symptoms and general psychiatric distress and increasing social adjustment among the 31 women studied. This study offers the first direct empirical extension of the DBT program for trauma survivors without borderline personality disorder. Indeed, in DBT, the distress tolerance module is conceptualized as facilitating the acquisition of skills related to greater adaptive tolerance of acute, high levels of distress. DBT groups are often conceptualized as a means to "achieve stabilization prior to initiating exposure-based interventions" (Wagner & Linehan, 2006, p. 117) or to provide a framework for emotion-related skill acquisition before embarking on PTSD-specific treatment.

In addition, emotion regulation skills training interventions for individuals with PTSD have demonstrated efficacy in attenuating symptoms of posttraumatic stress, anxiety, and general well-being in various trauma-exposed populations and among individuals with PTSD (Cloitre, Stovall-McClough, Miranda, & Chemtob, 2004; Iverson et al., 2009; Trappler & Newville, 2007; Zlotnick et al., 1997). For example, Zlotnick and colleagues (1997) found support for a 15-week affect-management group treatment program, compared with a wait-list control, in reducing symptoms of posttraumatic stress and dissociation among women with PTSD and a history of childhood sexual abuse. In a similar sample, Cloitre and colleagues (2004) found evidence for the mediating role of negative mood regulation (during prolonged exposure therapy) with regard to the association between positive therapeutic relationship and reduced PTSD symptoms at the end of treatment. The treatment, skills training in affect and interpersonal regulation, was composed of two phases: (1) enhancement of interpersonal and emotion regulation skills (eight sessions) and (2) modified prolonged exposure (eight sessions). In other work, improvements in emotion regulation abilities, via skills-based intervention, significantly predicted decreases in PTSD symptoms following exposure-based treatment among childhood sexual abuse survivors (Cloitre, Koenen, Cohen, & Han, 2002). As yet another example, Gratz and Gunderson's (2006) acceptance-based emotion regulation group therapy, for individuals with borderline personality disorder and often a history of trauma, is designed to target distress tolerance by promoting emotional willingness, broadly, and teaching patients impulse control behaviors and strategies to use in affectively distressing contexts.

It may be that levels of distress tolerance are indirectly or inadvertently changed in empirically supported treatments for PTSD, such as cognitive processing therapy (Monson et al., 2006; Resick, Nishith, Weaver, Astin, & Feuer, 2002; Resick & Schnicke, 1992) and prolonged exposure (Foa, Hembree, & Rothbaum, 2007; Foa et al., 2005; Foa & Kozak, 1986; Foa, Molnar, & Cashman, 1995). Facilitating the cognitive and emotional processing of trauma memories via cognitive restructuring exercises, imaginal exposure, or *in vivo* exposure may teach individuals to tolerate emotional stress generally and increase their ability to tolerate posttraumatic stress symptoms more specifically. Therefore, it might be useful for ongoing treatment trials to measure distress tolerance, using self-report and/or behavioral indices, over time (1) to note whether changes in the construct are noted in the context of treatment, (2) to determine at what points in treatment (and in relation to what treatment component) change in distress tolerance may be most salient, and (3) to explore whether changes in distress tolerance may be linked to treatment–outcomes relations.

## SUMMARY

Distress tolerance is a meaningful, though significantly understudied, construct that is theoretically germane to traumatic stress. We attempted to highlight the relations between theoretically related factors linked to posttraumatic stress for the purpose of advancing more critical thought and empirical study of the distress tolerance construct. Although in the early stages of development, study of distress tolerance may lead to a better understanding of the mechanisms underlying the etiology and maintenance of traumatic stress and, ultimately, its prevention/treatment.

## REFERENCES

Amdur, R. L., Larsen, R., & Liberzon, I. (2000). Emotional processing in combat-related posttraumatic stress disorder: A comparison with traumatized and normal controls. *Journal of Anxiety Disorders, 14,* 219–238.

American Psychiatric Association. (2000). *Diagnostic and statistical manual of mental disorders* (4th ed., text rev.). Washington, DC: Author.

Amstadter, A. (2008). Emotion regulation and anxiety disorders. *Journal of Anxiety Disorders, 22,* 211–221.

Ansorge, S., Litz, B. T., & Orsillo, S. M. (1996). Thinking about feelings: The role of meta-mood in PTSD. *NCP: Clinical Quarterly, 6,* 38–41.

Asmundson, G. J. G., & Stein, M. B. (1994). Triggering the false suffocation alarm in panic disorder patients by using a voluntary breath-holding procedure. *American Journal of Psychiatry, 151,* 264–266.

Baer, R. A., Smith, G. T., & Allen, K. B. (2004). Assessment of mindfulness by self-report: The Kentucky Inventory of Mindfulness Skills. *Assessment, 11,* 191–206.

Barlow, D., Allen, L., & Choate, M. (2004). Toward a unified treatment for emotional disorders. *Behavior Therapy, 35,* 205–230.

Bernstein, A., Tanay, G., & Vujanovic, A. A. (in press). Concurrent relations between mindful attention and awareness and psychopathology among trauma-exposed adults: Preliminary evidence of transdiagnostic resilience. *Journal of Cognitive Psychotherapy.*

Bernstein, A., Zvolensky, M. J., Feldner, M. T., Lewis, S. F., & Leen-Feldner, E. W. (2005). Anxiety sensitivity taxonicity: A concurrent test of cognitive vulnerability for post-traumatic stress symptomatology among young adults. *Cognitive Behaviour Therapy, 34,* 229–241.

Bernstein, A., Zvolensky, M. J., Norton, P. J., Schmidt, N. B., Taylor, S., Forsyth, J. P., et al. (2007). Taxometric and factor analytic models of anxiety-sensitivity: Integrating approaches to latent structural research. *Psychological Assessment, 19,* 74–87.

Bernstein, A., Zvolensky, M. J., Vujanovic, A. A., & Moos, R. (2009). Integrating anxiety sensitivity, distress tolerance, and discomfort intolerance: A hierarchical model of affect sensitivity and tolerance. *Behavior Therapy, 40,* 291–301.

Bishop, S. R., Lau, M., Shapiro, S., Carlson, L., Anderson, N. D., Carmody, J., et al. (2004). Mindfulness: A proposed operational definition. *Clinical Psychology: Science and Practice, 11,* 230–241.

Blake, D. D., Weathers, F. W., Nagy, L. M., Kaloupek, D. G., Gusman, F. D.,

Charney, D. S., et al. (1995). The development of a clinician-administered PTSD scale. *Journal of Traumatic Stress, 8,* 75–90.

Bleich, A., Koslowsky, M., Dolev, A., & Lerer, B. (1997). Post-traumatic stress disorder and depression. An analysis of comorbidity. *British Journal of Psychiatry, 170,* 479–482.

Boelen, P. A., & Reijntjes, A. (2009). Intolerance of uncertainty and social anxiety. *Journal of Anxiety Disorders, 23,* 130–135.

Bonn-Miller, M. O., Zvolensky, M. J., & Bernstein, A. (2009). Discomfort intolerance: Evaluation of incremental validity for panic-relevant symptoms using 10% carbon dioxide-enriched air provocation. *Journal of Anxiety Disorders, 23,* 197–203.

Breslau, N., & Davis, G. C. (1992). Posttraumatic stress disorder in an urban population of young adults: Risk factors for chronicity. *American Journal of Psychiatry, 149,* 671–675.

Breslau, N., Davis, G., Andreski, P., Federman, B., & Anthony, J. C. (1998). Epidemiological findings on posttraumatic stress disorder and co-morbid disorders in the general population. In B. P. Dohrenwend (Ed.), *Adversity, stress, and psychopathology* (pp. 319–330). New York: Oxford University Press.

Briere, J. N. (1997). Treating adults severely abused as children: The self-trauma model. In D. A. Wolfe, R. J. McMahon, & R. D. Peters (Eds.), *Child abuse: New directions in prevention and treatment across the lifespan* (pp. 177–204). Thousand Oaks, CA: Sage.

Brown, K. W., & Ryan, R. M. (2003). The benefits of being present: Mindfulness and its role in psychological well-being. *Journal of Personality and Social Psychology, 84,* 822–848.

Brown, R. A., Lejuez, C. W., Kahler, C. W., Strong, D. R., & Zvolensky, M. J. (2005). Distress tolerance and early smoking lapse. *Clinical Psychology Review, 25,* 713–733.

Bryant, R. A., & Harvey, A. G. (1995). Processing threatening information in posttraumatic stress disorder. *Journal of Abnormal Psychology, 104,* 537–541.

Burriss, L., Ayers, E., & Powell, D. A. (2007). Combat veterans show normal discrimination during differential trace eyeblink conditioning, but increased responsivity to the conditioned and unconditioned stimulus. *Journal of Psychiatric Research, 41,* 785–794.

Cloitre, M., Koenen, K. C., Cohen, L. R., & Han, H. (2002). Skills training in affective and interpersonal regulation followed by exposure: A phase-based treatment for PTSD related to childhood abuse. *Journal of Consulting and Clinical Psychology, 70,* 1067–1074.

Cloitre, M., Stovall-McClough, K., Miranda, R., & Chemtob, C. M. (2004). Therapeutic alliance, negative mood regulation, and treatment outcome in child abuse-related posttraumatic stress disorder. *Journal of Consulting and Clinical Psychology, 72,* 411–416.

Cook, J. W., McFall, M. M., Calhoun, P. S., & Beckham, J. C. (2007). Posttraumatic stress disorder and smoking relapse: A theoretical model. *Journal of Traumatic Stress, 20,* 989–998.

Dalgleish, T., Rolfe, J., Golden, A.-M., Dunn, B. D., & Barnard, P. J. (2008).

Reduced autobiographical memory specificity and posttraumatic stress: Exploring the contributions of impaired executive control and affect regulation. *Journal of Abnormal Psychology, 117,* 236–241.

Daughters, S. B., Reynolds, E. K., McPherson, L., Kahler, C. W., Danielson, C. K., Zvolensky, M., et al. (2009). Distress tolerance and early adolescent externalizing and internalizing symptoms: The moderating role of gender and ethnicity. *Behaviour Research and Therapy, 47,* 198–205.

Ehlers, A., & Clark, D. M. (2000). A cognitive model of posttraumatic stress disorder. *Behaviour Research and Therapy, 38,* 319–345.

Engelhard, I. M., Macklin, M. L., McNally, R. J., van den Hout, M. A., & Arntz, A. (2001). Emotion- and intrusion-based reasoning in Vietnam veterans with and without chronic posttraumatic stress disorder. *Behaviour Research and Therapy, 39,* 1339–1348.

Fedoroff, I. C., Taylor, S., Asmundson, G. J. G., & Koch, W. J. (2000). Cognitive factors in traumatic stress reactions: Predicting PTSD symptoms from anxiety sensitivity and beliefs about harmful events. *Behavioral and Cognitive Psychotherapy, 28,* 5–15.

Feldner, M. T., Lewis, S. F., Leen-Feldner, E. W., Schnurr, P. P., & Zvolensky, M. J. (2006). Anxiety sensitivity as a moderator of the relation between trauma exposure and posttraumatic stress symptomatology. *Journal of Cognitive Psychotherapy, 20,* 201–213.

Foa, E. B. (1995). *Posttraumatic Stress Diagnostic Scale manual.* Minneapolis, MN: National Computer Systems.

Foa, E. B., Hembree, E. A., Cahill, S. P., Rauch, S. A. M., Riggs, D. S., Feeny, N. C., et al. (2005). Randomized trial of prolonged exposure for posttraumatic stress disorder with and without cognitive restructuring: Outcome at academic and community clinics. *Journal of Consulting and Clinical Psychology, 73,* 953–964.

Foa, E. B., Hembree, E. A., & Rothbaum, B. O. (2007). *Prolonged exposure therapy for PTSD: Emotional processing of traumatic experiences: Therapist guide.* New York: Oxford University Press.

Foa, E. B., & Kozak, M. J. (1986). Emotional processing of fear: Exposure to corrective information. *Psychological Bulletin, 99,* 20–35.

Foa, E. B., Molnar, C., & Cashman, L. (1995). Change in rape narratives during exposure therapy for posttraumatic stress disorder. *Journal of Traumatic Stress, 8,* 675–690.

Gratz, K. L., & Gunderson, J. G. (2006). Preliminary data on acceptance-based emotion regulation group intervention for deliberate self-harm among women with borderline personality disorder. *Behavior Therapy, 37,* 25–35.

Gratz, K. L., & Roemer, L. (2004). Multidimensional assessment of emotion regulation and dysregulation: Development, factor structure, and initial validation of the difficulties in emotion regulation scale. *Journal of Psychopathology and Behavioral Assessment, 26,* 41–54.

Gross, J. J. (1998). Antecedent- and response-focused emotion regulation: Divergent consequences for experience, expression, and physiology. *Journal of Personality and Social Psychology, 74,* 224–237.

Gross, J. J., & Levenson, R. W. (1993). Emotional suppression: Physiology, self-report, and expressive behavior. *Journal of Personality and Social Psychology, 64,* 970–986.

Gross, J. J., & Levenson, R. W. (1997). Hiding feelings: The acute effects of inhibiting negative and positive emotion. *Journal of Abnormal Psychology, 106,* 95–103.

Hajek, P., Belcher, M., & Stapleton, J. (1987). Breath-holding endurance as a predictor of success in smoking cessation. *Addictive Behaviors, 12,* 285–288.

Hayes, S. C., Strosahl, K. D., & Wilson, K. G. (1999). *Acceptance and commitment therapy: An experiential approach to behavior change.* New York: Guilford Press.

Horowitz, M. J. (1986). Stress-response syndromes: A review of posttraumatic and adjustment disorders. *Hospital and Community Psychiatry, 37,* 241–249.

Hyer, L., Woods, M. G., & Boudewyns, P. A. (1991). A three tier evaluation of PTSD among Vietnam combat veterans. *Journal of Traumatic Stress, 4,* 165–194.

Iverson, K. M., Shenk, C., & Fruzzetti, A. E. (2009). Dialectical behavior therapy for women victims of domestic abuse: A pilot study. *Professional Psychology: Research and Practice, 40,* 242–248.

Keane, T. M., & Barlow, D. H. (2002). Posttraumatic stress disorder. In D. H. Barlow (Ed.), *Anxiety and its disorders* (pp. 418–453). New York: Guilford Press.

Kessler, R. C., Sonnega, A., Bromet, E., Hughes, M., & Nelson, C. B. (1995). Posttraumatic stress disorder in the National Comorbidity Survey. *Archives of General Psychiatry, 52,* 1048–1060.

Khantzian, E. J. (1997). The self-medication hypothesis of substance use disorders: A reconsideration and recent applications. *Harvard Review of Psychiatry, 4,* 231–244.

Kilpatrick, D. G., & Resnick, H. S. (1993). PTSD associated with exposure to criminal victimization in clinical and community populations. In J. R. T. Davidson & E. B. Foa (Eds.), *PTSD in review: Recent research and future directions* (pp. 113–143). Washington, DC: American Psychiatric Press.

Kimbrough, E., Magyari, T., Langenberg, P., Margaret, C., & Berman, B. (2010). Mindfulness intervention for child abuse survivors. *Journal of Clinical Psychology, 66,* 17–33.

King, D. W., Leskin, G. A., King, L. A., & Weathers, F. W. (1998). Confirmatory factor analysis of the clinician-administered PTSD scale: Evidence for the dimensionality of posttraumatic stress disorder. *Psychological Assessment, 10,* 90–96.

Lanius, R. A., Williamson, P. C., Hopper, J., Densmore, M., Boksman, K., Gupta, M. A., et al. (2003). Recall of emotional states in posttraumatic stress disorder: An fMRI investigation. *Biological Psychiatry, 53,* 204–210.

Linehan, M. M. (1993). *Cognitive-behavioral treatment of borderline personality disorder.* New York: Guilford Press.

Litz, B. T. (1992). Emotional numbing in combat-related post-traumatic stress disorder: A critical review and reformulation. *Clinical Psychology Review, 12,* 417–432.

Litz, B. T., Orsillo, S. M., Kaloupek, D., & Weathers, F. (2000). Emotional processing in posttraumatic stress disorder. *Journal of Abnormal Psychology, 109*, 26–39.

Litz, B. T., Schlenger, W. E., Weathers, F. W., Caddell, J. M., Fairbank, J. A., & LaVange, L. M. (1997). Predictors of emotional numbing in posttraumatic stress disorder. *Journal of Traumatic Stress, 10*, 607–618.

Luterek, J. A., Orsillo, S. M., & Marx, B. P. (2005). An experimental examination of emotional experience, expression, and disclosure in women reporting a history of childhood sexual abuse. *Journal of Traumatic Stress, 18*, 237–244.

Marshall, E. C., Vujanovic, A. A., Bonn-Miller, M. O., Bernstein, A., & Zvolensky, M. J. (2010). *Multi-method study of distress tolerance and posttraumatic stress symptom severity in a trauma-exposed community sample.* Manuscript submitted for publication.

Marshall, E. C., Zvolensky, M. J., Vujanovic, A. A., Gregor, K., Gibson, L. E., & Leyro, T. M. (2008). Panic reactivity to voluntary hyperventilation challenge predicts distress tolerance to bodily sensations among daily cigarette smokers. *Experimental and Clinical Psychopharmacology, 16*, 313–321.

Marx, B. P., & Sloan, D. M. (2005). Peritraumatic dissociation and experiential avoidance as predictors of posttraumatic stress symptomatology. *Behaviour Research and Therapy, 43*, 569–583.

McNally, R. J. (1998). Experimental approaches to cognitive abnormality in posttraumatic stress disorder. *Clinical Psychology Review, 18*, 971–982.

McNally, R. J. (2002). Anxiety sensitivity and panic disorder. *Biological Psychiatry, 52*, 938–946.

McNally, R. J., English, G. E., & Lipke, H. J. (1993). Assessment of intrusive cognition in PTSD: Use of the modified Stroop paradigm. *Journal of Traumatic Stress, 6*, 33–41.

McNally, R. J., Metzger, L. J., Lasko, N. B., Clancy, S. A., & Pitman, R. K. (1998). Directed forgetting of trauma cues in adult survivors of childhood sexual abuse with and without posttraumatic stress disorder. *Journal of Abnormal Psychology, 107*, 596–601.

Michal, M., Beutel, M. E., Jordan, J., Zimmermann, M., Wolters, S., & Heidenreich, T. (2007). Depersonalization, mindfulness, and childhood trauma. *Journal of Nervous and Mental Disease, 195*, 693–696.

Milanak, M. E., & Berenbaum, H. (2009). The relationship between PTSD symptom factors and emotion. *Journal of Traumatic Stress, 22*, 139–145.

Miller, M. W., & Litz, B. T. (2004). Emotional-processing for posttraumatic stress disorder: II. Startle reflex modulation during picture processing. *Journal of Abnormal Psychology, 113*, 451–463.

Miller, M. W., Vogt, D. S., Mozley, S. L., Kaloupek, D. G., & Keane, T. M. (2006). PTSD and substance-related problems: The mediating roles of disconstraint and negative emotionality. *Journal of Abnormal Psychology, 115*, 369–379.

Monson, C. M., Price, J. L., Rodriguez, B. F., Ripley, M. P., & Warner, R. A.

(2004). Emotional deficits in military-related PTSD: An investigation of content and process disturbances. *Journal of Traumatic Stress, 17,* 275–279.

Monson, C. M., Schnurr, P. P., Resick, P. A., Friedman, M. J., Young-Xu, Y., & Stevens, S. P. (2006). Cognitive processing therapy for veterans with military-related posttraumatic stress disorder. *Journal of Consulting and Clinical Psychology, 74,* 898–907.

Morey, R. A., Petty, C. M., Cooper, D. A., LaBar, K. S., & McCarthy, G. (2008). Neural systems for executive and emotional processing are modulated by symptoms of posttraumatic stress disorder in Iraq war veterans. *Psychiatry Research: Neuroimaging, 162,* 59–72.

New, A. S., Fan, J., Murrough, J. W., Liu, X., Liebman, R. E., Guise, K. G., et al. (2009). A functional magnetic resonance imaging study of deliberate emotion regulation in resilience and posttraumatic stress disorder. *Biological Psychiatry, 66,* 656–664.

O'Cleirigh, C., Ironson, G., & Smits, J. A. J. (2007). Does distress tolerance moderate the impact of major life events on psychosocial variables and behaviors important in the management of HIV? *Journal of Behavior Therapy and Experimental Psychiatry, 38,* 314–323.

Orsillo, S. M., & Roemer, L. (2005). *Acceptance and mindfulness-based approaches to anxiety.* New York: Springer.

Pitman, R. K., van der Kolk, B. A., Orr, S. P., & Greenberg, M. S. (1990). Naloxone-reversible analgesic response to combat-related stimuli in posttraumatic stress disorder: A pilot study. *Archives of General Psychiatry, 47,* 541–544.

Polusny, M. A., Dickinson, K. A., Murdoch, M., & Thuras, P. (2008). The role of cumulative sexual trauma and difficulties identifying feelings in understanding female veterans' physical health outcomes. *General Hospital Psychiatry, 30,* 162–170.

Price, J. L., Monson, C. M., Callahan, K., & Rodriguez, B. F. (2006). The role of emotional functioning in military-related PTSD and its treatment. *Journal of Anxiety Disorders, 20,* 661–674.

Reiss, S., Peterson, R. A., Gursky, D. M., & McNally, R. J. (1986). Anxiety sensitivity, anxiety frequency and the predictions of fearfulness. *Behaviour Research and Therapy, 24,* 1–8.

Resick, P. A., & Miller, M. W. (2009). DSM-V: Should PTSD be in a class of its own? *British Journal of Psychiatry, 194,* 90.

Resick, P. A., Nishith, P., Weaver, T. L., Astin, M. C., & Feuer, C. A. (2002). A comparison of cognitive-processing therapy with prolonged exposure and a waiting condition for the treatment of chronic posttraumatic stress disorder in female rape victims. *Journal of Consulting and Clinical Psychology, 70,* 867–879.

Resick, P. A., & Schnicke, M. K. (1992). Cognitive processing therapy for sexual assault victims. *Journal of Consulting and Clinical Psychology, 60,* 748–756.

Roemer, L., Litz, B. T., Orsillo, S. M., & Wagner, A. W. (2001). A preliminary investigation of the role of strategic withholding of emotions in PTSD. *Journal of Traumatic Stress, 14,* 149–156.

Rothbaum, B. O., Foa, E. B., Riggs, D. S., Murdock, T., & Walsh, W. (1992). A prospective examination of post-traumatic stress disorder in rape victims. *Journal of Traumatic Stress, 5,* 455–475.

Rottenberg, J., & Gross, J. J. (2003). When emotion goes wrong: Realizing the promise of affective science. *Clinical Psychology: Science and Practice, 10,* 227–232.

Schmidt, N. B., Richey, J. A., & Fitzpatrick, K. K. (2006). Discomfort intolerance: Development of a construct and measure relevant to panic disorder. *Journal of Anxiety Disorders, 20,* 263–280.

Simons, J. S., & Gaher, R. M. (2005). The Distress Tolerance Scale: Development and validation of a self-report measure. *Motivation and Emotion, 29,* 83–102.

Staiger, P. K., Melville, F., Hides, L., Kambouropoulos, N., & Lubman, D. I. (2009). Can emotion-focused coping help explain the link between post-traumatic stress disorder severity and triggers for substance use in young adults? *Journal of Substance Abuse Treatment, 36,* 220–226.

Strong, D. R., Lejuez, C. W., Daughters, S. B., Marinello, M., Kahler, C. W., & Brown, R. A. (2003). *Computerized mirror tracing task version 1.* Unpublished manual.

Taylor, S., Koch, W. J., & McNally, R. J. (1992). How does anxiety sensitivity vary across the anxiety disorders? *Journal of Anxiety Disorders, 6,* 249–259.

Telch, M. J., Jacquin, K., Smits, J. A. J., & Powers, M. B. (2003). Respiratory hypersensitivity as a predictor of agoraphobia status among individuals suffering from panic disorder. *Journal of Behavior Therapy and Experimental Psychiatry, 34,* 161–170.

Thompson, B. L., & Waltz, J. (2010). Mindfulness and experiential avoidance as predictors of posttraumatic stress disorder avoidance symptom severity. *Journal of Anxiety Disorders, 24,* 409–415.

Thrasher, S. M., Dalgleish, T., & Yule, W. (1994). Information processing in posttraumatic stress disorder. *Behaviour Research and Therapy, 32,* 247–254.

Timpano, K. R., Buckner, J. D., Richey, J. A., Murphy, D. L., & Schmidt, N. B. (2009). Exploration of anxiety sensitivity and distress tolerance as vulnerability factors for hoarding behaviors. *Depression and Anxiety, 26,* 343–353.

Trappler, B., & Newville, H. (2007). Trauma healing via cognitive behavior therapy in chronically hospitalized patients. *Psychiatric Quarterly, 78,* 317–325.

Tull, M. T., Barrett, H. M., McMillan, E. S., & Roemer, L. (2007). A preliminary investigation of the relationship between emotion regulation difficulties and posttraumatic stress symptoms. *Behavior Therapy, 38,* 303–313.

Tull, M. T., Gratz, K. L., Salters, K., & Roemer, L. (2004). The role of experiential avoidance in posttraumatic stress symptoms and symptoms of depression, anxiety, and somatization. *Journal of Nervous and Mental Disease, 192,* 754–761.

Tull, M. T., Jakupcak, M., McFadden, M. E., & Roemer, L. (2007). The role of negative affect intensity and the fear of emotions in posttraumatic stress symptom severity among victims of childhood interpersonal violence. *Journal of Nervous and Mental Disease, 195,* 580–587.

Tull, M. T., & Roemer, L. (2003). Alternative explanation of emotional numbing of posttraumatic stress disorder: An examination of hyperarousal and experiential avoidance. *Journal of Psychopathology and Behavioral Assessment, 25,* 147–154.

Van der Kolk, B., Greenberg, M., Boyd, H., & Krystal, J. (1985). Inescapable shock, neurotransmitters, and addiction to trauma: Toward a psychobiology of post traumatic stress. *Biological Psychiatry, 20,* 314–325.

Van der Kolk, B. A. (1987). *Psychological trauma.* Arlington, VA: American Psychiatric Publishing.

Vujanovic, A. A., Bonn-Miller, M. O., Bernstein, A., McKee, L. G., & Zvolensky, M. J. (in press). Incremental validity of mindfulness skills in relation to emotional dysregulation among a young adult community sample. *Cognitive Behaviour Therapy.*

Vujanovic, A. A., Bonn-Miller, M. O., Potter, C. M., Marshall, E. C., & Zvolensky, M. J. (2010). *An evaluation of the association between distress tolerance and posttraumatic stress within a trauma-exposed sample.* Manuscript submitted for publication.

Vujanovic, A. A., Marshall, E. C., Gibson, L. E., & Zvolensky, M. J. (2010). Cognitive-affective characteristics of smokers with and without posttraumatic stress disorder and panic psychopathology. *Addictive Behaviors, 35,* 419–425.

Vujanovic, A. A., Youngwirth, N. E., Johnson, K. A., & Zvolensky, M. J. (2009). Mindfulness-based acceptance and posttraumatic stress symptoms among trauma-exposed adults without axis I psychopathology. *Journal of Anxiety Disorders, 23,* 297–303.

Vujanovic, A. A., Zvolensky, M. J., & Bernstein, A. (2008). The interactive effects of anxiety sensitivity and emotion dysregulation in predicting anxiety-related cognitive and affective symptoms. *Cognitive Therapy and Research, 32,* 803–817.

Wagner, A. W., & Linehan, M. M. (2006). Applications of dialectical behavior therapy to posttraumatic stress disorder and related problems. In V. M. Follette & J. I. Ruzek (Eds.), *Cognitive-behavioral therapies for trauma* (2nd ed., pp. 117–145). New York: Guilford Press.

Walser, R. D., & Westrup, D. (2007). *Acceptance and commitment therapy for the treatment of post-traumatic stress disorder and trauma-related problems: A practitioner's guide to using mindfulness and acceptance strategies.* Oakland, CA: New Harbinger.

Zlotnick, C., Shea, T. M., Rosen, K., Simpson, E., Mulrenin, K., Begin, A., et al. (1997). An affect-management group for women with posttraumatic stress disorder and histories of childhood sexual abuse. *Journal of Traumatic Stress, 10,* 425–436.

# 7

## Major Depressive Disorder

Shauna L. Clen, Douglas S. Mennin,
*and* David M. Fresco

$\text{M}$ajor depressive disorder (MDD) is one of the most prevalent psychiatric disorders (Kessler, Chiu, Demler, Merikangas, & Walters, 2005) and foremost public health threats of the 21st century (Judd & Kunovac, 1997). Emotionality is central to the diagnosis of MDD (American Psychiatric Association, 2000), as the disorder is characterized by both high levels of negative emotions and low levels of positive emotions (see Morris, Bylsma, & Rottenberg, 2009, for a discussion). Despite the central role of emotionality in MDD and other forms of psychopathology, emotional functioning has historically been a neglected research area in psychology (Greenberg, 2002; Samoilov & Goldfried, 2000). However, in the past 10 years, emotion-based psychological research is growing as researchers turn toward emotion regulation research and affective neuroscience to gain a greater understanding of psychological disorders, including MDD (e.g., Davidson, Pizzagalli, Nitschke, & Putnam, 2002; Rottenberg, Gross, & Gotlib, 2005; Teasdale, 1999).

Emotions are integral to human functioning as they promote behaviors that ensure survival. Emotional responding is the result of the activation of motivational systems that have been triggered in response to punishment, reward, or the need for current action (i.e., fight-or-flight system; Carver & Scheier, 1998; Gray & McNaughton, 2000; Higgins, 1997). Emotional responses include physiological responses (e.g., heart rate), behavioral responses (e.g., facial expressions; moving to escape danger), and subjective responses (e.g., thoughts and "feelings") (LeDoux, 1996). In addition to relaying motivational information, emotions also convey information regarding one's values and goals in a given situation (Keltner & Haidt, 1999). For instance, negative emotions can focus us in a specific direction so that we can clarify a goal or solve a problem (Parrott, 2001). Positive emotions can expand the array of thoughts and actions and, in turn, create new approach behaviors (Fredrickson, 2001).

Emotions have generative (e.g., motivational, functional) as well as regulatory (e.g., modulating responses according to contextual demands; see Cole, Martin, & Dennis, 2004) characteristics. Emotions respond to environmental demands and personal values by regulating processes such as cognition and behavior. Emotions also respond to personal and environmental contexts by being regulated or changed by processes such as cognition and behavior, which may result in emotional responses being enhanced or diminished in a given situation (see Cole et al., 2004). Although emotions are integral to our survival and functioning, they can take harmful forms when characterized by invariable excesses, deficits, or lability. Emotions can also take harmful forms when regulatory strategies aimed at modulating emotions are deficient or are used excessively, rigidly, or not at all (Kring & Werner, 2004).

Dysfunction in executive responses to emotions is a growing area of study in psychopathology and MDD research (e.g., Leahy, 2002). Mennin and Fresco (2009) argued that executive responses to emotions can involve awareness/understanding of emotions (i.e., clarifying, labeling, and understanding the informational conveyed by emotions as well as distinguishing between different emotions), metacognitive reactions to emotions (i.e., thinking about one's own inner experiences in terms of appraising, interpreting, or implementing beliefs about emotions), and poor management of emotions (i.e., knowing how and when to diminish or enhance an emotional experience in a manner that is appropriate for a given context). Whereas lack of ability to describe and identify emotions (e.g., alexithymia; Bagby, Parker, & Taylor, 1994) and poor emotion management (i.e., regulation; Gross & John, 2003) have received increasing attention, detrimental metacognitive reactions to emotions have received less attention.

Metacognition entails one's knowledge about one's own cognitive processes or "thinking about thinking" (see Flavell, 1978). Metacognitive reactions refer to one's beliefs about one's own inner experiences and one's appraisal of one's own experiences. One construct reflecting metacognitive reactions to emotions is *emotional distress tolerance*. Emotional distress tolerance is a theoretical derivation of the construct of distress tolerance, an individual-difference variable representing the degree to which an individual tolerates a form of experiential discomfort (see Otto, Powers, & Fischmann, 2005). Emotional distress tolerance represents the degree to which an individual tolerates the experience of any of the following families of negative emotions: sadness, fear, anger and disgust (basic negative emotions; Williams, Teasdale, Segal, & Kabat-Zinn, 2007; see also Zvolensky & Otto, 2007, for a discussion of similar constructs such as affect intolerance or emotional sensitivity).

Emotional distress tolerance may be a useful framework for integrating findings and theory regarding emotional dysfunction that occurs after an emotion has been generated but before emotion regulation strategies have been employed. In particular, emotional distress tolerance may help to clarify one's appraisals, beliefs, and willingness to experience negative emotions. Although cognitive or behavioral regulatory actions (e.g., emotional suppression) can result, in part, from appraisals, beliefs, and willingness to experience negative emotions, emotional distress tolerance, as defined herein, will only refer to the metacognitive processes of appraisals, beliefs, and willingness to experience negative emotions as opposed to these latter management actions.

Emotional distress tolerance may be of particular relevance to MDD as the manner in which an individual experiences, interprets, and cognitively responds to negative emotions, specifically sadness or lack of happiness, has been identified as a possible source of vulnerability to MDD (e.g., Segal, Williams, & Teasdale, 2002; Williams et al., 2007). MDD treatments that include a focus on emotional appraisals and willingness to experience emotions have also emerged (e.g., Hayes, Strosahl, & Wilson, 1999; Segal et al., 2002). Emotional distress tolerance may be a helpful way of integrating somewhat disparate findings regarding emotional processes and MDD. Emotional distress tolerance may also help to highlight relevant findings regarding emotional processes and other forms of psychopathology that can be extended to MDD research. Although we are focusing on emotional distress tolerance as it relates to MDD, emotional distress tolerance is likely relevant to many other forms of psychopathology. However, such a comprehensive review is beyond the scope of this chapter.

In this chapter, we (1) provide a definition of emotional distress tolerance, including explication of three components of emotional distress tolerance (i.e., negativity and/or threat appraisals, coping beliefs, and willingness to experience negative emotions) and how they relate to psychopathology and MDD in particular; (2) examine the relationship between emotion regulation strategies and MDD and propose a possible contributory role for emotional distress tolerance in the relationship between emotion regulation strategies and MDD; and (3) briefly review clinical assessments and treatments that reflect our definition of emotional distress tolerance and are relevant to MDD.

# EMOTIONAL DISTRESS TOLERANCE

## Defining Emotional Distress Tolerance

An individual's level of emotional distress tolerance denotes how one perceives negative emotional experiences in terms of his or her (1) appraisals of the negativity and/or threat value of negative emotions, (2) beliefs regarding his or her coping ability in a given negative emotional situation, and (3) resulting willingness to experience negative emotions. The three components of emotional distress tolerance are mutually influential, as a given component is unlikely to be present in the absence of the other two components. Although we refer to negative emotions in general, an individual's emotional distress tolerance could theoretically differ among various negative emotions (e.g., one could have a particularly low emotional distress tolerance to sadness but not to fear). It should be noted that the term *emotional distress tolerance* was originally defined by Simons and Gaher (2005). Our definition of emotional distress tolerance is a theoretical expansion of Simons and Gaher but also incorporates our prior theorizations of the related construct of negative metacognitive reactions to emotions (i.e., negative cognitive reactivity; Mennin & Fresco, 2009).

Although the three components of emotional distress tolerance overlap with the construct of negative cognitive reactivity, the latter has been solely discussed as one of four aspects of a larger emotion dysregulation model of anxiety and mood pathology (e.g., Mennin, Heimberg, Turk, & Fresco, 2005). Accordingly, negative cognitive reactivity has not received specific attention and detailed delineation of its components. In fact, after finding a unique relationship between negative cognitive reactivity and MDD symptoms, Mennin, Holaway, Fresco, Moore, and Heimberg (2007) advocated for the breakdown of negative cognitive reactivity into separate components so that a more detailed examination of negative cognitive reactivity and MDD could be conducted. Emotional distress tolerance fulfills this need by conceptually expanding on the construct of negative cognitive reactivity, providing a detailed definition as well as a framework for integrating findings and theory regarding the three components—appraisals of the negativity and/or threat value of negative emotions, beliefs regarding coping ability in a given negative emotional situation, and resulting willingness to experience negative emotions—as they relate to psychopathology.

Our emotional distress tolerance definition does not include any form of cognitive regulatory action (e.g., suppression) or behavioral regulatory action (e.g., avoidance of social activities). As previously mentioned, one of the purposes of our emotional distress tolerance framework is to extricate metacognitive reactions from regulatory actions, as beliefs and appraisals are related to but separable from regulatory actions (e.g., appraising an emotion as harmful does not de facto produce a certain behavior).

According to our operational definition, an individual with low emotional distress tolerance appraises negative emotions as aversive, threatening, or harmful, sees himself or herself as unable to effectively cope with negative emotions, and is resultantly unwilling to experience negative emotions (i.e., is intolerant of negative emotions). Low emotional distress tolerance denotes a rigid and inflexible view of negative emotions (e.g., negative emotions are always harmful; one is never able to cope effectively with negative emotions; one is consistently unwilling to experience negative emotions). Inflexibility in metacognitive appraisals may be detrimental to well-being, given that low flexibility in metacognitive appraisals of causality (i.e., low explanatory flexibility; see Fresco, Rytwinski, & Craighead, 2007) predicts MDD symptoms in college students both concurrently (Fresco, Williams, & Nugent, 2006) and longitudinally (Fresco, Rytwinski, et al., 2007).

Although we view low emotional distress tolerance as detrimental and high emotional distress tolerance as beneficial to well-being, it is possible that being rigidly, overly tolerant of negative emotions (e.g., viewing oneself as extremely capable of coping effectively with all negative emotions) could be detrimental to well-being. However, in this chapter we mainly focus on the association among low emotional distress tolerance, psychopathology, and MDD.

## Appraisals of the Negativity and/or Threat Value of Negative Emotions

The first component of emotional distress tolerance involves appraisal of the negativity of negative emotions and/or appraisal of the threat value of negative emotions. Appraisal of the negativity of negative emotions specifically relates to the extent to which negative emotions are perceived as aversive (e.g., highly aversive: "I hate this feeling"). Williams and colleagues (2007) proposed that initial patterns of reactions to negative emotions are characterized by aversion or the desire to avoid or eliminate an experience, which can be arousing and lead individuals to report that they "hate" their emotions. Appraisal of the threat value of negative emotions relates to the extent to which an individual assigns harmful meanings (e.g., highly harmful meanings: "Feeling sad means I am a failure") and/or harmful consequences (e.g., highly harmful consequences: "Sadness is dangerous") to negative emotions.

Individuals interpret or appraise their inner experiences (see Clore & Ortony, 2000; Wells, 1995), including their emotions (see Leahy, 2002).

Leahy (2002) argued that an individual's tendency to interpret her or his emotions as problematic (e.g., "Anxiety will make me go crazy") may lead to detrimental consequences. Leahy found that emotional appraisals were related to self-reported MDD symptoms in adult psychiatric patients. Specifically, higher levels of MDD symptoms were associated with viewing emotions as difficult to understand, difficult to control, and different than the emotions that other people experience. Leahy also found guilt over emotions, expectations that negative mood would be of a longer duration, and greater rumination to be associated with MDD symptoms.

Anxiety sensitivity would be expected to relate strongly to appraisals of the negativity and/or threat value of negative emotions. Anxiety sensitivity refers to the fear of anxiety sensations due to the belief that anxiety produces negative social, psychological, or somatic consequences (Reiss, 1991). Anxiety sensitivity has been found to longitudinally predict the presence of panic attacks in college students (Maller & Reiss, 1992) and military personnel, even after controlling for trait anxiety and history of panic attacks (Schmidt, Lerew, & Jackson, 1999). Anxiety sensitivity is associated with self-reported anxiety symptoms (McNally & Eke, 1996; Zvolensky et al., 2002) and bodily sensations (McNally & Eke, 1996) in college students during laboratory-induced hyperventilation challenges.

More generally, the fear of emotions construct (Williams, Chambless, & Ahrens, 1997), which refers to apprehension about losing control over emotions or reacting negatively to emotions, also relates to the first component of emotional distress tolerance. Fear of emotions originated with the fear of fear phenomenon found in individuals with agoraphobia (Goldstein & Chambless, 1978) and was later extended to include fear of anxious arousal in anxiety disorders, fear of sadness in MDD (Barlow, 1991; Reiss, 1991; Taylor & Rachman, 1991), as well as fear of anger and happiness (Williams et al., 1997). Fear of emotions as assessed by the Affective Control Scale (ACS; Williams et al., 1997) was found to be associated with fear of laboratory-induced panic sensations (e.g., breathlessness, heart palpitations) in college students with no history of panic attacks (Williams et al., 1997), even when accounting for state and trait anxiety (Berg, Shapiro, Chambless, & Ahrens, 1998). Also, Roemer, Salters, Raffa, and Orsillo (2005) found that fear of anxiety was related to self-reported anxiety and MDD symptoms, and fear of depression was related to self-reported MDD symptoms, in patients with generalized anxiety disorder (GAD). Research regarding anxiety sensitivity and fear of emotions indicates that individuals differ in their appraisals of the negativity and/or threat value of negative emotions, and that appraising emotions as aversive or harmful in meaning or consequences may be related to psychopathology.

## Beliefs Regarding Coping Ability in a Given Negative Emotional Situation

The second component of emotional distress tolerance, beliefs regarding coping ability in a given negative emotional situation, relates to individuals' expectations regarding their ability to experience negative emotions without undue disruption in their lives (e.g., high negative expectations about disruptions: "I am going to freak out if I keep feeling this way") or without slowing or ceasing progress toward important goals (e.g., high negative expectations about goals: " I cannot get anything done when I feel sad").

Lazarus and Folkman (1984) argued that individuals hold outcome expectancies, or beliefs about the outcomes of given behaviors, as well as self-efficacy expectancies, or beliefs about whether one is capable of producing the necessary behaviors to achieve the desired outcomes. Following this line of reasoning, Catanzaro and Mearns (1990) developed the Negative Mood Rating Scale (NMR) to evaluate individuals' beliefs regarding their ability to alleviate negative moods (e.g., "When I'm upset, I believe that it won't be long before I can calm myself down"). Negative expectancies regarding ability to alleviate negative moods, as measured by the NMR, are associated with self-reported MDD symptoms in college students (Catanzaro, 1993; Kirsch, Mearns, & Catanzaro, 1990), level of active coping strategies in college students (Kirsch et al., 1990), self-reported MDD symptoms in older adults, and avoidant coping strategies in older adults (Catanzaro, Horaney, & Creasey, 1995). In addition, recovered depressed individuals were found to endorse more difficulties engaging in goal-directed behavior when "upset," as measured by the Goals scale of the Difficulties with Emotion Regulation Scale (DERS; Gratz & Roemer, 2004), than never-depressed control (Ehring, Fischer, Schnulle, Bosterling, & Tuschen-Caffier, 2008). Findings regarding perceived ability to regulate negative mood and perceived ability to engage in goal-directed behavior when distressed imply that individuals hold beliefs regarding their coping ability in a given negative emotional situation. However, items on the NMR and DERS evaluate one's beliefs about how one will cope with being "upset" rather than one's beliefs about how one will cope with specific negative emotions per se.

Negative cognitive reactivity, originally defined as a discomfort with emotional experiences and holding negative beliefs about emotions (see Mennin et al., 2007), has been examined using items from the ACS (Williams et al., 1997). The ACS addresses both the first and the second components of emotional distress tolerance. For instance, an item on the ACS reads "When I get 'the blues,' I worry that they will pull me down too far," which implies that one has appraised sadness as highly harmful in terms of consequences (i.e., first component of emotional distress tolerance) and as an experience that one is not capable of experiencing without undue disruption in his or her life (i.e., second component of emotional distress tolerance). Mennin and colleagues (2007) found an association between negative cognitive reactivity and self-reported MDD symptoms in college students, even after accounting for symptom overlap with GAD and social anxiety disorder (SAD). Findings regarding negative cognitive reactivity support a possible relationship among appraisals of the negativity of negative emotions and/or appraisals of the threat value of negative emotions, beliefs regarding coping ability in a given negative emotional situation, and symptoms of MDD.

## Willingness to Experience Negative Emotions

Willingness to experience negative emotions derives in part from the other components of emotional distress tolerance (i.e., appraisals of the negativity and/or threat value of negative emotions and beliefs regarding ability to cope with negative emotions; see Table 7.1). The beliefs about willingness to experience negative emotions component denotes the extent to which an individual accepts negative emotions as valid experiences (e.g., high nonacceptance of emotions: "I should not feel sad right now" or "It is stupid to feel sad").

Unwillingness to experience negative emotions, or nonacceptance of emotions, has been examined as it relates to experiential avoidance. Hayes, Wilson, Gifford, Follette, and Strosahl (1996) defined experiential avoidance as a phenomenon in which an individual is unwilling to remain in contact with inner experiences, such as bodily sensations and emotions, and attempts to alter the quality or frequency of the experiences or the situations that produce them. Hayes and colleagues (1999) argued that emotional nonacceptance is influenced by the negative connotations of "difficult" emotions that are inherent in our language. The verbal label given to an emotion (e.g., "sadness") can include an inherent evaluation of "badness" in our language (Hayes et al., 1999). The bidirectionality of human language makes badness seem to be an innate quality of a negative emotion such as sadness rather than a subjective evaluation. Therefore, individuals in our society view difficult emotions as inherently bad experiences that should be avoided (Hayes et al., 1999).

Nonacceptance of emotions is relevant to psychopathology. For instance, Campbell-Sills, Barlow, Brown, and Hofmann (2006) found a clinical sample of patients with mood disorders and anxiety disorders to be less accepting of induced emotions as compared to a sample of control participants. Hayes, Strosahl, and colleagues (2004) found a measure of experiential avoidance, an aspect of which is nonacceptance of emotions,

**TABLE 7.1. Delineating the Components of Emotional Distress Tolerance**

|  | Component 1: Appraisals of the negativity and/or threat value of negative emotions | Component 2: Beliefs regarding coping ability in a given negative emotional situation | Component 3: Willingness to experience negative emotions |
|---|---|---|---|
| Definition | Appraisals of negativity: the extent to which negative emotions are perceived as aversive Appraisals of threat value: the extent to which an individual assigns harmful meanings and/or harmful consequences to negative emotions | Expectations regarding ability to experience negative emotions without undue disruption in one's life or without slowing or ceasing progress toward important goals | The extent to which an individual accepts negative emotions as valid experiences |
| Distinct aspects of component | Perceived aversiveness; assigning harmful meanings | Expectations for undue disruptions; expectations for goal progress | Nonacceptance |
| Overlap with other components | Assigning highly harmful consequences is more likely to occur if one has negative expectations about goal progress and undue disruptions (i.e., Component 2). | High negative expectations about disruptions or goal progress are more likely to occur if negative emotions are appraised as harmful and/or aversive (i.e., Component 1). | High nonacceptance of negative emotions is unlikely to occur in the absence of negative emotional appraisals and/or negative coping beliefs (i.e., Components one and two). |
| Relevant assessments | Fear of Anxiety, fear of Depression, and fear of Anger subscales of the ACS (Williams et al., 1997) | NMR (Catanzaro & Mearns 1990); Goals subscale of the DERS (Gratz & Roemer, 2004) | Nonacceptance subscale of the DERS (Gratz & Roemer, 2004) |

to be associated with self-reported MDD symptoms in clinical and non-clinical samples. Mennin, McLaughlin, and Flanagan (2009) found non-acceptance of emotions, as measured by the Nonacceptance subscale of the DERS (Gratz & Roemer, 2004), to predict the presence of comorbid SAD and GAD, as assessed by diagnostic interviews, in college students. Salters-Pedneault, Roemer, Tull, Rucker, and Mennin (2006) found that nonacceptance of emotions, as measured by the Nonacceptance subscale of the DERS (e.g., "When I'm upset, I become embarrassed for feeling that way"; Gratz & Roemer, 2004), was associated with self-reported levels of worry and GAD.

Ehring and colleagues (2008) found that recovered depressed individuals endorsed less emotional acceptance, as measured by the Nonacceptance subscale of the DERS (Gratz & Roemer, 2004), than never-depressed control participants. Findings and theory regarding nonacceptance of emotions indicate that individuals can differ in their willingness to experience negative emotions and that a cognitive set of nonacceptance of emotions may produce detrimental consequences.

## EMOTION DYSREGULATION, MAJOR DEPRESSIVE DISORDER, AND THE ROLE OF EMOTION DISTRESS TOLERANCE

### Emotion Dysregulation Strategies in Major Depressive Disorder

Emotion regulation strategies involve actions aimed at changing, eliminating, or preventing an emotional experience (see Gross, 1998). The ability to engage in emotion regulation strategies that allow one to adaptively conform to a situation is important to well-being and mental health (e.g., Kring & Werner, 2004; Mayer, Salovey, & Caruso, 2004). Several theorists have proposed a link between emotion dysregulation and MDD such that the employment of maladaptive emotion regulation strategies may confer a vulnerability to MDD (e.g., Campbell-Sills & Barlow, 2007; Gross & Muñoz, 1995; Kring & Werner, 2004; Rude & McCarthy, 2003). Theorists have also proposed a bidirectional relationship between emotion regulation strategies and MDD in which utilization of emotion regulation strategies could be influenced by acute depression, but may also be a risk factor for experiencing a major depressive episode (e.g., Gross & Muñoz, 1995; Kring & Werner, 2004). Indeed, compared with healthy controls, individuals with symptoms of MDD use more dysfunctional emotion regulation strategies (Garnefski & Kraaij, 2006; Gross & John, 2003; Mennin et al., 2007; Rude & McCarthy, 2003) and have a poorer understanding of their emotions (Mennin et al., 2007; Rude & McCarthy, 2003).

Cicchetti, Ackerman, and Izard (1995) proposed that difficulties with emotional regulation strategies fall into two categories: (1) difficulty modulating emotional experiences and/or expressing emotions (e.g., difficulty self-soothing) and (2) frequently or automatically attempting to control or suppress emotional experiences or expressions. Both categories may be relevant to MDD, although difficulties in emotional modulation may be of particular importance to MDD. For example, self-reported MDD symptoms have been associated with self-reported difficulty repairing negative moods (Salovey, Stroud, Woolery, & Epel, 2002) and self-reported difficulty managing emotions (Mennin et al., 2007). Similarly, Ehring and colleagues (2008) found that recovered depressed individuals endorsed more difficulties regulating emotions than never-depressed controls.

## Depressive Rumination

Maladaptive cognitive strategies may be an important factor in MDD (e.g., Garnefski & Kraaij, 2006). Depressive rumination, or "behaviors and thoughts that focus one's attention on one's depressive symptoms and on the implications of these symptoms" (Nolen-Hoeksema, 1991, p. 569), is perhaps the most well-known emotion regulation strategy that reflects difficulty modulating emotions in individuals with MDD. Depressive rumination, as opposed to distraction, has been found to predict the onset of major depressive episodes in adults (Nolen-Hoeksema, 2000) and college students (Just & Alloy, 1997) and the presence of past and current symptoms of MDD in college students (Roberts, Gilboa, & Gotlib, 1998).

Individuals who tend to engage in depressive rumination may believe that they are fixing their emotional experiences by finding an "answer" to the "problem" of sadness or lack of happiness (Williams et al., 2007). A study by Watkins and Baracaia (2001) found that 80% of depressive ruminators believed there was a positive benefit to rumination, such as problem solving or understanding depressed mood, in a self-selected sample of adults who reported suffering from depressive rumination. Although depressive ruminators think that they are problem solving, they may be passively brooding about their problems, which could lead to more detrimental consequences than actual problem solving. A study by Armey and colleagues (2009) found that brooding (i.e., directing one's attention to one's problems and the consequences of one's problems) was more strongly associated with MDD symptoms than pondering, or actively seeking to understand and solve one's problems. Findings from studies on depressive rumination imply that this well-known factor in MDD may be a maladaptive emotion regulation strategy aimed at reducing negative mood.

## Emotional Suppression

Emotional suppression may also be a relevant factor in MDD. Campbell-Sills and colleagues (2006) found that individuals with mood disorders and anxiety disorders engaged in more emotional suppression in response to induced emotion than controls. Also, engaging in emotional suppression was associated with an increase in negative emotions in both clinical and nonclinical participants (Campbell-Sills et al., 2006), suggesting that emotional suppression may be a relevant emotion regulation strategy difficulty in mood disorders, including MDD.

Gross and John (2003) found that college students who endorsed the tendency to suppress emotional expressions experienced more negative emotions and less positive emotions, expressed less positive emotions to others, had less social support, engaged in less emotional disclosure, had more discomfort with sharing in close relationships, and endorsed more MDD symptoms, less life satisfaction, lower self-esteem, and less optimism, in comparison with nonsuppressors on a battery of self-report measures and peer-report measures. Likewise, Gross and Levenson (1997) found that suppressing sadness was more taxing on the body than simply experiencing sadness (e.g., increased sympathetic activation of the cardiovascular system) in female college students. Participants instructed to suppress also endorsed less positive emotions than individuals who were not instructed to suppress (Gross & Levenson, 1997). Lynch, Robins, Morse, and Krause (2001) found that emotional inhibition, a construct related to emotional suppression, was associated with self-reported MDD symptoms and emotional inhibition mediated the relationship between negative affect intensity and self-reported MDD symptoms in both clinical and nonclinical samples.

## Behavioral Avoidance

Behavioral avoidance, as it relates to MDD, entails avoiding activities because of their emotionally eliciting nature. Specifically, Ferster (1973) argued that individuals' life spaces can become constricted when they are concerned about the possible rise of negative emotions because they feel that emotions cannot be managed. Behavioral avoidance can involve not taking the risks necessary to facilitate goal attainment due to the possibility that mistakes or failure could produce negative emotions (Blackledge & Hayes, 2001). Researchers have theorized that the onset and maintenance of MDD is the result of people orienting their lives around emotional avoidance and the avoidance of other aversive stimuli to the detriment of seeking out positive reinforcement, which leads to a reduced behavioral repertoire (Ferster, 1973; Jacobson, Martell, & Dimidjian, 2001; Martell, Addis, & Jacobson, 2001). Consistent with this line of reasoning, Ottenbreit and Dobson (2004) found that self-reported cognitive and behavioral avoidance in both social and nonsocial domains were related to self-reported MDD symptoms in college students.

## Emotional Distress Tolerance and Emotion Dysregulation in Major Depressive Disorder

Metacognitive reactions to emotions have received less attention than emotional regulation strategies in general and in MDD research specifically. Consequently, the relationship between emotional distress tolerance and emotion regulation strategies requires further examination. Could low emotion distress tolerance be a variable that affects the likelihood of engaging in certain maladaptive emotion regulation strategies? Logically, if an individual had low emotional distress tolerance regarding certain negative emotions, the likelihood of engaging in any emotion regulation strategy in response to the negative emotions could increase, and the likelihood of engaging in maladaptive emotional regulation strategies specifically could increase due to the individual exploring strategies that provide temporary or quick relief.

In relation to MDD, if an individual was generally unwilling to experience sadness or lack of happiness because of the perception that sadness, or lack of happiness, is highly aversive, harmful, and causes undue disruptions in his or her life (i.e., low emotional distress tolerance regarding sadness or lack of happiness), the likelihood of engaging in depressive rumination in order to "fix" the emotion, emotional suppression in order to end the emotion, or behavioral avoidance in order to avoid situations that produce the emotion could increase. For instance, Williams and colleagues (2007) theorized that viewing sadness or lack of happiness as a "problem" (i.e., the fist component of emotional distress tolerance) could lead to engaging in depressive rumination (i.e., maladaptive emotional regulation) and, subsequently, contribute to the onset and maintenance of MDD.

Indeed, Campbell-Sills and colleagues (2006) found that viewing emotions as unacceptable mediated the relationship between the intensity of negative emotions and the use of emotional suppression in patients with mood disorders, including MDD, and anxiety disorders. Mennin and colleagues (2007) found self-reported MDD symptoms to be associated with a latent factor of emotion dysregulation as well as the specific factors of negative cognitive reactivity (i.e., the first and second components of emotions distress tolerance) and maladaptive management of emotions (i.e., knowing how and when to diminish or enhance an emotional experience in a manner that is appropriate for a given context) in college students. Future research is needed to investigate possible relationships among low emotional distress tolerance, maladaptive emotion regulation strategies, and MDD.

## ASSESSMENTS, TREATMENT, AND EMOTIONAL DISTRESS TOLERANCE

### Clinical Assessments

Although there is no form of clinical assessment that reflects our definition of emotional distress tolerance, there are several self-report assessments that are relevant to the constructs that compose emotional distress tolerance.

The Acceptance and Action Questionnaire (AAQ; Hayes, Strosahl, et al., 2004) is a nine-item self-report measure of different aspects of experiential avoidance. The AAQ is related to measures of depressive symptoms, anxiety symptoms, and other measures of psychopathology and well-being (Hayes, Luoma, Bond, Masuda, & Lillis, 2006). The AAQ has only modest internal consistency ($\alpha$ = .7; Hayes, Strosahl, et al., 2004), and a second version, the 10-item AAQ-II ($\alpha$ = .85; Bond et al., 2009), was developed because of psychometric concerns regarding the first version. The ACS (Williams et al., 1997) is a 42-item self-report measure of fear of emotions and attempts to control emotions. It has four subscales that assess fear of anxiety, fear of depression, fear of anger, and fear of positive emotions. The ACS is internally consistent ($\alpha$ = .94), reliable (test–retest reliability over 2 weeks: $r$ = .78), related to emotional control, and related to fear of laboratory-induced bodily sensations (Williams et al., 1997).

The DERS (Gratz & Roemer, 2004) is a 36-item self-report measure that assesses six aspects of emotional regulation: ability to modulate emotions, emotional awareness, emotional understanding, emotional acceptance, impulse control, and ability to engage in goal-directed behavior during an emotional experience. The DERS is internally consistent ($\alpha$ = .93), and the subscales (i.e., Strategies, Awareness, Clarity, Nonacceptance, Goals, and Impulse) are differentially related to measures of experiential avoidance, emotional expressivity, self-injury, and partner abuse (Gratz & Roemer, 2004). Emotional distress tolerance is most relevant to the nonacceptance (i.e., the third component of emotional distress tolerance) and the Goals (i.e., the second component of emotional distress tolerance) subscales.

The Distress Tolerance Scale (DTS; Simons & Gaher, 2005) is a 15-item self-report measure of the toleration of emotional distress in terms of emotional aversiveness, emotion appraisal, attentional absorption as a result of emotions, and emotion regulation strategies. The DTS is internally consistent ($\alpha$ = .82) and reliable (test–retest reliability over 6 months: $r$ = .61) and is related to a measure of alcohol-related problems (Simons & Gaher, 2005).

Fresco, Moore, and colleagues' (2007) Experiences Questionnaire includes an 11-item self-report subscale to measure decentering. Decentering involves being able to view one's thoughts and emotions as temporary, objective events in the mind that do not necessarily constitute true information about the self (Fresco, Moore, et al., 2007). Decentering involves taking a present-moment, accepting, and nonjudgmental stance in regards to thoughts and emotions (Fresco, Segal, Buis, & Kennedy, 2007). Thus, decentering from one's emotions may be viewed as the converse of emotional distress intolerance. The Decentering subscale is internally consistent ($\alpha$ = .81 at pretreatment and $\alpha$ = .84 at posttreatment in a sample of patients with MDD; Fresco, Segal, et al., 2007) and is related to measures of MDD symptoms, depressive rumination, experiential avoidance, and emotion regulation in college students (Fresco, Moore, et al., 2007), MDD symptoms in remitted MDD patients (Fresco, Moore, et al., 2007), and likelihood of posttreatment relapse in MDD patients (Fresco, Segal, et al., 2007).

The 30-item NMR (Catanzaro & Mearns, 1990) is a self-report measure, which includes a Cognitive scale assessing beliefs about the ability to use cognitive strategies to alleviate negative mood, a Behavior scale assessing beliefs about the ability to use actions to alleviate negative mood, and a General scale assessing beliefs about the ability to alter negative mood. The NMR is internally consistent (Cronbach alphas range from $\alpha$ = .86–.92; Catanzaro & Mearns, 1990), reliable (test–retest reliability over 6–8 weeks range from .67 in men to .78 in women; Catanzaro & Mearns, 1990), and related to self-reported MDD symptoms in college students (Catanzaro, 1993; Kirsch et al., 1990), level of active coping strategies in college students (Kirsch et al., 1990), self-reported MDD symptoms in older adults, and avoidant coping strategies in older adults (Catanzaro et al., 1995).

## Treatment of Major Depressive Disorder

Many therapies targeting MDD address constructs related to low emotional distress tolerance, including lack of emotional acceptance (e.g., acceptance and commitment therapy [ACT]; Hayes et al., 1999), lack of emotional awareness (e.g., mindfulness-based cognitive therapy [MBCT]; Segal et al., 2002), lack of understanding of the functional nature of emotions (emotionally-focused therapy [EFT]; Greenberg & Watson, 2005), and maladaptive action tendencies stemming from negative emotions (e.g., Behavioral Activation [BA]; Jacobson et al., 2001). In addition, emotion regulation therapy (ERT; Mennin & Fresco, 2009) applies the emotional dysregulation model to the treatment of GAD, which includes increasing emotional awareness, emotional acceptance, and understanding of the functional nature of emotions. As the emotional dysregulation model has been shown to be associated with MDD and SAD as well as GAD (Mennin et al., 2007), ERT will likely be adapted to more specifically address co-occurring MDD in the future.

Incorporating research and theory regarding emotional processes in MDD is showing promise for the treatment of this recurrent disorder, as support has been found for the efficacy of MBCT (e.g., Teasdale et al., 2000), ACT (e.g., Hayes, Masuda, Bissett, Luoma, & Guerrero, 2004), EFT (e.g., Watson, Gordon, Stermac, Kalogerakos, & Steckley, 2003), and BA (e.g., Dimidjian et al., 2006) in treating MDD.

## DISCUSSION, LIMITATIONS, AND FUTURE DIRECTIONS

MDD conceptualizations (e.g., Teasdale, 1999) and treatment (e.g., Hayes et al., 1999) have increasingly paid attention to the role of emotion in the onset and maintenance of MDD. In this chapter, we strived to demonstrate the usefulness of emotional distress tolerance as a framework for integrating findings regarding metacognitive reactions to emotions, psychopathology, and MDD. Specifically, appraisals of the negativity and/or threat value of negative emotional experiences, beliefs regarding ability to cope with negative emotional experiences, and willingness to undergo negative emotional experiences may be important components of emotion distress tolerance that, with further research, may show relevance to understanding emotional factors in MDD. This chapter also discussed maladaptive emotion regulation strategies in MDD such as depressive rumination (e.g., Just & Alloy, 1997), emotional suppression (e.g., Gross & John, 2003) and behavioral avoidance (e.g., Ottenbreit & Dobson, 2004), which may contribute to the onset and maintenance of MDD.

Although speculative, low emotional distress tolerance may be a relevant variable in understanding why individuals with MDD utilize certain maladaptive emotion regulation strategies. Future research is needed to examine whether low emotional distress tolerance is a characteristic of MDD, a causal factor in MDD, a characteristic of the employment of maladaptive emotion regulation strategies, and/or a causal factor in employment of maladaptive emotion regulation strategies. Conceptually, low emotional distress tolerance may be a vulnerability factor that may directly or indirectly increase the likelihood of MDD through the employment of maladaptive emotion regulation strategies.

Future research is also needed to examine the mutual interactions between the three components of emotion distress tolerance. Certain components may lead to more detrimental consequences, or may be more relevant to certain forms of psychopathology, than other components. Emotional distress tolerance can be examined in the context of sadness, fear, anger, and disgust to investigate whether people can have differing levels of emotional distress tolerance for different negative emotions. Currently, there is no single assessment measure that would allow for the separate examination of the three components as well as an examination of a general factor of emotional distress tolerance. After such an assessment measure has been identified/developed, emotional distress tolerance would be best examined by assessing how individuals tend to view negative emotions in general as well as how they view the negative emotions they are currently experiencing (e.g., in response to an emotional induction in the laboratory).

## REFERENCES

American Psychiatric Association. (2000). *Diagnostic and statistical manual of mental disorders* (4th ed., text rev.). Washington, DC: Author.

Armey, M. F., Moore, M. T., Fresco, D. M., Mennin, D. S., Turk, C. L., Heimberg, R. G., et al. (2009). Brooding and pondering: Isolating the active ingredients of depressive rumination with confirmatory factor analysis. *Assessment, 16,* 315–327.

Bagby, R. M., Parker, J. D., & Taylor, G. J. (1994). The twenty-item Toronto Alexithymia Scale: I. Item selection and cross-validation of the factor structure. *Journal of Psychosomatic Research, 38,* 23–32.

Barlow, D. H. (1991). Disorders of emotion. *Psychological Inquiry, 2,* 58–71.

Berg, C. Z., Shapiro, N., Chambless, D. L., & Ahrens, A. H. (1998). Are emotions frightening? II: An analogue study of fear of emotion, interpersonal conflict, and panic onset. *Behaviour Research and Therapy, 36,* 3–15.

Blackledge, J. T., & Hayes, S. C. (2001). Emotion regulation in acceptance and commitment therapy. *Journal of Clinical Psychology, 57,* 243–255.

Bond, F. W., Hayes, S. C., Baer, R. A., Carpenter, K. M., Orcutt, H. K., Waltz, T, et al. (2009). *Preliminary psychometric properties of the Acceptance and Action Questionnaire—II: A revised measure of psychological flexibility and acceptance.* Manuscript submitted for publication.

Campbell-Sills, L., & Barlow, D. H. (2007). Incorporating emotion regulation into conceptualizations and treatments of anxiety and mood disorders. In J. J. Gross (Ed.), *Handbook of emotion regulation* (pp. 542–559). New York: Guilford Press.

Campbell-Sills, L., Barlow, D. H., Brown, T. A., & Hofmann, S. G. (2006). Acceptability and suppression of negative emotion in anxiety and mood disorders. *Emotion, 6,* 587–595.

Carver, C. S., & Scheier, M. F. (1998). *On the self-regulation of behavior.* New York: Cambridge University Press.

Catanzaro, S. J. (1993). Mood regulation expectancies, anxiety sensitivity, and emotional distress. *Journal of Abnormal Psychology, 102,* 327–330.

Catanzaro, S. J., Horaney, F., & Creasey, G. (1995). Hassles, coping, and depressive symptoms in an elderly community sample: The role of mood regulation expectancies. *Journal of Counseling Psychology, 42,* 259–265.

Catanzaro, S. J., & Mearns, J. (1990). Measuring generalized expectancies for negative mood regulation: Initial scale development and implications. *Journal of Personality Assessment, 54,* 546–565.

Cicchetti, D., Ackerman, B. P., & Izard, C. E. (1995). Emotions and emotion regulation in developmental psychopathology. *Development and Psychopathology, 7,* 1–10.

Clore, G. L., & Ortony, A. (2000). Cognition in emotion: Always, sometimes, or never? In R. D. Lane & L. Nadel (Eds.), *Cognitive neuroscience of emotion* (pp. 13–24). New York: Oxford University Press.

Cole, P. M., Martin, S. E., & Dennis, T. A. (2004). Emotion regulation as a scientific construct: Methodological challenges and directions for child development research. *Child Development, 75,* 317–333.

Davidson, R. J., Pizzagalli, D., Nitschke, J. B., & Putnam, K. (2002). Depression: Perspectives from affective neuroscience. *Annual Review of Psychology, 53,* 545–574.

Dimidjian, S., Hollon, S. D., Dobson, K. S., Schmaling, K. B., Kohlenberg, R. J., Addis, M. E., et al. (2006). Randomized trial of behavioral activation, cognitive therapy, and antidepressant medication in the acute treatment of adults with major depression. *Journal of Consulting and Clinical Psychology, 74,* 658–670.

Ehring, T., Fischer, S., Schnulle, J., Bosterling, A., & Tuschen-Caffier, B. (2008). Characteristics of emotion regulation in recovered depressed versus never depressed individuals. *Personality and Individual Differences, 44,* 1574–1584.

Ferster, C. B. (1973). A functional analysis of depression. *American Psychologist, 28,* 857–870.

Flavell, J. H. (1978). Metacognitive development. In J. M. Scandura & C. J. Brainerd (Eds.), *Structural/process theories of complex human behavior* (pp. 34–78). Alphen an den Rijn, the Netherlands: Sijthoff & Noordhoff.

Fredrickson, B. L. (2001). The role of positive emotions in positive psychology: The broaden-and-build theory of positive emotions. *American Psychologist, 56,* 218–226.

Fresco, D. M., Moore, M. T., van Dulmen, M., Segal, Z. V., Ma, S. H., Teasdale, J. D., et al. (2007). Initial psychometric properties of the Experiences Questionnaire: A self-report survey of decentering. *Behavior Therapy, 38,* 234–246.

Fresco, D. M., Rytwinski, N. K., & Craighead, L. W. (2007). Explanatory flexibility and negative life events interact to predict depression symptoms. *Journal of Social and Clinical Psychology, 26,* 595–608.

Fresco, D. M., Segal, Z. V., Buis, T., & Kennedy, S. (2007). Relationship of posttreatment decentering and cognitive reactivity to relapse in major depression. *Journal of Consulting and Clinical Psychology, 75,* 447–455.

Fresco, D. M., Williams, N. L., & Nugent, N. R. (2006). Flexibility and negative affect: Examining the associations of explanatory flexibility and coping flexibility to each other and to depression and anxiety. *Cognitive Therapy and Research, 30,* 201–210.

Garnefski, N., & Kraaij, V. (2006). Relationships between cognitive emotion regulation strategies and depressive symptoms: A comparative study of five specific samples. *Personality and Individual Differences, 40,* 1659–1669.

Goldstein, A. J., & Chambless, D. L. (1978). A reanalysis of agoraphobia. *Behavior Therapy, 9,* 47–59.

Gratz, K. L., & Roemer, L. (2004). Multidimensional assessment of emotion regulation and dysregulation: Development, factor structure, and initial validation of the difficulties in emotion regulation scale. *Journal of Psychopathology and Behavioral Assessment, 26,* 41–54.

Gray, J. A., & McNaughton, N. (2000). *The neuropsychology of anxiety: An enquiry into the functions of the septo-hippocampal system* (2nd ed.). New York: Oxford University Press.

Greenberg, L. S. (2002). *Emotion-focused therapy: Coaching clients to work through their feelings.* Washington, DC: American Psychological Association.

Greenberg, L. S., & Watson, J. (2005). *Emotion-focused therapy of depression.* Washington, DC: American Psychological Association.

Gross, J. J. (1998). The emerging field of emotion regulation: An integrative review. *Review of General Psychology, 2,* 271–299.

Gross, J. J., & John, P. (2003). Individual differences in two emotion regulation processes: Implications for affect, relationships, and well-being. *Journal of Personality and Social Psychology, 85,* 348–362.

Gross, J. J., & Levenson, R. W. (1997). Hiding feelings: The acute effects of inhibiting positive and negative emotions. *Journal of Abnormal Psychology, 106,* 95–103.

Gross, J. J., & Muñoz, R. F. (1995). Emotion regulation and mental health. *Clinical Psychology: Science and Practice, 2,* 151–164.

Hayes, S. C., Luoma, J., Bond, F., Masuda, A., & Lillis, J. (2006). Acceptance and commitment therapy: Model, processes, and outcomes. *Behaviour Research and Therapy, 44,* 1–25.

Hayes, S. C., Masuda, A., Bissett, R., Luoma, J., & Guerrero, L. F. (2004). DBT, FAR and ACT: How empirically oriented are the new behavior therapy technologies? *Behavior Therapy, 35,* 35–54.

Hayes, S. C., Strosahl, K. D., & Wilson, K. G. (1999). *Acceptance and commitment therapy: An experimental approach to behavior change.* New York: Guilford Press.

Hayes, S. C., Strosahl, K. D., Wilson, K. G., Bissett, R. T., Pastorally, J., Taormina, D., et al. (2004). Measuring experiential avoidance: A preliminary test of a working model. *Psychological Record, 54,* 553–578.

Hayes, S. C., Wilson, K. G., Gifford, E. V., Follette, V. M., & Strosahl, K. (1996). Experiential avoidance and behavioral disorders: A functional dimensional approach to diagnosis and treatment. *Journal of Consulting and Clinical Psychology, 64,* 1152–1168.

Higgins, E. T. (1997). Beyond pleasure and pain. *American Psychologist, 52,* 1280–1300.

Jacobson, N. S., Martell, C. R., & Dimidjian, S. (2001). Behavioral activation treatment for depression: Returning to contextual roots. *Clinical Psychology: Science and Practice, 8,* 255–270.

Judd, L. L., & Kunovac, J. L. (1997). Diagnosis and classification of depression. In A. Honig & H. M van Praag (Eds.), *Depression: Neurobiological, psychopathological, and therapeutic advances* (pp. 3–16). Hoboken, NJ: Wiley.

Just, N., & Alloy, L. B. (1997). The response styles theory of depression: Tests and an extension of the theory. *Journal of Abnormal Psychology, 106,* 221–229.

Keltner, D., & Haidt, J. (1999). Social functions of emotions at four levels of analysis. *Cognition and Emotion, 13,* 505–521.

Kessler, R. C., Chiu, W. T., Demler, O., Merikangas, K. R., & Walters, E. E. (2005). Prevalence, severity, and comorbidity of 12-month DSM-IV disorders in the National Comorbidity Survey replication. *Archives of General Psychiatry, 62,* 617–627.

Kirsch, I., Mearns, J., & Catanzaro, S. J. (1990). Mood-regulation expectancies as determinants of dysphoria in college students. *Journal of Counseling Psychology, 37,* 306–312.

Kring, A. M., & Werner, K. H. (2004). Emotion regulation and psychopathology. In P. Philippot & R. S. Feldman (Eds.), *The regulation of emotion* (pp. 359–385). Mahwah, NJ: Erlbaum.

Lazarus, R. S., & Folkman, S. (1984). *Stress, appraisal, and coping.* New York: Springer.

Leahy, R. L. (2002). A model of emotional schemas. *Cognitive and Behavioral Practice, 9,* 177–190.

LeDoux, J. E. (1996). *The emotional brain: The mysterious underpinnings of emotional life.* New York: Simon & Schuster.

Lynch, T. R., Robins, C. J., Morse, J. Q., & Krause, E. D. (2001). A mediational model relating affect intensity, emotion inhibition, and psychological distress. *Behavior Therapy, 32,* 519–536.

Maller, R. G., & Reiss, S. (1992). Anxiety sensitivity in 1984 and panic attacks in 1987. *Journal of Anxiety Disorders, 6,* 241–247.

Martell, C. R., Addis, M. E., & Jacobson, N. S. (2001). *Depression in context: Strategies for guided action.* New York: W. W. Norton.

Mayer, J. D., Salovey, P., & Caruso, D. (2004). Emotional intelligence: Theory, findings, and implications. *Psychological Inquiry, 15,* 197–215.

McNally, R. J., & Eke, M. (1996). Anxiety sensitivity, suffocation fear, and breath-holding duration as predictors of response to carbon dioxide challenge. *Journal of Abnormal Psychology, 105,* 146–149.

Mennin, D. S., & Fresco, D. M. (2009). Emotion regulation as an integrative framework for understanding and treating psychopathology. In A. M. Kring & D. M. Sloan (Ed.), *Emotion regulation and psychopathology: A trans-*

*diagnostic approach to etiology and treatment* (pp. 356–379). New York: Guilford Press.

Mennin, D. S., Heimberg, R., Turk, C., & Fresco, D. (2005). Preliminary evidence for an emotion dysregulation model of generalized anxiety disorder. *Behaviour Research and Therapy, 43,* 1281–1310.

Mennin, D. S., Holaway, R. M., Fresco, D. M., Moore, M. T., & Heimberg, R. G. (2007). Delineating components of emotion and its dysregulation in anxiety and mood psychopathology. *Behavior Therapy, 38,* 284–302.

Mennin, D. S., McLaughlin, K. A., & Flanagan, T. J. (2009). Emotion regulation deficits in generalized anxiety disorder, social anxiety disorder, and their co-occurrence. *Journal of Anxiety Disorders, 23,* 866–871.

Morris, B. H., Bylsma, L. M., & Rottenberg, J. (2009). Does emotion predict the course of major depressive disorder?: A review of prospective studies. *British Journal of Clinical Psychology, 48,* 255–273.

Nolen-Hoeksema, S. (1991). Responses to depression and their effects on the duration of depressive episodes. *Journal of Abnormal Psychology, 100,* 569–582.

Nolen-Hoeksema, S. (2000). The role of rumination in depressive disorders and mixed anxiety/depressive symptoms. *Journal of Abnormal Psychology, 109,* 504–511.

Ottenbreit, N. D., & Dobson, S. (2004). Avoidance and depression: The construction of the Cognitive-Behavioral Avoidance Scale. *Behaviour Research and Therapy, 42,* 293–313.

Otto, M., Powers, M., & Fischmann, D. (2005). Emotional exposure in the treatment of substance use disorders: Conceptual model, evidence, and future directions. *Clinical Psychology Review, 25,* 824–839.

Parrott, W. G. (2001). Implications of dysfunctional emotions for understanding how emotions function. *Review of General Psychology, 5,* 180–186.

Reiss, S. (1991). Expectancy model of fear, anxiety, and panic. *Clinical Psychology Review, 11,* 141–153.

Roberts, J. E., Gilboa, E., & Gotlib, I. H. (1998). Ruminative response style and vulnerability to episodes of dysphoria: Gender, neuroticism, and episode duration. *Cognitive Therapy and Research, 22,* 401–423.

Roemer, L., Salters, K., Raffa, S. D., & Orsillo, S. M. (2005). Fear and avoidance of internal experiences in GAD: Preliminary tests of a conceptual model. *Cognitive Therapy and Research, 29,* 71–88.

Rottenberg, J., Gross, J. J., & Gotlib, I. H. (2005). Emotion context insensitivity in major depressive disorder. *Journal of Abnormal Psychology, 114,* 627–639.

Rude, S. S., & McCarthy, T. (2003). Emotional functioning in depressed and depression-vulnerable college students. *Cognition and Emotion, 17,* 799–806.

Salovey, P., Stroud, L. R., Woolery, A., & Epel, E. S. (2002). Perceived emotional intelligence, stress reactivity, and symptom reports: Further explorations using the trait meta-mood scale. *Psychology and Health, 17,* 611–627.

Salters-Pedneault, K., Roemer, L., Tull, M. T., Rucker, L., & Mennin, D. S. (2006). Evidence of broad deficits in emotion regulation associated with chronic worry and generalized anxiety disorder. *Cognitive Therapy and Research, 30,* 469–480.

Samoilov, A., & Goldfried, M. R. (2000). Role of emotion in cognitive-behavior therapy. *Clinical Psychology: Science and Practice, 7,* 373–385.

Schmidt, N. B., Lerew, D. R., & Jackson, R. J. (1999). Prospective evaluation of anxiety sensitivity in the pathogenesis of panic: Replication and extension. *Journal of Abnormal Psychology, 108,* 532–537.

Segal, Z. V., Williams, M. G., & Teasdale, J. D. (2002). *Mindfulness-based cognitive therapy for depression.* New York: Guilford Press.

Simons, J., & Gaher, R. (2005). The Distress Tolerance Scale: Development and validation of a self-report measure. *Motivation and Emotion, 29,* 83–102.

Taylor, S., & Rachman, J. (1991). Fear of sadness. *Journal of Anxiety Disorders, 5,* 375–381.

Teasdale, J. D. (1999). Emotional processing, three modes of mind and the prevention of relapse in depression. *Behaviour Research and Therapy, 37,* S53–S77.

Teasdale, J. D., Segal, Z. V., Williams, J. M. G., Ridgeway, V. A., Soulsby, J. M., & Lau, M. A. (2000). Prevention of relapse/recurrence in major depression by mindfulness-based cognitive therapy. *Journal of Consulting and Clinical Psychology, 68,* 615–623.

Watkins, E., & Baracaia, S. (2001). Why do people ruminate in dysphoric moods? *Personality and Individual Differences, 30,* 723–734.

Watson, J. C., Gordon, L. B., Stermac, L., Kalogerakos, F., & Steckley, P. (2003). Comparing the effectiveness of process-experiential with cognitive-behavioral psychotherapy in the treatment of depression. *Journal of Consulting and Clinical Psychology, 71,* 773–781.

Wells, A. (1995). Meta-cognition and worry: A cognitive model of generalized anxiety disorder. *Behavioural and Cognitive Psychotherapy, 23,* 301–320.

Williams, J. M. G., Teasdale, J. D., Segal, Z. V., & Kabat-Zinn, J. (2007). *The mindful way through depression: Freeing yourself from chronic unhappiness.* New York: Guilford Press.

Williams, K. E., Chambless, D. L., & Ahrens, A. (1997). Are emotions frightening?: An extension of the fear of fear construct. *Behaviour Research and Therapy, 35,* 239–248.

Zvolensky, M. J., Goodie, J. L., Ruggiero, K. J., Black, A. L., Larkin, K. T., & Taylor, B. K. (2002). Perceived stress and anxiety sensitivity in the prediction of anxiety-related responding: A multichallenge evaluation. *Anxiety, Stress, and Coping, 15,* 211–229.

Zvolensky, M. J., & Otto, M. (2007). Affective intolerance, sensitivity, and processing: Advances in clinical science introduction. *Behavior Therapy, 38,* 228–233.

# 8

# Substance Use Disorders

Jessica M. Richards, Stacey B. Daughters,
Marina A. Bornovalova, Richard A. Brown,
*and* Carl W. Lejuez

Substance use disorders are chronically relapsing disorders characterized by continued use of alcohol or drugs despite negative consequences, tolerance to drug effects, and withdrawal symptoms upon cessation. These disorders are associated with serious public health and economic consequences, including increases in unemployment (Luck, Elifson, & Sterk, 2004), homelessness (e.g., Nyamathi, Wenzel, Keenan, Leake, & Gelberg, 1999), crime (e.g., Friedman, Glassman, & Terras, 2001), and rates of sexually transmitted diseases such as HIV (e.g., Avants, Marcotte, Arnold, & Margolin, 2003; Ensminger, Anthony, & McCord, 1997; Miller & Neaigus, 2002). Despite the high costs of substance use, 22.3 million people ages 12 years and older were classified with substance dependence or abuse as of 2007 (9% of this population; Substance Abuse and Mental Health Services Administration, 2008), and relapse rates remain high (e.g., Monti, Rohsenow, Michalec, Martin, & Abrams, 1997; Morgenstern, Blanchard, Morgan, Labouvie, & Hayaki, 2001).

Given the high cost and prevalence of substance use disorders, researchers have examined potential mechanisms that may serve as targets for assessment and intervention. The goal of this chapter is to examine distress tolerance as a potential mechanism. Distress tolerance has received considerable attention recently and appears to be an important variable for understanding substance use development and relapse. We begin with background information and theoretical rationale for examining distress tolerance in substance use. Next, we review the empirical literature on distress tolerance among substance users, discuss theoretical implications of extant findings, review clinical interventions that have been developed to treat substance users with low distress tolerance, and provide a case example to illustrate the application of specific clinical strategies to increase distress tolerance among substance users.

## BACKGROUND

In examining the potential mechanisms that may underlie substance use and relapse, a long history of evidence implicates the role of environmental stressors and subsequent affective distress. For example, exposure to chronic and acute stressors such as childhood emotional, physical, and sexual abuse as well as trauma experiences are associated with increased risk for addiction and with early initiation of substance use (e.g., Bender, Ferguson, Thompson, Komlo, & Pollio, 2010; Bensley, Spieker, Van Eenwyk, & Schoder, 1999; Najavits et al., 1998; Widom, Weiler, & Cottler, 1999). Additionally, high levels of social and environmental stress have been associated with a rapid progression in tobacco, marijuana, and alcohol use (Kaplan & Johnson, 1992; Wills, McNamara, Vaccaro, & Hirky, 1996). Furthermore, direct exposure to acute stress has been shown to increase desire to smoke and the subsequent number and duration of puffs in smokers (Payne, Schare, Levis, & Colletti, 1991) and to increase drug craving among cocaine users (Sinha, Catapano, & O'Malley, 1999).

Specific to relapse, affective distress also may be elicited by withdrawal symptoms during early abstinence, which themselves can serve as significant stressors. Negative affect often arises in addicted individuals as a result of withdrawal syndromes, which cause feelings of irritability, anxiety, stress, and depression (Baker, Japuntich, Hogle, McCarthy, & Curtin, 2006), and the severity of these withdrawal symptoms predicts treatment outcome and relapse across drug classes (Carroll, Power, Bryant, & Rounsaville, 1993; Doherty, Kinnunen, Militello, & Garvey, 1995; McLellan, Luborsky, Woody, O'Brien, & Druley, 1983; Mulvaney, Alterman, Boardman, & Kampman, 1999; Tennant, Shannon, Nork, Sagherian, & Berman, 1991).

Despite the utility of considering affective distress as a predictor of substance use from initiation through relapse, many individuals who experience heightened negative affect can resist the urge to initiate or relapse to substance use. Conversely, some individuals resort to substance use following only slight elevations in negative affect. As such, affective distress alone is not an adequate predictor of substance use initiation or treatment outcomes. An alternative perspective suggests that, in addition to severity of affective distress, one's ability to tolerate distress may impact substance use outcomes (Brown, Lejuez, Kahler, Strong, & Zvolensky, 2005). That is, individuals with a diminished ability to tolerate distress may use substances to escape from distress, thereby maintaining substance use through negative reinforcement, or the reduction or avoidance of aversive internal states. This vulnerability is particularly relevant to substance use, as Baker, Piper, McCarthy, Majeskie, and Fiore (2004) concluded from their review of a wealth of theory and data, suggesting that "escape or avoidance of negative affect is the principal motive for addictive drug use" (p. 33). Thus, a comprehensive understanding of substance use development and relapse requires investigation not only of individual differences in affective distress but also differences in individuals' ability to tolerate distress without resorting to negative reinforcement behaviors, including substance use.

One construct that may provide a useful index of negative reinforcement vulnerability is distress tolerance, defined as the ability to persist in goal-directed activity in the face of aversive psychological and/or physical stress. The construct of distress tolerance has particular relevance as an index of negative reinforcement processes in the field of substance use and relapse because many addictive substances are effective in alleviating both physical and psychological distress (e.g., Mello & Mendelson, 1970; Parrott, 1999; Wikler, 1977; Zinser, Baker, Sherman, & Cannon, 1992). Thus, individuals with high distress tolerance may be most capable of persisting in their long-term goal of abstinence from substance use, even when abstinence is accompanied by physical and psychological distress. Conversely, individuals who have low distress tolerance may be at the greatest risk of terminating their goal-directed behavior (i.e., abstinence) in times of psychological stress and giving in to the negative reinforcing effects of most drugs of abuse.

## MEASUREMENTS OF DISTRESS TOLERANCE

To assess one's ability to tolerate affective distress, researchers first developed performance-based challenge tasks to examine the role of psychological distress tolerance in substance use and relapse. In brief, participants are asked to engage in a task that gradually increases in difficulty, to the point where the task becomes virtually impossible to complete successfully. Furthermore, participants are inundated with constant negative feedback, including aversive noises and repeated failure, which is designed to increase emotional distress. Participants have the option to persist in order to receive a small reward or to terminate the task, thereby reducing affective distress in the short term but losing out on potential long-term rewards. Distress tolerance is measured continuously as latency in seconds to task termination or categorically as high distress tolerance (i.e., persisting for the entire task duration) versus low distress tolerance (i.e., premature task termination).

The earliest work linking persistence through with tolerance of a psychologically stressful task utilized the anagram persistence task (APT), in which participants are asked to solve a series of difficult anagrams, and the mirror-tracing persistence task (MTPT), in which participants must trace difficult geometric shapes while looking at the shape only through a mirror, rendering all aspects of the shapes reversed (e.g., Quinn, Brandon, & Copeland, 1996). Later, computerized versions of challenge tasks were developed, including the paced auditory serial addition task (PASAT-C; Lejuez, Kahler, & Brown, 2003), which is a difficult mathematical processing task, and the MTPT-C (Strong et al., 2003). All of the tasks are extremely challenging and include an option to terminate the tasks before their scheduled end time to allow for assessment of distress tolerance.

In addition to performance-based challenge tasks, physical challenges have also been utilized to assess distress tolerance. For example, Hajek and colleagues (Hajek, 1989; Hajek, Belcher, & Stapleton, 1987) measured breath-holding duration among smokers in order to assess one's ability to tolerate uncomfortable physical sensations. Other physical challenges that have been used to assess distress tolerance include cold-pressor tasks (e.g., Daughters, Lejuez, Bornovalova, et al., 2005), inhalation of carbon dioxide ($CO_2$)–enriched air (e.g., Brown, Lejuez, Kahler, & Strong, 2002), and voluntary hyperventilation (e.g., Marshall et al., 2008). Physical distress tolerance is generally measured continuously as persistence in seconds on the tasks or categorically as low or high distress tolerance (i.e., quit or persist on the tasks).

Several lines of evidence support the construct validity of performance-based and physiological challenge tasks as measures of distress tolerance among substance users. First, performance-based challenge tasks, including the PASAT-C and MTPT-C, have consistently been shown to increase self-reported ratings of affective distress, including feelings of anger, frustration, irritability, and anxiety across a wide range of samples (e.g., Bornovalova et al., 2008; Brown et al., 2002; Daughters, Lejuez, Bornovalova, et al., 2005; Daughters, Lejuez, Kahler, et al., 2005; Lejuez et al., 2003). Furthermore, subjective feelings of distress during performance-based challenge tasks have been corroborated using physiological measures such as heart rate and skin conductance (e.g.,

Lejuez et al., 2003), thus emphasizing the ability of the tasks to induce an elevation in distress. Additionally, performance on both physical and performance-based challenge tasks has been shown to prospectively predict theoretically relevant substance use outcomes such as smoking relapse and substance use treatment dropout, as outlined later in the chapter (e.g., Brandon et al., 2003; Brown et al., 2009; Daughters, Lejuez, Bornovalova, et al., 2005), suggesting that willingness to remain in contact with aversive internal experiences while persisting on the tasks is predictive of one's ability to withstand aversive sensations in the context of substance use abstinence, thereby supporting the construct validity of these tasks.

Despite the available evidence supporting the construct validity of distress tolerance tasks among substance users, some have proposed that these assessments may actually assess persistence (i.e., propensity to maintain a behavior related to reward contingencies) (Cloninger, Przybeck, & Švrakic, 1991) rather than distress tolerance because investigators frequently utilize rewards for persistence. However, performance incentives (usually small monetary sums) that are most commonly utilized in these tasks are small and intentionally described vaguely (e.g., "Your compensation is dependent on your performance") in order to mirror the real world, in which persistence toward a goal, such as abstinence from substance use, may only result in small or vague rewards, such as a smile or other small signs of approval from a family member. An alternative explanation may be that performance-based tasks measure distress tolerance by assessing one's motivation to seek negative reinforcement by terminating the task, relative to one's motivation to seek positive reinforcement by persisting in the hope of earning vague rewards (Leyro, Zvolensky, & Bernstein, 2010). Given the abundant behavioral, self-report, and physiological data in support of the tasks, as well as the ecological validity of the administration procedures that are used, performance-based and physiological measures of distress tolerance appear to be promising tools for assessing distress tolerance among substance users. More research is needed to clarify how performance on these tasks relates to other constructs that are theoretically related to distress tolerance, such as stress reactivity, emotion regulation, and coping, in order to provide further support for their validity.

More recently, self-report measures have also been developed to assess distress tolerance. Specifically, the Distress Tolerance Scale (DTS; Simons & Gaher, 2005) was developed as an index of one's ability to withstand negative emotional states, and the Discomfort Intolerance Scale (DIS; Schmidt, Richey, & Fitzpatrick, 2006) was developed to assess one's capacity to tolerate uncomfortable physical sensations. Self-report measures are somewhat new, yet there are promising data indicating high internal consistency, adequate test–retest reliability (Schmidt et al., 2006; Simons & Gaher, 2005), and validity as evidenced by relationships between the DTS and theoretically relevant affect-related factors, including positive affect ($r = .26$), mood acceptance ($r = .47$), and mood regulation expectancies ($r = .54$), as well as modest inverse relationships with both alcohol ($r = -.23$) and marijuana ($r = -.20$) coping motives, suggesting that low distress tolerance is associated with an increased propensity to use substances to alleviate negative affect (all $ps < .05$; Simons & Gaher, 2005). Similarly, the DIS has been related to anxious and fearful responding to bodily sensations among nonclinical populations (e.g., Schmidt & Trakowski, 1999) as well as motives to use tobacco specifically for habitual, addictive, and negative affect reduction reasons, but not other types of motives (Leyro, Zvolensky, Vujanovic, & Bernstein, 2008). As such, the limited available work has provided initial support for the construct validity of the DTS and DIS as measures of distress tolerance among substance users.

Despite the growing body of work supporting the validity of both performance-based and self-report methods of assessing distress tolerance, several unpublished studies from our laboratory as well as others suggest that self-report measures of distress tolerance are rarely related to persistence on performance-based and physiological challenge tasks. As such, additional research is needed to clarify the relationships between these two methodological approaches to assessing distress tolerance among substance users and to understand the extent to which they are all capturing the construct of distress tolerance.

## REVIEW OF RELEVANT EMPIRICAL LITERATURE

### Substance Use Initiation

Evidence suggests that distress tolerance plays a significant role across the stages of substance use, beginning with initiation. For example, Daughters and colleagues (2009) used an adolescent version of the PASAT-C, the Behavioral Indicator of Resilience to Distress (BIRD), to examine the relationship between distress tolerance and past year internalizing symptoms and externalizing behavior among a sample of 231 European American and African American preadolescents (age range at study enrollment = 9–13 years; $M = 10.9$ years). Findings suggested interesting moderating relationships such that low distress tolerance was associated with an increased risk of alcohol use among European Americans (odds ratio [OR] = 0.37, 95% [confidence interval [CI] = 0.17–0.79, $p < .01$), delinquent behavior among African Americans ($B = 1.24$, $sr^2 = 0.09$, $p <$

.001), and internalizing symptoms among females ($\beta$ = 9.40, $sr^2$ = 0.05, $p < .05$). Thus, findings from this study suggest that low distress tolerance may increase the risk of early alcohol use initiation among some populations and increase the prevalence of factors such as delinquency and internalizing symptoms that may increase the risk of future engagement in substance use among other populations. The relatively small effects observed in this study may be explained by the low base rates of alcohol use, delinquent behaviors, and internalizing symptoms that were reported in this young sample, thus emphasizing the need to extend research to older adolescents, who may report higher rates of negative outcomes.

Next, MacPherson and colleagues (2009) examined the combined influence of appetitive and negative reinforcement processes on risk-taking behaviors in a prospective study involving a larger sample from which the Daughters data were collected ($n$ = 277). Using the BIRD as well as a behavioral assessment of risk-taking propensity, researchers found that risk-taking propensity interacted with distress tolerance, such that levels of self-reported risky behaviors, including cigarette smoking and alcohol use, were highest among individuals with high risk-taking propensity and low distress tolerance ($\beta$ = 0.29, $\Delta R^2$ = .04, $p < .001$). Results from this study highlighted the importance of considering both positive and negative reinforcement processes when investigating vulnerability factors for early risk behavior engagement in youth. Additionally, these findings provide further support for a theoretical framework for substance use initiation that includes distress tolerance as an important mechanism underlying substance use prior to the development of drug dependence. Furthermore, these two studies emphasize the need for additional research to explore the moderating relationships between distress tolerance and other individual difference factors in predicting substance use initiation among children and adolescents.

## Substance-Use Engagement and Previous Abstinence Durations

As individuals progress from early experimentation to drug dependence, ample evidence suggests that both physical and psychological distress tolerance may be crucial for distinguishing substance users from nonusers. Quinn and colleagues (1996) administered two difficult paper-and-pencil challenge tasks (the APT and MTPT), with persistence serving as the index of distress tolerance, to 52 heavy smokers and 57 nonsmokers. Nonsmokers were more persistent than smokers on both tasks (APT: $F(1, 93)$ = 12.26, $p < .001$; MTPT: $F(1, 91)$ = 7.24, $p < .05$), even after controlling for cognitive ability, levels of drug and alcohol use, and positive and negative affect. Furthermore, individuals with substance abuse histories tended to be less persistent than those without such histories, even after controlling for smoking status, supporting the premise that substance abusers evidence higher rates of distress intolerance than the general population.

In addition to distinguishing smokers from nonsmokers, distress tolerance paradigms also have been used to identify individuals within substance-using populations who report a history of early lapse to substance use. For example, Brown and colleagues (2002) utilized two physical challenges, including inhalations of $CO_2$-enriched air and a timed breath-holding procedure, as well as one performance-based challenge task (i.e., the PASAT-C) to examine the differences between current smokers who reported a quit history of immediate relapses (abstinence durations of < 24 hours; $n$ = 16) versus delayed relapses (quit for at least 3 months; $n$ = 16). Immediate relapsers were characterized by higher baseline levels of affective vulnerability, greater levels of dysphoria and urge to smoke following 12-hour nicotine deprivation, and less persistence on the PASAT-C compared with delayed relapsers (adjusted OR [AOR] = 4.6, $p$ = .03). Immediate relapsers were also significantly more likely to quit the $CO_2$ challenge (AOR = 12.2, $p$ = .03) and had shorter breath-holding durations, $t(30)$ = 2.46, $p$ = .02, compared with delayed relapsers. The larger observed effect size using the $CO_2$ challenge as opposed to the PASAT-C may suggest that among smokers persistence on physical challenge tasks may be a more accurate index of one's ability to persist in a smoking abstinence attempt. Although these findings conflicted with one earlier study examining breath-holding among smokers (Zvolensky, Feldner, Eifert, & Brown, 2001), this may have been due to the smaller sample size and methodological differences in the earlier study.

Applying performance-based measures of distress tolerance to illicit drug users, Daughters, Lejuez, Kahler, and colleagues (2005) utilized the PASAT-C to assess the relationship between distress tolerance and self-reported relapse history among 89 illicit drug-abusing individuals in an inner-city residential substance abuse treatment facility. Distress intolerance was related to shorter previous abstinence durations beyond the influence of demographics, substance use level, and negative affect ($B$ = 0.002, $SE$ = 0.001, $R^2\Delta$ = .06, $p$ = .02), thus extending previous findings to inner-city illicit substance users and providing support for distress tolerance as a common mechanism underlying abstinence duration across drug classes.

## Predicting Substance Use Outcomes

In addition to retrospective examinations of distress tolerance among substance users, researchers have also examined the utility of distress tolerance tasks in prospectively predicting relapse across drug classes. Specifically, Hajek and colleagues utilized breath-holding duration as an index of tolerance for physical discomfort (Hajek, 1991, 1989; West, Hajek, & Belcher, 1989), and reported positive relationships between pretreatment breath-holding endurance and end-of-treatment smoking abstinence outcome ($r = .44$, $p < .001$) (Hajek et al., 1987). Extending these findings to psychological distress tolerance, Brandon and colleagues (2003) assessed the utility of persistence on two performance-based challenge tasks in predicting relapse following smoking cessation treatment. These authors assessed cognitive ability, negative affect, and persistence on two performance-based challenge tasks (i.e., APT and MTPT) in 144 smokers just before participating in a smoking cessation treatment. Persistence on the MTPT, but not the APT, predicted sustained abstinence following treatment, above and beyond severity of nicotine dependence and gender (Wald = 4.25, $p = .04$, hazard ratio [HR] = .998, 95%CI = 0.996–1.000), indicating that for each additional minute of persistence on the MTPT, relapse risk decreased by 11.3%. Furthermore, mean persistence times on the MTPT increased monotonically across treatment noncompleters, lapsers, and abstainers.

A more recent study extended earlier findings by combining two physical challenge tasks (i.e., breath-holding duration and inhalation of $CO_2$-enriched air) with a performance-based challenge task (i.e., the PASAT-C) to predict relapse among current smokers ($n = 81$) following an unaided quit attempt (Brown et al., 2009). As hypothesized, results showed that persistence on both physical challenge tasks was associated with a reduced risk of relapse. These effects were above and beyond the risk associated with levels of nicotine dependence, education, and history of major depressive disorder, suggesting that distress tolerance may operate independently of other previously identified risk factors. Additionally, the authors created a composite score for the two physical challenges by adding the two dichotomous variables together to form three groups (low persistence on both tasks, low persistence on one task and high persistence on the other, and high persistence on both tasks). After controlling for significant covariates, those in the low persistence group had a 3.27 times higher risk of relapsing during the 28-day follow-up than those in the high persistence group ($p = .006$). Persistence on the PASAT-C was not prospectively related to smoking relapse.

Physical and psychological distress tolerance tasks have also been utilized to prospectively predict substance use outcomes among illicit drug users. Specifically, 122 illicit drug users in residential treatment completed two physical challenge tasks (breath holding and a cold-pressor task) and two psychological distress tolerance tasks (PASAT-C and MTPT-C) within their first few days of treatment to examine distress tolerance as a predictor of early treatment dropout (Daughters, Lejuez, Bornovalova, et al., 2005). As hypothesized, lower distress tolerance (shorter persistence time) on both the MTPT-C ($B = -0.72$, $SE = 0.27$; HR = .49; $p < .01$) and the PASAT-C ($B = -0.57$, $SE = 0.27$; HR = .56; $p < .05$) predicted an increased likelihood of 30-day treatment dropout above and beyond relevant social-cognitive predictors of residential substance use treatment dropout (e.g., comorbid psychopathology, treatment readiness), supporting the unique utility of psychological distress tolerance in predicting one's ability to complete a residential substance use treatment program. However, unlike previous studies among smokers, persistence on the physical challenge tasks did not significantly predict treatment outcome among illicit drug users. The authors reason that participants in this study were enrolled in a residential drug treatment center that required 72-hour abstinence or detoxification before entering treatment. As such, the recruitment procedures utilized in this study may have excluded individuals with the lowest levels of physical distress tolerance who were unable to persist through the first 72 hours of abstinence, when physical withdrawal symptoms are strongest. Thus, among illicit drug users who are able to maintain the earliest stages of abstinence, premature termination of residential substance use treatment is predicted specifically by one's ability to tolerate psychological distress as opposed to physical distress.

## Mechanisms Underlying Distress Tolerance among Substance Users

Some initial work has also examined affective mechanisms underlying distress tolerance and its relationship with early smoking lapse. Marshall and colleagues (2008) recruited 95 daily smokers to participate in two voluntary hyperventilation procedures and examined the effects of panic reactivity during the first hyperventilation procedure on distress tolerance during the second procedure. As hypothesized, smokers who experienced a panic attack during the first hyperventilation procedure showed lower levels of distress tolerance during the second procedure above and beyond the effects of other relevant factors, including anxiety sensitivity, negative affectivity, number of cigarettes per day, and self-reported discomfort intolerance ($t = -2.44$, $p < .05$, $\beta = -0.26$). In terms of predicting relapse, Abrantes and colleagues (2008) examined the combined influence of both negative affect on quit day and distress tolerance as measured by two physical challenge tasks (breath-holding and $CO_2$ challenge) to predict early smoking lapse. Consistent with previous findings, participants in the low-persistence group (i.e., low persistence on both tasks; $n = 21$) were significantly more likely to lapse on quit day compared with smokers in the high-persistence group (i.e., high persistence on both tasks; $n = 23$; OR = 9.22, 95%CI = 1.41–60.41, $p < .03$). Furthermore, smokers in the low-persistence group reported higher levels of negative affect ($B = 0.58$, $SE = 0.21$; $p < .01$) and urges to smoke on quit day ($B = 0.52$, $SE = 0.23$; $p < .03$), and those in the low-persistence group who reported elevated levels of negative affect upon cessation were at the highest risk of lapsing on quit day ($B = 1.36$, $SE = 0.67$; $p < .05$). These findings suggest that a tendency to experience panic reactivity and elevated negative affect in response to uncomfortable bodily sensations may be two mechanisms underlying one's inability to tolerate distress and, therefore, may increase one's risk of early smoking lapse.

Despite promise across all measures of psychological and physical distress tolerance, contradictory findings exist, with some tasks showing inconsistent relationships with substance use outcomes from one study to the next. Additional research is needed to clarify the relationships between different performance-based measures of psychological and physical distress tolerance and the mechanisms that may underlie their differential ability to predict smoking relapse.

## The Influence of Contextual Factors on Distress Tolerance among Substance Users

Although distress tolerance has largely been conceptualized as a stable trait-like construct, initial research has also begun to examine the context-specific nature of distress tolerance among smokers. Bernstein, Trafton, Ilgen, and Zvolensky (2008) examined breath-holding duration among a sample of 43 smokers two times: once during a smoking-as-usual condition and once immediately after 12 hours of smoking deprivation. Breath-holding duration was significantly shorter following 12 hours of smoking deprivation compared with the smoking-as-usual condition above and beyond the effects of changes in self-reported stress between Sessions 1 and 2 ($F(1, 40) = 19.9$, $p < .001$, partial $\eta^2 = .33$). Furthermore, they found a significant negative correlation between psychiatric symptoms (a composite of anxiety, depression, paranoid ideation, and psychoticism symptoms) and breath-holding duration during the smoking deprivation condition ($r = -.35$, $p = .025$) but not during smoking as usual ($r = -.18$, $p = .24$). These findings suggest that one's capacity to withstand physical discomfort may be a malleable trait that is influenced by contextual factors such as smoking deprivation. Furthermore, among individuals with a preexisting vulnerability (i.e., psychiatric symptoms), contextual factors may have a stronger influence on one's ability to persist in the face of distress. Notably, in an unpublished master's thesis, Trotman (2004) found that 12 hours of smoking deprivation did not result in a significant decrease in distress tolerance across two behavioral measures.

## Initial Findings from Self-Report Measures of Distress Tolerance

In addition to performance-based assessments of distress tolerance, limited work utilizing self-report assessments of distress tolerance among substance users has also emerged. For example, in a prospective study over a 6-month interval, distress tolerance, as indicated by DTS scores, interacted with gender to prospectively predict alcohol problems among men, but not women, even after controlling for other relevant variables, including negative affectivity, problems at baseline, and use frequency at follow-up ($B = -0.05$, $SE = 0.02$; $p = .012$; Simons & Gaher, 2005). Additionally, DTS scores have been found to mediate the relationship between depression and alcohol and cannabis problems among young adults (Buckner, Keough, & Schmidt, 2007) and to moderate the relationship between negative life events and substance use coping, alcohol use, and cocaine use among HIV-positive individuals, such that individuals with lower distress tolerance and higher stressful life events were significantly more vulnerable to substance use than others (O'Cleirigh, Ironson, & Smits, 2007). Specific to physical distress tolerance, work using the DIS suggests that discomfort intolerance moderates the relationship between depression and marijuana use problems such that individuals high in both depression and discomfort intolerance are at the greatest risk for marijuana-related problems (Buckner et al., 2007). At the same time, individuals who are high in discomfort intolerance but low in depression showed the least marijuana-related problems, suggesting that discomfort intolerance may serve as a protective factor against marijuana use in non-depressed individuals. Further research replicating and extending existing findings utilizing the DTS and DIS is needed to understand how one's perceived capacity to withstand physical and psychological distress may influence other substance use outcomes.

## Gender Differences

Gender has been found to moderate the relationship between distress tolerance and substance use outcomes across studies. Specifically, Simons and Gaher (2005) found that men reported significantly higher levels of distress tolerance than women on the DTS ($p < .001$) even after controlling for negative affectivity. Furthermore, DTS scores predicted alcohol use-related problems at 6-month follow-up among men but not women ($p = .01$) even after controlling for other relevant factors, including negative affectivity and alcohol problems at baseline, as well as use frequency at 6-month follow-up, suggesting that men with low distress tolerance may be more likely to turn specifically to alcohol to cope with affective distress as opposed to other escape or avoidance strategies.

Among active substance users, significant gender differences have been found on performance-based measures of physical distress tolerance. Specifically, Brown and colleagues (2002) found that among smokers, women were significantly more likely to terminate a $CO_2$ challenge task than men (AOR = 30.0, $p$ = .005). Additionally, Daughters Lejuez, Bornovalova, and colleagues (2005) found that female illicit substance users in residential treatment showed significantly lower distress tolerance on a cold-pressor task compared with males. Gender differences in one's ability to withstand physical discomfort may have implications for quit success, particularly during the early stages of abstinence when physical withdrawal symptoms are strongest.

In addition to differences in distress tolerance across gender among active substance users, MacPherson, Stipelman, Duplinsky, Brown, and Lejuez (2008) reported on the moderating role of gender in the relationship between physical and psychological distress tolerance and smoking cessation outcomes among depressed smokers. Specifically, physical distress tolerance, as measured by breath-holding duration and persistence on a cold-pressor task, was significantly lower among men who dropped out of a behavioral activation treatment for smoking before quit day compared with men who remained in treatment, above and beyond the effects of anxiety sensitivity and current depressive symptoms, but this effect was not observed among women. Conversely, psychological distress tolerance, as measured by persistence on the PASAT-C, was significantly lower for women who dropped out of treatment before quit day compared with women who remained in treatment. This effect was significant above and beyond other affect-related factors, including anxiety sensitivity and current depressive symptoms, and was not significant among men. As such, physical and psychological distress tolerance may play differential roles in substance use treatment outcomes across genders, suggesting the potential need for differential treatment approaches across gender.

## THEORETICAL IMPLICATIONS AND FUTURE DIRECTIONS

Taken together, evidence indicates that beyond the magnitude of distress that individuals experience, how one responds to both physical and psychological distress is important in predicting substance use and relapse. In line with negative reinforcement models of substance use, current research examining the relationship between distress tolerance and substance use provides support for the escape or avoidance of aversive internal states (i.e., physical and psychological distress) as a driving motivational force in substance use and relapse.

Despite the contributions that have been made through the use of distress tolerance measures, many questions remain. First, the extent to which various measures of distress tolerance genuinely measure the same underlying construct remains unclear. Evidence suggests that some measures are better at predicting certain substance use outcomes than others. For example, relapse to smoking is most consistently predicted through the use of physical distress tolerance tasks, while treatment dropout among illicit substance users is more closely related to performance on psychological distress tolerance tasks. Although this may reflect differing distress tolerance vulnerabilities across drug class, it remains unclear whether physical and psychological distress tolerance tasks are measuring different facets of the same construct or fundamentally different constructs. Second, it is unclear how the different measures of distress tolerance relate to one another. Finally, the extant literature regarding the relationship between distress tolerance and substance use is largely descriptive and cross-sectional in nature. Therefore, the developmental origins of distress tolerance have yet to be elucidated. Specifically, it is unclear whether low distress tolerance precedes substance use or whether engagement in substance use leads to low distress tolerance. There is likely a dynamic interplay between distress tolerance and substance use such that low distress tolerance serves as a risk factor for substance use engagement, and chronic substance use then functions to lower one's willingness to withstand physical and psychological distress over time. Future research should aim to clarify the direction of the relationship between distress tolerance and substance use.

Given the utility of multimodal assessment batteries, including performance-based and self-report measures of distress tolerance, to predict substance use outcomes, a next step will be to increase understanding of the mechanisms underlying individual differences in distress tolerance. Specifically, investigations of the physiological and neurobiological mechanisms that may modulate one's ability to tolerate distress could substantially inform pharmacological and behavioral interventions that are targeted toward substance users with low distress tolerance. Additionally, a greater understanding of the biological basis of distress tolerance may inform prevention efforts by targeting the specific physiological and neurobiological deficits that may put individuals at risk for low distress tolerance and, thus, substance use initiation and addiction. Examination of mechanisms that may be driving differences in distress tolerance will be a fruitful field for future research.

## CLINICAL IMPLICATIONS AND APPLICATIONS

As noted, the available evidence indicates that it is not the intensity of distress that is important in substance use initiation and relapse but rather how one reacts to this distress. For example, greater tolerance of environmental and social pressures to experiment with addictive substances may reduce vulnerability to substance use initiation or progression to problem use. Specific to dependent substance users, a number of challenges that individuals must face during the early stages of abstinence may serve to increase their subjective levels of affective distress, including physical and psychological withdrawal symptoms, potential social pressures to continue use, and in the case of illicit drug use dealing with the legal system, reconnecting with loved ones, and finding employment and housing. Thus, the ability to tolerate distress during the early stages of abstinence and persist in an abstinence attempt is a crucial factor in obtaining positive long-term outcomes. As such, the development of novel prevention and intervention strategies for individuals with low distress tolerance may be useful for reducing the rates of substance use disorders and improving substance use outcomes following cessation.

In developing treatments to address distress tolerance among substance users, it is important to consider the contribution of specific mechanisms that may underlie distress intolerance. A recent theoretical conceptualization of distress tolerance and early lapse to smoking emphasized the role of anxiety sensitivity and experiential avoidance in smoking withdrawal and cessation (Brown et al., 2005). Specifically, the authors suggest that the extent to which one tolerates discomfort is likely to be influenced by specific factors, including one's appraisal of internal states and one's motivation to avoid them. As such, a focus on the clinical constructs of anxiety sensitivity and experiential avoidance may have some relevance to treatments aimed at increasing distress tolerance among substance users (Brown et al., 2005).

### Issues of Psychiatric Comorbidity

Psychiatric comorbidity is highly prevalent among individuals with substance use disorders (Kessler et al., 1996; Regier, Narrow, & Rae, 1990) and is often associated with poorer drug treatment outcomes across psychiatric conditions (Greenfield et al., 1998; Thomas, Melchert, & Banken, 1999; Tomasson & Vaglum, 1998). Furthermore, many psychiatric disorders have been associated with low distress tolerance, including generalized anxiety disorder (Roemer & Orsillo, 2002), depression (Buckner et al., 2007), and personality disorders (Bornovalova et al., 2008; Daughters, Sargeant, Bornovalova, Gratz, & Lejuez, 2008; Gratz, Rosenthal, Tull, Lejuez, & Gunderson, 2006). Thus, clinical approaches that aim to increase distress tolerance provide promising avenues for treating substance users with comorbid psychopathology.

Acceptance-based psychotherapy approaches may be beneficial for comorbid substance users with low distress tolerance. As one example, dialectical behavior therapy (DBT; Linehan, 1993) for individuals with comorbid borderline personality disorder and substance use has been found to significantly reduce the rates of premature treatment termination (Linehan et al., 1999) and significantly improve the rates of posttreatment abstinence (Linehan, Dimeff, & Reynolds, 2002). Furthermore, a recent randomized controlled trial compared methadone maintenance alone to 16 weeks of either acceptance and commitment therapy (ACT; Hayes, Strosahl, & Wilson, 1999) or intensive twelve-step facilitation among opiate users, many of whom had comorbid personality (52%), mood (40%), or anxiety (42%) disorders (Hayes et al., 2004). Both treatment groups evidenced less substance use at 6-month follow-up than the methadone-alone group (Hayes et al., 2004), providing further support for acceptance-based approaches for treating substance users with comorbid psychopathology. Despite the encouraging preliminary findings on the effectiveness of acceptance-based interventions, these studies included small sample sizes ($n = 12$ for Linehan et al., 2002; $n = 24$ for Hayes et al., 2004) and continued to yield high relapse rates (e.g., 57% and 50% positive urine tests, respectively). As such, the research examining the utility of acceptance-based approaches to treating substance users with comorbid psychopathology is currently limited; however, initial findings are promising and emphasize the need for further investigations.

## Clinical Techniques and Therapeutic Tactics

Two treatments that borrow strategies from acceptance-based therapies, including DBT and ACT, have been developed that specifically aim to increase distress tolerance among substance users. As a first line of work in this field, a distress tolerance treatment for smokers with a history of early lapses (i.e., individuals with no quit attempts lasting longer than

72 hours in the last 10 years) was developed (Brown et al., 2008). The treatment includes six 50-minute individual sessions, nine 2-hour group sessions, and 8 weeks of nicotine replacement therapy over the course of 10 weeks. Specific treatment components include psychoeducation about triggers, self-management strategies for dealing with external triggers, withdrawal-based exposure exercises, nicotine replacement therapy, and a large collection of ACT-based acceptance strategies. The treatment was piloted with a sample of 16 smokers with a history of early lapses, and follow-up assessments were conducted at 8, 13, and 26 weeks postquit. By the end of treatment (4 weeks postquit), the 7-day point prevalence of abstinence was 31.25%. By 8, 13, and 26 weeks postquit, 7-day point prevalence abstinence rates were 25%, 18%, and 0%, respectively. Despite the low abstinence rates, these participants, who reported a history of no quit attempts lasting longer than 3 days in the last 10 years, achieved a median of 24 days of continuous abstinence and 40.5 days of non-continuous abstinence. Furthermore, although most participants lapsed relatively quickly, they did not evidence full-blown relapse (7 consecutive days of smoking) until much later (median = 45.5 days), and many continued to make efforts to quit smoking even after lapsing (median number of quit attempts = 2.5). Taken together, initial testing of a distress tolerance treatment for smokers with a history of early lapse suggested that, compared with past efforts to quit smoking, participants exhibited increased persistence at maintaining smoking abstinence. These initial findings are promising given that a greater number and longer duration of past quit attempts have predicted maintenance of cessation at 6-month follow-up (Garvey, Bliss, Hitchcock, Heinold, & Rosner, 1992; Ockene et al., 2000). A small randomized controlled trial is now underway comparing the distress tolerance treatment for early-lapse smokers with a standard CBT smoking cessation treatment.

A second, novel technique that specifically addresses distress tolerance among substance users is Bornovalova, Trotman, Daughters, Gratz, and Lejuez's (2007) skills for improving distress intolerance (SIDI) treatment, which was developed with the aim of increasing distress tolerance and treatment retention among inner-city minority substance users in residential treatment. The six-session treatment protocol included strategies from both ACT and DBT as well as mood induction procedures that allowed clients the opportunity to practice new acceptance-based skills in the presence of negative affect. The treatment was pilot-tested with 78 illicit substance users who exhibited low distress tolerance by quitting at least one of two distress tolerance tasks (MTPT-C and/or PASAT-C) upon entering the residential drug treatment center. Participants were randomly assigned to receive SIDI, a time-matched supportive counseling condition, or treatment as usual. Early findings from this study showed that participants in the SIDI group showed significantly greater improvement in distress tolerance (as evidenced by persistence on the distress tolerance tasks at the end of treatment) than the two comparison groups, and treatment condition accounted for 24% of the variance in distress tolerance scores ($F(2, 58) = 7.37$, $p < .001$; $\eta^2 = .21$). Current work is examining the extent to which changes in distress tolerance are related to treatment dropout and relapse. Taken together, the evidence from this preliminary examination of a novel treatment for distress intolerance in inner-city substance users suggests that exposure- and acceptance-based approaches may be useful for increasing distress tolerance among substance users in residential treatment.

## Future Clinical Directions

Although existing treatments targeting distress tolerance among substance users appear promising, methodological issues, including small sample sizes and lack of control groups, limit the conclusions that can be drawn at present. As such, there is a need for larger randomized controlled trials to examine the utility of acceptance-based treatments for low distress tolerance among current substance users. Additionally, given the relevance of distress tolerance in earlier stages of substance use, including initiation and the progression to problem use, there is a need to examine the utility of treatments aimed at increasing distress tolerance with the goal of preventing substance use initiation or reducing the likelihood that occasional substance use will progress to abuse or dependence. As of yet, it is unclear whether a similar acceptance-based approach to increasing distress tolerance would be effective at preventing early initiation of substance use.

# CASE CONCEPTUALIZATION ILLUSTRATION

Leo J., a 43-year-old male, entered a residential substance use treatment facility reporting a history of regular marijuana use beginning at age 13 and progressing to heroin use by age 20. Leo was diagnosed with past marijuana dependence and current heroin dependence; symptoms included continued use despite problems, increased tolerance to drug effects, multiple failed attempts to quit using, and withdrawal symptoms upon cessation from both substances.

Leo reported that his first real exposure to drugs was from friends, many of whom started smoking marijuana when they were about 12 years old. At first, there was little pressure from his friends to smoke with them, but as more and more of his peers began to use marijuana, the pressure began to mount. Leo reported feeling angry with his friends for pressuring him but also shameful when they accused him of being "scared to smoke." Soon enough, Leo gave into the pressure and began smoking marijuana socially because he could not stand the anger and isolation he felt when he refused.

Although Leo initially only smoked at parties, he quickly noticed that smoking would bring a sense of relief and comfort when things were not going well. It wasn't long before Leo recognized that marijuana was the most effective strategy to deal with stress. At age 20, he was offered a "special blunt" that was laced with heroin and experienced the most profound sense of relief and relaxation he had ever felt. Although Leo continued to smoke marijuana, he moved on to heroin when he really needed to relax, which became more and more common as academic pressures increased. Eventually, he began experiencing symptoms of physical withdrawal. Initially, he tried to ignore the symptoms, but he simply wasn't able to tolerate this type of physical discomfort, and his heroin use progressively increased.

Unlike marijuana, under the influence of which Leo believed he could continue to live a productive life, fulfill his responsibilities, and maintain healthy relationships, heroin started to cause impairments across multiple domains in his life. Starting to feel out of control, he tried several times to stop or even cut down on his heroin use, but the withdrawal symptoms, such as diarrhea, vomiting, muscle cramps, and sweating, would lead him to go back to using heroin almost immediately. Before long, Leo had maxed out two credit cards and felt he had no choice but to make a few deliveries for his drug dealer in order to afford his habit. Soon he started dealing himself, which occupied much of his time and fueled his drug use. As Leo's grades worsened, he eventually dropped out of college and began selling drugs full time.

Over the next 20 years, Leo continued dealing drugs to support his heroin habit, which he never successfully stopped for more than a day. He has never experienced any legal consequences but has been unable to sustain a meaningful relationship, and he has not held a legitimate job for more than 3 months because of his tendency to quit when work became too stressful. Following the death of his mother, Leo vowed to quit using heroin. The first time he sought treatment, he was unable to complete the medicated detoxification period, citing overwhelming physical pain. During his second abstinence attempt, Leo was able to persist through the physical withdrawal syndrome with appropriate medical assistance in a residential inpatient treatment center, but he began experiencing intense anger because of the strict rules and his belief that he was smarter than the counselors at the treatment center. Following an intense confrontation with a member of the treatment staff, Leo immediately left the treatment facility and lapsed to heroin use within 2 hours.

Following these two failures, Leo recently entered a 90-day residential substance use treatment program affiliated with a university-based research team, which provided an individualized intervention for Leo based in the SIDI treatment approach outlined previously, which includes both exposure-based exercises and acceptance-based approaches to coping with affective distress. In terms of exposure, imaginal exposure to negative affective experiences via mood induction procedures is an effective behavioral approach to addressing Leo's appraisal of anxiety symptoms as unbearable, which has served to lower his threshold for tolerating distress. Given that the early stages of abstinence are marked by situations that frequently induce naturally occurring distress, exposure to negative affective states was easily achieved through prolonged and repeated descriptions of recent distressing situations in Leo's life, described in extensive detail. In addition to in-session exposure, Leo was also directed to apply acceptance-based strategies that were learned in session to the distressing situations that occurred between sessions, providing *in vivo* exposure to the negative affective experiences that have served to trigger substance use in the past as well as opportunities to utilize new, more adaptive means of coping with the distress. As such, the use of imaginal and *in vivo* exposures provided a theoretically consistent approach to increasing Leo's ability to tolerate distress by inducing systematic and repeated exposure to negative mood states, during which he was able to practice strategies that facilitate emotional acceptance (rather than avoidance) and distress tolerance.

Based on conceptually relevant research examining treatments for anxiety-related disorders, exposure exercises are significantly more effective when clients are fully engaged in the procedure and refrain from using avoidant behaviors (e.g., Craske, Street, & Barlow, 1989; Grayson, Foa, & Steketee, 1982). In line with this perspective, the use of acceptance-based strategies is also seen as integral to any effective treatment of substance users with low distress tolerance. In the case of Leo, treatment incorporated strategies specifically targeted at increasing acceptance and willingness to experience aversive sensations, including mindfulness exercises, tips for using healthy distraction to regulate emotions in the moment and to use problem-focused approaches to address upsetting situations later, and interpersonal effectiveness training. Taken together, a combination of exposure and acceptance-based techniques served as an integrated approach to treating both the cognitive and behavioral factors that have contributed to Leo's unwillingness to tolerate distress in the past and his subsequent pattern of substance use in the face of both physical withdrawal symptoms and affective distress. As a result of the treatment described previously, Leo was able to remain in residential treatment for his full contracted period of 90 days and was hopeful about his ability to maintain abstinence upon treatment completion.

## SUMMARY

Distress tolerance, defined as the ability to persist in goal-directed activity in the face of distress, is a clinical construct of significance in both theoretical and empirical work on substance use. Specifically, one's ability to persist in the face of physical and psychological distress has been implicated as a key mechanism across the stages of addiction, from substance use initiation among adolescents to relapse following cessation among dependent individuals. As such, researchers have begun to apply findings from basic laboratory research to the development of novel clinical approaches to treating substance users with low distress tolerance. Preliminary findings are promising based on pilot studies both in smokers with a history of early lapses and in illicit drug users entering residential treatment. Therefore, research on distress tolerance among substance users has not only improved our knowledge of the basic mechanisms underlying substance use and relapse, but it also has contributed to the development of novel interventions that have the potential to improve substance use outcomes. Future researchers should aim to elucidate mechanisms underlying the relationship between distress tolerance and substance use, examine individual difference factors that may serve as moderators in this relationship, clarify the directionality of the relationship between distress tolerance and substance use disorders, and design larger randomized controlled trials to examine the utility of psychotherapy interventions aimed at increasing distress tolerance among substance users.

## REFERENCES

Abrantes, A. M., Strong, D. R., Lejuez, C. W., Kahler, C. W., Carpenter, L. L., Price, L. H, et al. (2008). The role of negative affect in risk for early lapse among low distress tolerance smokers. *Addictive Behaviors, 33,* 1394–1401.
Avants, S. K., Marcotte, D., Arnold, R., & Margolin, A. (2003). Spiritual beliefs,

world assumptions, and HIV risk behavior among heroin and cocaine users. *Psychology of Addictive Behaviors, 17,* 159–162.

Baker, T. B., Japuntich, S. J., Hogle, J. M., McCarthy, D. E., & Curtin, J. J. (2006). Pharmacologic and behavioral withdrawal from addictive drugs. *Current Directions in Psychological Science, 15,* 232–236.

Baker, T. B., Piper, M. E., McCarthy, D. E., Majeskie, M. R., & Fiore, M. C. (2004). Addiction motivation reformulationed: An affective processing model of negative reinforcement. *Psychological Review, 111,* 33–51.

Bender, K., Ferguson, K., Thompson, S., Komlo, C., & Pollio, D. (2010). Factors associated with trauma and posttraumatic stress disorder among homeless youth in three U.S. cities: The importance of transience. *Journal of Traumatic Stress, 23*(1), 161–168.

Bensley, L. S., Spieker, S. J., Van Eenwyk, J., & Schoder, J. (1999). Self-reported abuse history and adolescent problem behaviors: II. Alcohol and drug use. *Journal of Adolescent Health, 24,* 173–180.

Bernstein, A., Trafton, J., Ilgen, M., & Zvolensky, M. J. (2008). An evaluation of the role of smoking context on a biobehavioral index of distress tolerance. *Addictive Behaviors, 33,* 1409–1415.

Bornovalova, M. A., Gratz, K. L., Daughters, S. B., Nick, B., Delany-Brumsey, A., Lynch, T. R., et al. (2008). A multimodal assessment of the relationship between emotion dysregulation and borderline personality disorder among inner-city substance users in residential treatment. *Journal of Psychiatric Research, 42,* 717–726.

Bornovalova, M. A., Trotman, A. J.-M., Daughters, S. B., Gratz, K. L., & Lejuez, C. W. (2007). *Skills for improving distress intolerance.* Unpublished manual.

Brandon, T. H., Herzog, T. A., Juliano, L. M., Irvin, J. E., Lazev, A. B., & Simmons, V. N. (2003). Pretreatment task persistence predicts smoking cessation outcome. *Journal of Abnormal Psychology, 112,* 448–456.

Brown, R. A., Lejuez, C. W., Kahler, C. W., & Strong, D. R. (2002). Distress tolerance and duration of past smoking cessation attempts. *Journal of Abnormal Psychology, 111,* 180–185.

Brown, R. A., Lejuez, C. W., Kahler, C. W., Strong, D. R., & Zvolensky, M. J. (2005). Distress tolerance and early smoking lapse. *Clinical Psychology Review, 25,* 713–733.

Brown, R. A., Lejuez, C. W., Strong, D. R., Kahler, C. W., Zvolensky, M. J., Carpenter, L. L., et al. (2009). A prospective examination of distress tolerance and early smoking lapse in adult self-quitters. *Nicotine and Tobacco Research, 11,* 493–502.

Brown, R. A., Palm, K. M., Strong, D. R., Lejuez, C. W., Kahler, C. W., Zvolensky, M. J., et al. (2008). Distress tolerance treatment for early-lapse smokers. *Behavior Modification, 32,* 302–332.

Buckner, J. D., Keough, M. E., & Schmidt, N. B. (2007). Problematic alcohol and cannabis use among young adults: The roles of depression on discomfort and distress tolerance. *Addictive Behaviors, 32,* 1957–1963.

Carroll, K. M., Power, M., Bryant, K., & Rounsaville, B. (1993). One year follow-up status of treatment-seeking cocaine abusers: Psychopathology and dependence severity as predictors of outcome. *Journal of Nervous and Mental Disease, 181,* 71–79.

Cloninger, C., Przybeck, T., & Švrakic, D. (1991). The Tridimensional Personality Questionnaire: U.S. normative data. *Psychological Reports, 69,* 1047–1057.

Craske, M. G., Street, L., & Barlow, D. H. (1989). Instructions to focus upon or distract from internal cues during exposure treatment of agoraphobic avoidance. *Behaviour Research and Therapy, 27,* 663–672.

Daughters, S. B., Reynolds, E. K., McPherson, L., Kahler, C. W., Danielson, C. K., Zvolensky, M., et al. (2009). Distress tolerance and early adolescent externalizing and internalizing symptoms: The moderating role of gender and ethnicity. *Behaviour Research and Therapy, 47,* 198–205.

Daughters, S. B., Lejuez, C. W., Bornovalova, M. A., Kahler, C. W., Strong, D. R., & Brown, R. A. (2005). Distress tolerance as a predictor of early treatment dropout in a residential substance abuse treatment facility. *Journal of Abnormal Psychology, 114,* 729–734.

Daughters, S. B., Lejuez, C. W., Kahler, C. W., Strong, D. R., & Brown, R. A. (2005). Psychological distress tolerance and duration of most recent abstinence attempt among residential treatment-seeking substance abusers. *Psychology of Addictive Behaviors, 19,* 208–211.

Daughters, S. B., Sargeant, M. N., Bornovalova, M. A., Gratz, K. L., & Lejuez, C. W. (2008). The relationship between distress tolerance and antisocial personality disorder among male inner-city treatment seeking substance users. *Journal of Personality Disorders, 22,* 509–524.

Doherty, K., Kinnunen, T., Militello, F., & Garvey, A. (1995). Urges to smoke during the first month of abstinence: Relationship to relapse and predictors. *Psychopharmacology, 119,* 171–178.

Ensminger, M. E., Anthony, J. C., & McCord, J. (1997). The inner city and drug use: Initial findings from an epidemiological study. *Drug and Alcohol Dependence, 48,* 175–184.

Friedman, A. S., Glassman, K., & Terras, A. (2001). Violent behavior as related to use of marijuana and other drugs. *Journal of Addictive Diseases, 20,* 49–72.

Garvey, A. J., Bliss, R. E., Hitchcock, J. L., Heinold, J. W., & Rosner, B. (1992). Predictors of smoking relapse among self-quitters: A report from the normative aging study. *Addictive Behaviors, 17,* 367–377.

Gratz, K. L., Rosenthal, M. Z., Tull, M. T., Lejuez, C. W., & Gunderson, J. G. (2006). An experimental investigation of emotion dysregulation in borderline personality disorder. *Journal of Abnormal Psychology, 115,* 850–855.

Grayson, J. B., Foa, E. B., & Steketee, G. (1982). Habituation during exposure treatment: Distraction vs attention-focusing. *Behaviour Research and Therapy, 20,* 323–328.

Greenfield, S. F., Weiss, R. D., Muenz, L. R., Vagge, L. M., Kelly, J. F., Bello, L. R., et al. (1998). The effect of depression on return to drinking: A prospective study. *Archives of General Psychiatry, 55,* 259–265.

Hajek, P. (1989). Breath holding and success in stopping smoking: What does breath holding measure? *International Journal of the Addictions, 24,* 633–639.

Hajek, P. (1991). Individual differences in difficulty quitting smoking. *British Journal of Addiction, 86,* 555–558.

Hajek, P., Belcher, M., & Stapleton, J. (1987). Breath-holding endurance as a predictor of success in smoking cessation. *Addictive Behaviors, 12,* 285–288.

Hayes, S. C., Strosahl, K. D., & Wilson, K. G. (1999). *Acceptance and commitment therapy: An experiential approach to behavior change.* New York: Guilford Press.

Hayes, S. C., Wilson, K. G., Gifford, E. V., Bissett, R., Piasecki, M., Batten, S. V., et al. (2004). A randomized controlled trial of twelve-step facilitation and acceptance and commitment therapy with polysubstance-abusing methadone-maintained opiate addicts. *Behavior Therapy, 35,* 667–688.

Kaplan, H. B., & Johnson, R. J. (1992). Relationships between circumstances surrounding initial illicit drug use and escalation of use: Moderating effects of gender and early adolescent experiences. In M. Glantz & R. Pickins (Eds.), *Vulnerability to drug abuse* (pp. 299–358). Washington, DC: American Psychological Association.

Kessler, R. C., Nelson, C. B., McGonagle, K. A., Edlund, M. J., Frank, R. G., & Leaf, P. J. (1996). The epidemiology of co-occurring addictive and mental disorders: Implications for prevention and service utilization. *American Journal of Orthopsychiatry, 66,* 17–31.

Lejuez, C. W., Kahler, C. W., & Brown, R. A. (2003). A modified computer version of the paced auditory serial addition task (PASAT) as a laboratory-based stressor. *The Behavior Therapist, 26,* 290–293.

Leyro, T. M., Zvolensky, M. J., & Bernstein, A. (2010). Distress tolerance and psychopathological symptoms and disorders: A review of the empirical literature among adults. *Psychological Bulletin, 136*(4), 576–600.

Leyro, T. M., Zvolensky, M. J., Vujanovic, A. A., & Bernstein, A. (2008). Anxiety sensitivity and smoking motives and outcome expectancies among adult daily smokers: Replication and extension. *Nicotine and Tobacco Research, 10,* 985–994.

Linehan, M. M. (1993). *Cognitive-behavioral treatment for borderline personality disorder: The dialectics of effective treatment.* New York: Guilford Press.

Linehan, M. M., Dimeff, L. A., & Reynolds, S. K. (2002). Dialectical behavior therapy versus comprehensive validation therapy plus 12-step for the treatment of opioid dependent women meeting criteria for borderline personality disorder. *Drug and Alcohol Dependence, 67,* 13–26.

Linehan, M. M., Schmidt, H., Dimeff, L. A., Craft, J. C., Kanter, J., & Comtois, K. A. (1999). Dialectical behavior therapy for patients with borderline personality disorder and drug-dependence. *American Journal on Addictions, 8,* 279–292.

Luck, P. A., Elifson, K. W., & Sterk, C. E. (2004). Female drug users and the welfare system: A qualitative exploration. *Drugs: Education, Prevention and Policy, 11,* 113–128.

MacPherson, L., Reynolds, E. K., Daughters, S. B., Wang, F., Cassidy, J., Mayes,

L., et al. (2009). *Positive and negative reinforcement underlying risk behavior in early adolescents.* Manuscript submitted for publication.

MacPherson, L., Stipelman, B. A., Duplinsky, M., Brown, R. A., & Lejuez, C. W. (2008). Distress tolerance and pre-smoking treatment attrition: Examination of moderating relationships. *Addictive Behaviors, 33,* 1385–1393.

Marshall, E., Zvolensky, M., Vujanovic, A., Gregor, K., Gibson, L., & Leyro, T. (2008). Panic reactivity to voluntary hyperventilation challenge predicts distress tolerance to bodily sensations among daily cigarette smokers. *Experimental and Clinical Psychopharmacology, 16,* 313–321.

McLellan, A., Luborsky, L., Woody, G., O'Brien, C., & Druley, K. (1983). Predicting response to drug and alcohol treatments: Role of psychiatric severity. *Archives of General Psychiatry, 40,* 620–625.

Mello, N. K., & Mendelson, J. H. (1970). Experimentally induced intoxication in alcoholics: A comparison between programmed and spontaneous drinking. *Journal of Pharmacology and Experimental Therapeutics, 173,* 101–116.

Miller, M., & Neaigus, A. (2002). Sex partner support, drug use and sex risk among HIV negative non-injecting heroin users. *AIDS Care, 14,* 801–813.

Monti, P. M., Rohsenow, D. J., Michalec, E., Martin, R. A., & Abrams, D. B. (1997). Brief coping skills treatment for cocaine abuse: Substance use outcomes at three months. *Addiction, 92,* 1717–1728.

Morgenstern, J., Blanchard, K. A., Morgan, T. J., Labouvie, E., & Hayaki, J. (2001). Testing the effectiveness of cognitive-behavioral treatment for substance abuse in a community setting: Within treatment and posttreatment findings. *Journal of Consulting and Clinical Psychology, 69,* 1007–1017.

Mulvaney, F. D., Alterman, A. I., Boardman, C. R., & Kampman, K. (1999). Cocaine abstinence symptomatology and treatment attrition. *Journal of Substance Abuse Treatment, 16,* 129–135.

Najavits, L. M., Gastfriend, D. R., Barber, J. P., Reif, S., Muenz, L. R., Blaine, J., et al. (1998). Cocaine dependence with and without PTSD among subjects in the National Institute on Drug Abuse Collaborative Cocaine Treatment Study. *American Journal of Psychiatry, 155,* 214–219.

Nyamathi, A., Wenzel, S., Keenan, C., Leake, B., & Gelberg, L. (1999). Associations between homeless women's intimate relationships and their health and well-being. *Research in Nursing and Health, 22,* 486–495.

Ockene, J. K., Emmons, K. M., Mermelstein, R. J., Perkins, K. A., Bonollo, D. S., Voorhees, C. C., et al. (2000). Relapse and maintenance issues for smoking cessation. *Health Psychology, 19*(1), 17–31.

O'Cleirigh, C., Ironson, G., & Smits, J. A. J. (2007). Does distress tolerance moderate the impact of major life events on psychosocial variables and behaviors important in the management of HIV? *Behavior Therapy, 38,* 314–323.

Parrott, A. C. (1999). Does cigarette smoking cause stress? *American Psychologist, 54,* 817–820.

Payne, T. J., Schare, M. L., Levis, D. J., & Colletti, G. (1991). Exposure to smoking-relevant cues: Effects on desire to smoke and topographical components of smoking behavior. *Addictive Behaviors, 16,* 467–479.

Quinn, E. P., Brandon, T. H., & Copeland, A. L. (1996). Is task persistence related to smoking and substance abuse?: The application of learned industrious-ness theory to addictive behaviors. *Experimental and Clinical Psychophar-macology, 4,* 186–190.

Regier, D. A., Narrow, W. E., & Rae, D. S. (1990). The epidemiology of anxiety disorders: The Epidemiologic Catchment Area (ECA) experience. *Journal of Psychiatric Research, 24*(Suppl. 2), 3–14.

Roemer, L., & Orsillo, S. M. (2002). Expanding our conceptualization of and treatment for generalized anxiety disorder: Integrating mindfulness/accep-tance-based approaches with existing cognitive-behavioral models. *Clinical Psychology: Science and Practice, 9,* 54–68.

Schmidt, N. B., Richey, J., & Fitzpatrick, K. (2006). Discomfort intolerance: Development of a construct and measure relevant to panic disorder. *Journal of Anxiety Disorders, 20,* 263–280.

Schmidt, N. B., & Trakowski, J. H. (1999). Attentional focus and fearful respond-ing in patients with panic disorder during a 35% $CO_2$ challenge. *Behavior Therapy, 30,* 623–640.

Simons, J. S., & Gaher, R. M. (2005). The Distress Tolerance Scale: Develop-ment and validation of a self-report measure. *Motivation and Emotion, 29,* 83–102.

Sinha, R., Catapano, D., & O'Malley, S. (1999). Stress-induced craving and stress response in cocaine dependent individuals. *Psychopharmacology, 142,* 343–351.

Strong, D. R., Lejuez, C. W., Daughters, S., Marinello, M., Kahler, C. W., & Brown, R. A. (2003). *The computerized mirror tracing task version 1.* Unpublished manual.

Substance Abuse and Mental Health Services Administration. (2008). *Results from the 2007 National Survey on Drug Use and Health: National findings* (Office of Applied Studies, NSDUH Series H-34, DHHS Publication No. SMA 08-4343). Rockville, MD: Author.

Tennant, F., Shannon, J. A., Nork, J. G., Sagherian, A., & Berman, M. (1991). Abnormal adrenal gland metabolism in opioid addicts: Implications for clinical treatment. *Journal of Psychoactive Drugs, 23,* 135–149.

Thomas, V. H., Melchert, T. P., & Banken, J. A. (1999). Substance depen-dence and personality disorders: Comorbidity and treatment outcome in an inpatient treatment population. *Journal of Studies on Alcohol, 60,* 271–277.

Tomasson, K., & Vaglum, P. (1998). The role of psychiatric comorbidity in the prediction of readmission for detoxification. *Comprehensive Psychiatry, 39,* 129–136.

Trotman, A. J.-M. (2004). *The effects of nicotine deprivation on behavioral task performance.* Unpublished master's thesis, University of Maryland, College Park.

West, R. J., Hajek, P., & Belcher, M. (1989). Severity of withdrawal symptoms as a predictor of outcome of an attempt to quit smoking. *Psychological Medicine, 19,* 981–985.

Wikler, A. (1977). The search for the psyche in drug dependence. *Journal of Ner-vous and Mental Disease, 165,* 29–40.

Widom, C. S., Weiler, B. L., & Cottler, L. B. (1999). Childhood victimization and drug abuse: A comparison of prospective and retrospective findings. *Journal of Consulting and Clinical Psychology, 67,* 867–880.

Wills, T. A., McNamara, G., Vaccaro, D., & Hirky, A. E. (1996). Escalated substance use: A longitudinal grouping analysis from early to middle adolescence. *Journal of Abnormal Psychology, 105,* 166–180.

Zinser, M. C., Baker, T. B., Sherman, J. E., & Cannon, D. S. (1992). Relation between self reported affect and drug urges and cravings in continuing and withdrawing smokers. *Journal of Abnormal Psychology, 101,* 617–629.

Zvolensky, M. J., Feldner, M. T., Eifert, G. H., & Brown, R. A. (2001). Affective style among smokers: Understanding anxiety sensitivity, emotional reactivity, and distress tolerance using biological challenge. *Addictive Behaviors, 26,* 901–915.

# 9

# Borderline Personality Disorder

Kim L. Gratz *and* Matthew T. Tull

Borderline personality disorder (BPD) is a serious mental illness characterized by instability and dysfunction across interpersonal, emotional, behavioral, and cognitive domains (Gunderson, 2001; Linehan, 1993; Skodol et al., 2002). Although BPD is found at rates of 1–6% in the general population (Grant et al., 2008; Lenzenweger, Lane, Loranger, & Kessler, 2007; Torgersen, Kringlen, & Cramer, 2001), individuals with BPD represent approximately 15% of clinical populations (Widiger & Frances, 1989; Widiger & Weissman, 1991) and are major consumers of health care resources (Bender et al., 2001; Zanarini, Frankenburg, Khera, & Bleichmar, 2001). Furthermore, BPD is associated with extensive functional impairment and heightened levels of self-destructive and health-compromising behaviors, including deliberate self-harm and suicidal behaviors, drug and alcohol abuse, risky sexual behavior, bingeing and purging, and misuse of prescribed medications (American Psychiatric Association, 1994; Frankenburg & Zanarini, 2004; Gunderson, 2001; Skodol et al., 2002; Trull, Sher, Minks-Brown, Durbin, & Burr, 2000; Zanarini et al., 1998). Given its clinical relevance and public health significance, the past two decades have seen a dramatic increase in theory and research on the development and maintenance of BPD, with the goal of identifying mechanisms underlying the pathogenesis of this disorder that may inform targeted prevention and intervention efforts. One such mechanism is distress tolerance.

Indeed, the role of distress tolerance in BPD has been discussed extensively within prominent theoretical and clinical literature on this disorder. In particular, Linehan's (1993) seminal theoretical work on the pathogenesis of BPD suggests that one of the central mechanisms underlying BPD is the unwillingness to tolerate emotional distress. According to the biosocial model of BPD (Linehan, 1993), distress intolerance results from the combination of a biologically based emotional vulnerability (including heightened sensitivity, greater intensity and reactivity, and a slower return to baseline emotional arousal; see Rosenthal et al., 2008) and an invalidating environment wherein the communication of private experiences is met by erratic, inappropriate, or extreme negative responses, including the punishment or trivialization of emotional expression. According to Linehan, an invalidating environment contributes to the development of distress intolerance by failing to teach children how to tolerate emotional distress or regulate emotional arousal, leading to both an unwillingness to experience emotional distress and rigid attempts to avoid such distress (Linehan, 1993). Indeed, it is the unwillingness to tolerate distress that is thought to lead to a variety of maladaptive behaviors commonly found among individuals with BPD, including deliberate self-harm, substance abuse, and eating disorder-related behaviors (e.g., bingeing, purging), all of which may function to escape or avoid unwanted emotional distress (Chapman, Gratz, & Brown, 2006; Hayes, Wilson, Gifford, Follette, & Strosahl, 1996).

In fact, many of the symptoms of BPD may best be understood within the framework of distress tolerance, with the behavioral symptoms of BPD (e.g., deliberate self-harm) functioning to alleviate or avoid intolerable distress and the emotional symptoms of BPD (e.g., affective instability and intense anger) emerging, in part, as a result of the paradoxical consequences of such attempts. Overall, Linehan's (1993) theoretical work highlights the role of distress intolerance in the pathogenesis of BPD and its associated behaviors. Furthermore, the empirically supported treatment for BPD developed on the basis of this theory, dialectical behavior therapy (DBT), specifically targets distress tolerance, seeking to increase the willingness to tolerate emotional distress without resorting to impulsive, emotionally avoidant behaviors (Linehan, 1993).

As a result of the emphasis on distress tolerance within this prominent theoretical and clinical literature on BPD, researchers have begun to examine the role of distress tolerance in BPD and related behaviors, including deliberate self-harm. Given the centrality of distress intolerance to the symptom presentation of BPD, this disorder provides an excellent context for examining distress tolerance as a mechanism underlying psychopathology.

## REVIEW OF EMPIRICAL RESEARCH

Although research on distress tolerance in BPD is in its infancy, findings to date provide support for the relevance of distress tolerance to this disorder. First, a small body of studies have examined the association between BPD pathology and the unwillingness to tolerate emotional distress utilizing a self-report measure of the related construct of experiential avoidance (defined as the unwillingness to remain in contact with internal experiences and related efforts to escape or avoid these experiences; Hayes et al., 1996). Although the construct of experiential avoidance encompasses all aspects of internal experience, the unwillingness to experience emotional distress is often considered the primary motivation for avoidance or escape (Hayes, Strosahl, & Wilson, 1999). Likewise, the motivation to avoid the experience of certain thoughts and bodily sensations is thought to occur as a result of the emotional distress associated with those experiences.

With regard to the association between experiential avoidance and BPD, Chapman, Specht, and Cellucci (2005) found that experiential avoidance was significantly associated with the severity of BPD symptoms among a sample of female inmates. Furthermore, Gratz, Tull, and Gunderson (2008) found that levels of experiential avoidance were significantly higher among a sample of outpatients with BPD, compared with a group of outpatients with no personality disorder diagnosis. The relationship between experiential avoidance and BPD status was robust, remaining even when controlling for various BPD-relevant aspects of emotional vulnerability, including affect intensity/reactivity, anxiety sensitivity, and negative affectivity.

In addition to self-report measures, studies have begun to examine the association between BPD and distress tolerance using behavioral measures of the unwillingness to tolerate emotional distress, most notably the Paced Auditory Serial Addition Task—Computerized Version (PASAT-C; Lejuez, Kahler, & Brown, 2003) and the Computerized Mirror-Tracing Persistence Task (MTPT-C; Quinn, Brandon, & Copeland, 1996; Strong et al., 2003; see later discussion for a more detailed description of these measures). For example, in a study examining the association between BPD and the willingness to experience emotional distress in order to pursue goal-directed behavior (as assessed with a modified version of the PASAT-C), Gratz, Rosenthal, Tull, Lejuez, and Gunderson (2006) found that BPD outpatients evidenced significantly less willingness to tolerate emotional distress than outpatients without a personality disorder (non-PD). Furthermore, these differences remained even when controlling for relevant covariates (e.g., task performance, mathematical skill, and level of distress induced by the task). Moreover, findings that the PASAT-C

resulted in comparable levels of distress for the BPD and non-PD participants suggest that differences in the willingness to experience emotional
distress are not due to group differences in the level of distress induced
by the task. Thus, findings suggest that individuals with BPD, compared
with those without a PD, have a lower tolerance for comparable levels of distress. Furthermore, providing evidence for the overlap between
distress tolerance and experiential avoidance, the willingness to experience emotional distress on the PASAT-C was strongly correlated with
self-reported experiential avoidance among the BPD patients ($r = -.76$;
Gratz et al., 2006).

Likewise, Bornovalova and colleagues (2008) examined the association between BPD and the willingness to tolerate emotional distress as
indexed by latency to termination scores on the PASAT-C and MTPT-C.
However, this study examined the association between BPD and the willingness to tolerate distress among a sample of inpatient residents in a drug
and alcohol abuse treatment center. Consistent with the findings of Gratz
and colleagues (2006), results demonstrated that substance users with a
diagnosis of BPD evidenced a greater unwillingness to tolerate emotional
distress than substance users without BPD, persisting for a shorter amount
of time on both behavioral tasks. Furthermore, the willingness to tolerate distress predicted BPD status above and beyond relevant covariates
(e.g., gender, racial background, major depression, bipolar disorder) and a
self-report measure of emotion regulation difficulties, suggesting the robust
nature of the relationship between distress tolerance and BPD.

Finally, although not directly relevant to BPD, a number of studies
have provided support for an association between distress tolerance and
a variety of BPD-relevant behaviors. Specifically, studies have found an
association between the unwillingness to tolerate emotional distress as
assessed via self-report measures and deliberate self-harm (Chapman et
al., 2005; Gratz, Breetz, & Tull, 2010), suicidal ideation (Lynch, Cheavens, Morse, & Rosenthal, 2004), substance abuse (Buckner, Keogh, &
Schmidt, 2007; Stewart, Zvolensky, & Eifert, 2002), disordered eating
behaviors (Anestis, Selby, Fink, & Joiner, 2007; Corstorphine, Mountford, Tomlinson, Waller, & Meyer, 2007), aggressive behavior (Tull, Jakupcak, Paulson, & Gratz, 2007), and risky sexual behavior (Batten, Follette, & Aban, 2001). Furthermore, deliberate self-harm has been found
to be associated with behavioral measures of distress tolerance, including
the MTPT-C (Gratz, Hepworth, et al., 2009) and a modified version of
the Wisconsin Card Sort Test (WCST; Heaton, Chelune, Talley, Kay, &
Curtis, 1993), in which participants were given the option to terminate
the task following the provision of false negative feedback regarding their
performance (which was expected to induce frustration and distress;
Nock & Mendes, 2008).

## The Temporal Relationship between Distress Tolerance and Borderline Personality Disorder

Theoretical literature on distress tolerance and BPD highlights the etiologic role of distress tolerance in BPD, implicating distress intolerance in the pathogenesis of this disorder and many BPD-relevant behaviors that are thought to function to escape from or alleviate intolerable distress (Linehan, 1993). Although research on the association between BPD and distress tolerance does not provide evidence contrary to the proposed etiologic role of distress tolerance in BPD, no studies to date have examined this association prospectively. As such, there is no direct evidence for the role of distress tolerance in the development and maintenance of BPD, and research cannot yet speak to the temporal order of the relationship between these phenomena.

Furthermore, it is likely that the relationship between distress tolerance and BPD is bidirectional. Indeed, theoretical and clinical literature suggests that distress intolerance can become a vicious cycle, with emotional intolerance leading to attempts to avoid those emotions, followed by the paradoxical consequences of these avoidance attempts (including greater emotional distress and arousal) and so on (see Chapman et al., 2006). Moreover, although not specific to BPD, research suggests that the unwillingness to experience certain emotions and subsequent avoidance of those emotions may paradoxically intensify emotional arousal and dysregulation. For example, Zvolensky and colleagues (2009) found that distress intolerance was predictive of experiencing a panic attack during a carbon dioxide ($CO_2$) challenge, a procedure wherein participants inhale $CO_2$-enriched air, producing physiological symptoms consistent with the most commonly reported physical sensations accompanying panic attacks (Zvolensky & Eifert, 2001). In addition, the instructed suppression of emotional expression in response to negative emotional film clips has been found to be associated with increased physiological arousal (Gross & Levenson, 1993, 1997). Finally, studies examining differences in emotional reactivity between individuals high and low in experiential avoidance have found that individuals with high (vs. low) levels of experiential avoidance report greater negative emotion in response to a $CO_2$ challenge (Karekla, Forsyth, & Kelly, 2004).

Although these studies are not specific to BPD, the consequence of emotional unwillingness among individuals with BPD is likely the same (i.e., heightened emotional distress and dysregulation). As a result, the chronic intolerance and avoidance of emotional distress may exacerbate distress intolerance, further decreasing one's tolerance of emotional distress and resulting in a greater reliance on maladaptive behaviors that function to avoid distress (consistent with models of experiential avoidance for BPD-related behaviors, such as deliberate self-harm; see Chapman et al., 2006).

## Strengths and Limitations of Extant Research

Although research on the role of distress tolerance in BPD is in its infancy, studies in this area have some notable strengths, including the use of a multimethod approach to the assessment of the willingness to tolerate distress, the use of behavioral measures and experimental designs, and the examination of diverse patient populations (Bornovalova et al., 2008; Gratz et al., 2006). With regard to the latter, in addition to providing support for the association between BPD and distress tolerance across general outpatient, substance-dependent, and inmate samples (Bornovalova et al., 2008; Chapman et al., 2005; Gratz et al., 2006), studies in this area have examined this association across diverse racial/ethnic groups, including a sample of predominantly African American inner-city substance users. As such, findings of the relevance of distress tolerance to BPD have been found to generalize across a range of populations. Furthermore, research in this area has examined the unique association between distress tolerance and BPD by controlling for relevant variables, including emotion dysregulation, affect intensity/reactivity, anxiety sensitivity, negative affectivity, impulsivity, and substance use disorder severity. Consequently, even though this area of research is relatively young, there is some preliminary evidence for the incremental validity of distress tolerance in relation to BPD, relative to other factors commonly found to be associated with this disorder.

Yet, despite the overall quality of the research in this area, a notable limitation is that all studies to date have been correlational and cross-sectional in nature, with no research examining the longitudinal or prospective pattern of associations between distress tolerance and BPD. Therefore, extant research cannot speak to the direction or temporal order of the relationship between these phenomena. Furthermore, the absence of a consistent or agreed-upon operational definition of distress tolerance has resulted in the use of a variety of behavioral measures of this construct, including the PASAT-C, MTPT-C, and modified WCST. Although these measures share the approach of providing participants with an option to terminate a distressing task, further research is needed to explore the validity of each, particularly with regard to their external validity for individuals with BPD.

## THEORETICAL IMPLICATIONS AND FUTURE DIRECTIONS

Research on the association between distress tolerance and BPD provides support for the relevance of this proposed mechanism to this disorder.

Evidence suggests that distress intolerance distinguishes individuals with BPD from those without BPD, even when taking into account the effect of co-occurring conditions (such as substance dependence; Bornovalova et al., 2008) that are also associated with heightened distress intolerance. Thus, findings have begun to provide some support for a unique association between distress intolerance and BPD.

However, further research is needed to explore the nature and extent of this association. For example, a recent study (Gratz et al., in press) examining the association between deliberate self-harm and the unwillingness to experience emotional distress on the MTPT-C found that self-harming women did not evidence a generalized unwillingness to experience emotional distress but an unwillingness to experience emotional distress under certain conditions (i.e., a context-dependent emotional unwillingness). In particular, findings suggested that self-harming women may evidence less willingness to experience emotional distress only following depletion of their self-regulatory resources (e.g., in the aftermath of an interpersonal stressor); conversely, deficits in emotional willingness may not be present under conditions of low stress when self-regulatory resources have not been taxed. Given the common co-occurrence of self-harm and BPD, future studies should examine if the willingness to tolerate distress among individuals with BPD is likewise context dependent and, if so, should explore the particular contexts in which deficits in distress tolerance are more likely to emerge. Indeed, findings of the context-dependent nature of distress intolerance in BPD may help explain the wide variation in functioning observed among individuals with BPD (who may, under low-stress conditions, function remarkably well and demonstrate few emotion-related deficits; Linehan, 1993).

Furthermore, research is needed to continue to explore the factors that may increase the risk for distress intolerance among individuals with BPD. Such research may highlight other potential mechanisms underlying the development of this disorder, as well as other useful targets of treatment. For example, one study examining the association between childhood abuse and the willingness to tolerate emotional distress among a sample of substance users found that self-reported emotional nonacceptance in the form of secondary emotional reactions to negative emotions predicted less willingness to tolerate distress on the MTPT-C and PASAT-C (Gratz, Bornovalova, Delany-Brumsey, Nick, & Lejuez, 2007). These findings provide preliminary empirical evidence that the tendency to negatively evaluate one's emotional responses may increase the likelihood that one will attempt to avoid or escape emotional distress. Likewise, Evans, Baer, and Segerstrom (2009) found that nonjudging of inner experience was associated with greater distress tolerance as indexed by persistence on a difficult and stressful task. Given the relevance of emotional nonacceptance to BPD (see Glenn & Klonsky, 2009; Linehan, 1993), the role of emotional nonacceptance in distress intolerance among individuals with BPD may be a productive avenue for future inquiry. Furthermore, such research may have important clinical implications, suggesting the utility of interventions aimed at decreasing judgmental, nonaccepting responses to emotions in order to decrease distress intolerance.

Research is also needed to explore the construct validity of extant behavioral assessments of the willingness to tolerate distress among individuals with BPD. Although Gratz and colleagues (2006) found evidence of a strong relationship between latency to terminate the PASAT-C and a widely used self-report measure of experiential avoidance (i.e., the Acceptance and Action Questionnaire; Hayes et al., 2004), further research is needed to examine the validity and reliability of these behavioral measures, in particular their external validity and the extent to which findings within the laboratory generalize to the ways in which individuals with BPD cope with emotional distress in their daily lives. Future research also should explore ways to modify or expand upon these tasks to increase their ecological validity. One potentially useful modification may be to assess the willingness to experience emotional distress through the use of more emotionally salient or personally relevant distressing stimuli, such as interpersonal distress or emotionally evocative film clips.

Furthermore, as noted previously, prospective longitudinal studies are needed to better establish the temporal relationship between distress intolerance and BPD. In particular, studies examining the interactive effect of an underlying trait emotional vulnerability and invalidating environment on distress intolerance among children are needed to provide support for the proposed interrelations among these phenomena. Research is also needed to examine the etiologic role of distress tolerance in BPD. Most of what is known about the development of BPD comes from retrospective and correlational studies of adult patients with this disorder, which are limited in their ability to address the risk factors for BPD. In particular, because BPD is associated with such extensive dysfunction, it is not clear whether the mechanisms found to be associated with BPD in adult patients, such as distress intolerance, are indeed risk factors for BPD or simply associated factors or consequences of this disorder. Consequently, longitudinal studies examining whether distress intolerance in childhood prospectively predicts the development of BPD pathology in adolescence and adulthood are needed to establish the etiologic role of distress tolerance in BPD.

# CLINICAL IMPLICATIONS
# AND APPLICATIONS

Findings of an association between distress tolerance and BPD, as well as the emphasis on distress tolerance in theories of the development and maintenance of BPD, suggest the importance of targeting distress tolerance in treatments for this disorder. Especially given findings of the relevance of distress tolerance to some of the most maladaptive and self-damaging symptoms of BPD (e.g., self-harm; see Gratz et al., 2010; Nock & Mendes, 2008), treatments that focus on increasing distress tolerance could arguably help stabilize some of the most clinically concerning behaviors associated with this disorder. Specifically, if many of the behaviors associated with BPD function to escape unwanted emotional distress, increasing an individual's willingness to tolerate that distress should decrease the need for these behaviors.

Furthermore, findings of an association between an unwillingness to tolerate distress and BPD symptom severity (Chapman et al., 2005), self-harm frequency (Gratz et al., 2010), and severity of substance use problems (Buckner et al., 2007) suggest that improvements in distress tolerance may be followed by corresponding reductions in BPD symptoms, particularly the use of maladaptive behaviors to escape from or alleviate emotional distress. Such findings support a focus on distress tolerance as a target of treatment, indicating that gradual improvements in this mechanism over time are likely to have benefits with regard to the symptoms and maladaptive behaviors of interest.

## Treatments for Distress Tolerance in Borderline Personality Disorder

Not surprisingly, behavioral treatments for BPD have incorporated a focus on distress tolerance. Most notably, Linehan's (1993) theoretical work on the pathogenesis of BPD (which implicates distress intolerance as one of the primary mechanisms underlying BPD and its related behaviors) provided the basis for the development of DBT, a comprehensive treatment for BPD among chronically self-harming and/or suicidal women. DBT is a third-wave behavioral therapy, combining traditional cognitive-behavioral approaches with acceptance- and mindfulness-based approaches stemming from Eastern philosophies like Zen. Consistent with theoretical and clinical literature emphasizing the role of distress tolerance in BPD, a central premise underlying this treatment is that increasing distress tolerance will decrease the need for maladaptive behaviors that function to escape or avoid unwanted distress.

In its empirically supported package, DBT consists of four treatment components: weekly group skills training, individual psychotherapy, and therapist consultation/supervision meetings, as well as telephone consultation as needed between clients and individual therapists. With regard to the skills training in particular, four particular sets of skills are emphasized, including emotion regulation, distress tolerance, mindfulness, and interpersonal effectiveness skills. Importantly, it is not just the skills within the distress tolerance module that may target distress intolerance; instead, some of the mindfulness skills are applicable as well.

In general, distress tolerance skills emphasize the importance of tolerating negative emotions without engaging in impulsive behaviors. These skills teach clients to tolerate emotional distress and emphasize the benefits of accepting one's emotions without trying to change or alter them, as well as accepting reality for what it is in the moment. Furthermore, mindfulness skills promote a nonjudgmental awareness of one's internal experiences (including emotions), teaching clients to observe internal experiences as they occur in the moment and to label these experiences objectively (e.g., letting go of evaluations such as "good" or "bad"). As such, clients are taught the importance of taking a nonjudgmental and nonevaluative stance toward their emotions, which is expected to facilitate emotional acceptance and increase emotional willingness.

In addition to DBT, a short-term acceptance-based emotion regulation group therapy for deliberate self-harm among women with BPD (developed by Gratz & Gunderson, 2006) targets distress tolerance as a dimension of emotion dysregulation. This 14-week, adjunctive group therapy was designed to treat self-harm by directly targeting the function of this behavior and teaching self-harming women with BPD more adaptive ways of responding to their emotions. Specifically, this group therapy was developed to systematically address several dimensions of emotion regulation, including the ability to control impulsive behaviors when experiencing negative emotions and the willingness to experience negative emotions as part of pursuing meaningful activities (both of which overlap with the construct of distress tolerance). In addition to drawing from DBT, this group therapy draws heavily from another acceptance-based behavioral therapy, acceptance and commitment therapy (Hayes et al., 1999), a primary focus of which is increasing the willingness to experience distress. Indeed, the following themes are emphasized throughout the 14 sessions: (1) the potentially paradoxical effects of emotional avoidance, (2) the emotion-regulating consequences of emotional acceptance and willingness (i.e., an active process of being open to emotional experiences as they arise), and (3) the importance of controlling behavior when emotions are present rather than controlling emotions themselves. Thus, increasing distress tolerance is one of the explicit targets of this group therapy.

## Managing Diagnostic Comorbidity

Arguably, issues of diagnostic comorbidity are of less concern in behavioral treatments that target the function of maladaptive behaviors and seek to modify mechanisms thought to underlie numerous symptom presentations. Indeed, given the putative role of distress intolerance in the development and maintenance of many of the disorders that commonly co-occur with BPD, including substance use disorders, eating disorders, and posttraumatic stress disorder (Anestis et al., 2007; Buckner et al., 2007; Hayes et al., 1996; Marx & Sloan, 2005; Plumb, Orsillo, & Luterek, 2004), treatments for BPD that seek to increase distress tolerance may have a positive effect on these disorders as well. Specifically, by targeting the distress intolerance thought to underlie BPD, these treatments will simultaneously target a key putative underlying mechanism of the co-occurring disorders, thereby providing an effective treatment for these disorders as well. Providing some support for this premise, DBT has been found to be useful in the concurrent treatment of BPD and co-occurring substance use disorders (Linehan et al., 1999, 2002) and eating disorders (Chen, Matthews, Allen, Kuo, & Linehan, 2008).

## Clinical Techniques

### Assessment

When it comes to assessing the role of distress intolerance in the symptom presentation of clients with BPD, the importance of a thorough functional analysis of all targeted behaviors cannot be overemphasized. Indeed, the primary assessment tool within DBT is a functional analysis of treatment targets, many of which function to escape intolerable distress. In DBT, functional analysis of treatment targets is accomplished through a comprehensive behavioral chain analysis. In a behavioral chain analysis, a specific maladaptive behavior (e.g., deliberate self-harm) is selected, and the prompting internal and external events for that behavior are identified. Next, clients identify vulnerability factors that may have increased their risk for the particular chain of behaviors that unfolded (e.g., stress, physical illness, lack of sleep, alcohol use). Clients are then assisted in recounting, in a detailed fashion, all of the antecedent events (both environmental and internal) that eventually culminated in the maladaptive behavior of interest, as well as its positive and negative consequences. This chain analysis is then followed by a solution analysis, wherein multiple places to intervene along the chain (i.e., to break the links in the chain) are identified with the goal of preventing the behavior in the future.

A notable strength of the chain analysis is that it is more comprehensive and specific than behavioral analysis, focusing on a specific behavioral occurrence as well as in-the-moment changes in clients' internal and external environments that may have contributed to the maladaptive behavior (Lynch, Chapman, Rosenthal, Kuo, & Linehan, 2006). Thus, the chain analysis provides a useful strategy for assessing the role of distress intolerance in problem behaviors. Furthermore, the chain analysis may also serve as an intervention in its own right, in that the repeated detailed analysis of the antecedents and consequences of problem behaviors may increase clients' awareness of the ways in which both emotional distress and the unwillingness to experience that distress may prompt a variety of choices that eventually lead to a maladaptive, emotionally avoidant behavior. Furthermore, through the process of recounting the details of an event, clients cannot help but be exposed to internal experiences that were previously avoided (Lynch et al., 2006).

Arguably, the most common manifestation of distress intolerance in BPD is the presence of maladaptive, impulsive, self-destructive behaviors that function to escape or alleviate emotional distress. Some of the most common of these are deliberate self-harm, substance misuse, eating-disordered behaviors, risky sexual behaviors, and aggressive behavior (American Psychiatric Association, 1994; Frankenburg & Zanarini, 2004; Skodol et al., 2002; Trull et al., 2000; Zanarini et al., 1998). Notably, all of these behaviors have been theoretically and empirically linked to distress intolerance (Anestis et al., 2007; Batten et al., 2001; Chapman et al., 2005; Corstorphine et al., 2007; Gratz et al., 2009; Tull et al., 2007) and are thought to serve an emotionally avoidant function (Batten et al., 2001; Chapman et al., 2006; Hayes et al., 1996; Tull et al., 2007).

## Treatment

With regard to specific skills that may promote distress tolerance, DBT distress tolerance skills seek to increase acceptance and willingness (distinguishing between acceptance and approval and viewing willingness as an active choice), as well as the ability to control behaviors when distressed (e.g., by using distraction and self-soothing techniques rather than acting impulsively). Other skills emphasize the importance of considering the short- and long-term consequences of one's behaviors, a process that is expected to increase contact with the negative long-term consequences of behaviors that function to regulate distress in the short-term, such as deliberate self-harm or substance misuse.

Furthermore, DBT mindfulness skills facilitate distress tolerance by focusing on observing and describing emotions (the "what" skills) in a nonjudgmental manner (a "how" skill). Specifically, mindfulness skills promote a nonjudgmental awareness of one's internal experiences (including emotions), teaching clients to observe internal experiences as they occur in the moment, and to label these experiences objectively by letting go of evaluations such as "good" or "bad." As such, clients are taught the importance of taking a nonjudgmental and nonevaluative stance toward their emotions, which is expected to facilitate emotional acceptance and increase emotional willingness (in addition to increasing emotional awareness and clarity).

Likewise, Gratz and Gunderson's (2006) acceptance-based emotion regulation group therapy targets distress tolerance by emphasizing the benefits of emotional willingness, as well as teaching clients strategies for controlling impulsive behaviors in the context of emotional distress. With regard to the former, this group therapy emphasizes the experiential benefits of emotional acceptance, as well as the potentially paradoxical long-term consequences of emotional avoidance. Clients are taught that emotional nonacceptance and avoidance may amplify emotions and make the experience of these emotions more distressing. A distinction is drawn between emotional pain, which is a necessary part of life, and emotional suffering, which includes secondary emotions and failed attempts at emotional control/avoidance. Clients also are taught that emotional acceptance results in less *suffering* than emotional avoidance, as it prevents the amplification of emotional arousal (despite not necessarily reducing the primary emotional response). Clients are asked to actively monitor and assess the different *experiential* consequences of emotional willingness versus emotional unwillingness.

With regard to the latter, clients are taught nonavoidant strategies to modulate the intensity or duration of emotions rather than escaping the emotion entirely. Such strategies include journaling, painting or drawing, sharing one's emotions with others, and healthy distraction techniques such as exercising, cleaning, or watching a movie. Furthermore, clients are taught to identify adaptive behaviors that may serve the same functions or meet the same needs as their impulsive behaviors, and to replace the impulsive behaviors with these adaptive behaviors. As in DBT, clients are also taught to weigh the positive and negative consequences associated with either tolerating (vs. not tolerating) distress and engaging in (vs. not engaging in) some impulsive behavior to escape that distress, with an emphasis on increasing awareness of the long-term consequences of behavioral choices.

## Tracking Changes over the Course of Treatment

The first evidence of improvement in distress tolerance is often the reduction in the frequency and severity of maladaptive, impulsive behaviors. In DBT, this would likely be evidenced by a decrease in the number of target behaviors reported on the weekly diary card, or by the report of urges to engage in maladaptive behaviors and/or the experience of significant emotional distress combined with the absence of, or reduction in, maladaptive behaviors often used to escape that distress. Indeed, it is the reduction in impulsive behaviors and substitution of more adaptive (i.e., nonavoidant) emotion regulation strategies that indicates treatment progress and improving distress tolerance.

Nonetheless, more objective measures of distress tolerance are available and could be incorporated into treatments to assess improvements in this treatment target directly. These include both self-report and behavioral measures, all of which have been used with BPD patients (Bornovalova et al., 2008; Gratz et al., 2006, 2008) or individuals with BPD-relevant impulsive behaviors (e.g., deliberate self-harm, disordered eating behaviors, and substance use; see Buckner et al., 2007; Corstorphine et al., 2007; Gratz et al., 2009). The AAQ (Hayes et al., 2004) is a nine-item self-report measure of experiential avoidance, with a particular emphasis on the avoidance of emotions. It has been used frequently with BPD patient samples (Gratz & Gunderson, 2006; Gratz et al., 2006, 2008) and has been found to be associated with a variety of BPD-relevant behaviors, including deliberate self-harm, substance use, risky sexual behaviors, and aggression (Batten et al., 2001; Gratz et al., 2009; Stewart et al., 2002; Tull et al., 2007). Furthermore, the AAQ has been found to be significantly correlated with an experimental measure of the willingness to experience distress among patients with BPD ($r = -.76$; Gratz et al., 2006). Finally, AAQ scores have been found to be sensitive to change over time (i.e., following short-term treatments) among patients with BPD, with Gratz and Gunderson (2006) finding significant improvements in self-reported emotional avoidance on the AAQ following their 14-week acceptance-based emotion regulation group therapy.

The 14-item Distress Tolerance Scale (DTS; Simons & Gaher, 2005) is another, relatively new self-report measure of distress tolerance, defined as the extent to which individuals are able to experience and withstand unpleasant psychological states. The DTS was found to consist of a single higher order factor of distress tolerance, as well as four lower-order factors: (1) the ability to tolerate distress, (2) the appraisal of distress, (3) attention absorbed by negative emotions, and (4) the use of regulation strategies to alleviate distress (Simon & Gaher, 2005). Although the DTS has been examined primarily within nonclinical populations, it has been found to be associated with a variety of BPD-relevant behaviors, including eating-disordered behavior (Corstorphine et al., 2007) and substance use (Buckner et al., 2007; Simons & Gaher, 2005; Zvolensky et al., 2009). No research to date has examined its sensitivity to change over time among individuals with BPD.

Two behavioral measures that may also be used to examine changes in distress tolerance over the course of treatment are the PASAT-C (Lejuez et al., 2003) and the MTPT-C (Quinn et al., 1996; Strong et al., 2003). In the MTPT-C, participants use a computer mouse to trace a red dot along the lines of a star on the computer screen; however, the mouse is programmed to move the red dot in the reverse direction. Moreover, to further increase the difficulty of the task and resultant frustration, moving the red dot outside of the lines of the star or stalling for more than 2 seconds causes a loud buzzing sound to occur and the red dot to move back to the starting position. In the PASAT-C, on the other hand, numbers are sequentially flashed on a computer screen, and participants are instructed to add the most recent number to the previously presented number before the next number appears on the screen (using the computer mouse to click on the correct answer). If participants give an incorrect answer or fail to provide an answer before the next number is presented, an "explosion" sound occurs and the score does not change. The PASAT-C consists of multiple levels with increasingly shorter latencies between number presentations; because the correct answer must be provided before the presentation of the next number in order to obtain a point, difficulty increases as latencies decrease. In both the MTPT-C and PASAT-C, participants are provided with the option to terminate the task, with latency in seconds to task termination used as a measure of the willingness to tolerate distress. Importantly, however, participants are also informed that although they may terminate the task at any time, their performance will influence how much money they receive as reimbursement for their participation (thereby providing an incentive to perform well on the task). Both the PASAT-C and MTPT-C have been used in samples of substance users with co-occurring BPD (Bornovalova et al., 2008), and the PASAT-C has been used in a sample of outpatients with BPD (Gratz et al., 2006). Furthermore, although no studies to date have examined the sensitivity of these measures to change over time among individuals with BPD, Bornovalova, Gratz, Daughters, and Lejuez (2009) did find significant improvements in the willingness to tolerate distress on the PASAT-C following a brief distress tolerance treatment for substance users in residential treatment.

Finally, the Difficulties in Emotion Regulation Scale (DERS; Gratz & Roemer, 2004), a 36-item self-report measure of the related construct of emotion dysregulation, may also be relevant for assessing changes in distress tolerance over the course of treatment. Specifically, in addition to assessing individuals' typical levels of emotion regulation difficulties in general, the DERS assesses a number of specific dimensions of emotion regulation, including the nonacceptance of negative emotions, difficulties engaging in goal-directed behaviors when experiencing negative emotions, limited access to effective emotion regulation strategies, lack of emotional awareness, lack of emotional clarity, and difficulties controlling impulsive behaviors when experiencing negative emotions. As noted previously, this latter dimension overlaps with the construct of distress tolerance. Both the DERS in general and the subscale assessing difficulties controlling impulsive behaviors when experiencing negative emotions in particular have been used with BPD patient samples (Gratz & Gunderson, 2006), and have been found to be associated with the BPD-relevant behavior of deliberate self-harm among young adults with clinically relevant levels of BPD pathology (Gratz et al., 2009). Furthermore, Gratz and Gunderson (2006) found that scores on this subscale were sensitive to change over time among BPD patients, with significant improvements in difficulties controlling impulsive behaviors when distressed reported following their acceptance-based emotion regulation group therapy.

## Clinical Future Directions

Evidence that treatments targeting distress tolerance (e.g., DBT and the aforementioned acceptance-based emotion regulation group therapy) lead to increases in the willingness to tolerate emotional distress (Gratz & Gunderson, 2006), as well as decreases in maladaptive behaviors that function to escape emotional distress (Gratz & Gunderson, 2006; Linehan, Armstrong, Suarez, Allmon, & Heard, 1991; Linehan et al., 2006), suggests that distress tolerance may be a mechanism of change in these treatments. However, more direct support for distress tolerance as a mechanism of change would be provided by findings that changes in distress tolerance mediate changes in BPD-relevant symptoms and maladaptive behaviors from pre- to posttreatment.

Although little research has specifically examined the mediating role of changes in the willingness to tolerate distress in symptom improvement following these treatments, preliminary data on the acceptance-based emotion regulation group therapy described previously (see Gratz & Gunderson, 2006) provide suggestive support for this possibility. Specifically, we examined whether changes in emotion dysregulation and the willingness to experience emotional distress mediated changes in self-harm frequency following completion of the emotion regulation group therapy. Mediation was examined using a cross-product test, which directly tests the significance of the difference between the direct and indirect (i.e., mediated) effects. In particular, these mediational analyses used the nonparametric method of bootstrapping (which does not assume normal distribution of the cross product), with parameter estimates based on 3,000 bootstrap samples specifically. Results of these analyses indicate that changes in self-harm were mediated by changes in emotion dysregulation and the willingness to experience emotional distress in total ($p < .05$). Furthermore, individual mediators of changes in self-harm at posttreatment included the willingness to tolerate emotional distress ($p < .05$) and the particular emotion dysregulation dimensions of lack of access to effective emotion regulation strategies ($p < .05$) and difficulties controlling impulsive behaviors when experiencing negative emotions ($p < .07$).

Although these findings provide suggestive support for the mediating role of changes in distress tolerance in symptom improvement following this short-term group therapy for self-harm in BPD, further research is needed to explore the role of distress tolerance as a mechanism of change in BPD treatments. Furthermore, dismantling studies are needed to identify whether the aspects of DBT focused on increasing distress tolerance are an active ingredient of the treatment. Given the emphasis on the centrality of distress tolerance to BPD and BPD-related behaviors within Linehan's (1993) theoretical work on the pathogenesis of BPD, as well as empirical research highlighting the strong associations between distress tolerance and BPD (Bornovalova et al., 2008; Gratz et al., 2006), it is reasonable to expect that increases in the willingness to tolerate distress would underlie many of the improvements in symptoms observed following DBT. Providing suggestive support for this possibility, Miller, Wyman, Huppert, Glassman, and Rathus (2000) found that subjective ratings of the perceived helpfulness of the DBT distress tolerance skill of radical acceptance were positively associated with improvements in interpersonal problems among a sample of suicidal adolescents with BPD pathology in DBT. Nonetheless, the extent to which the aspects of DBT that target distress tolerance are active ingredients of the treatment remains to be tested.

Finally, future research should examine the utility of brief targeted treatments focused on increasing distress tolerance among individuals with BPD, as well as those with BPD and co-occurring disorders. Such treatments may provide a useful way to target the impulsive behaviors associated with BPD directly and immediately and could also be used to augment standard treatments for BPD or its co-occurring disorders. For example, preliminary data provide support for the utility of a 6-week adjunctive treatment for substance users in residential treatment targeting distress tolerance (Bornovalova et al., 2009). This adjunctive treatment was found to result in greater distress tolerance (as indexed by persistence on the PASAT-C) than either an adjunctive supportive counseling condition or the standard substance use treatment without an adjunctive intervention added. These findings highlight the potential utility of brief treatments targeting the mechanisms thought to underlie particular behaviors or disorders, and could be applied to the treatment of BPD and related behaviors as well.

## SUMMARY

Consistent with theories implicating distress intolerance in the development and maintenance of BPD, a growing body of literature provides support for the relevance of distress tolerance to BPD and its associated behaviors, with findings indicating an association between the willingness to tolerate distress and BPD, deliberate self-harm, substance use, eating-disordered behavior, aggressive behavior, and risky sexual behavior. Furthermore, research provides support for the unique role of distress tolerance in BPD, above and beyond known risk factors for this disorder, as well as when controlling for other disorders known to have a strong association with distress tolerance (e.g., substance use disorders).

This research, although still in its infancy, suggests the utility of targeting distress tolerance in the treatment of BPD. Indeed, increasing distress tolerance among individuals with BPD is expected to decrease the need for maladaptive behaviors that function to escape or avoid unwanted distress. Extant behavioral treatments for BPD, most notably DBT, do indeed target distress tolerance directly throughout the treatment. Distress tolerance skills and mindfulness skills alike teach clients to practice radical acceptance and the willingness to experience distress, to control their behaviors in the face of distress (e.g., by using self-soothing or distraction skills or focusing on the long-term negative consequences of maladaptive impulsive behaviors), and to take an accepting and non-judgmental stance toward their internal experiences, including their emotions. Likewise, Gratz and Gunderson's acceptance-based emotion regulation group therapy for self-harm among women with BPD targets distress tolerance as a dimension of emotion dysregulation, seeking to increase emotional acceptance, the willingness to experience emotional distress, and the ability to control behaviors when distressed. These treatments have been found to be efficacious in the treatment of BPD, and preliminary evidence suggests that improvements in distress tolerance may be one of the mechanisms of change in these treatments. Further research is needed to explore this more directly, however.

Future research is also needed to explore the factors that may increase the risk for distress intolerance among individuals with BPD (including the potential genetic underpinnings of distress tolerance), as well as the ways in which distress intolerance may contribute to the pathogenesis or exacerbation of BPD symptoms. Such research may provide insight into additional promising treatment and prevention targets. For example, findings that emotional nonacceptance and judging of one's internal experiences are associated with greater unwillingness to tolerate distress highlight the utility of targeting emotional acceptance and nonjudging in treatments for BPD, and suggest the potential utility of mindfulness training in treating the distress intolerance prominent within this disorder.

## REFERENCES

American Psychiatric Association. (1994). *Diagnostic and statistical manual of mental disorders* (4th ed.). Washington, DC: Author.

Anestis, M. D., Selby, E. A., Fink, E. L., & Joiner, T. E. (2007). The multifaceted role of distress tolerance in dysregulated eating behaviors. *International Journal of Eating Disorders, 40*, 718–726.

Batten, S. V., Follette, V. M., & Aban, I. B. (2001). Experiential avoidance and high-risk sexual behavior in survivors of child sexual abuse. *Journal of Child Sexual Abuse, 10*, 101–120.

Bender, D. S., Dolan, R. T., Skodol, A. E., Sanislow, C. A., Dyck, I. R., McGlasgan, T. H., et al. (2001). Treatment utilization by patients with personality disorders. *American Journal of Psychiatry, 158*, 295–302.

Bornovalova, M. A., Gratz, K. L., Daughters, S. B., & Lejuez, C. W. (2009). *Distress tolerance treatment for inner-city drug users: A preliminary trial.* Manuscript in preparation.

Bornovalova, M. A., Gratz, K. L., Daughters, S. B., Nick, B., Delany-Brumsey, A., Lynch, T. R., et al. (2008). A multimodal assessment of the relationship between emotion dysregulation and borderline personality disorder among inner-city substance users in residential treatment. *Journal of Psychiatric Research, 42*, 717–726.

Buckner, J. D., Keogh, M. E., & Schmidt, N. B. (2007). Problematic alcohol and cannabis use among young adults: The roles of depression and discomfort and distress tolerance. *Addictive Behaviors, 32*, 1957–1963.

Chapman, A. L., Gratz, K. L., & Brown, M. Z. (2006). Solving the puzzle of deliberate self-harm: The experiential avoidance model. *Behaviour Research and Therapy, 44*, 371–394.

Chapman, A. L., Specht, M. W., & Cellucci, T. (2005). Borderline personality disorder and deliberate self-harm: Does experiential avoidance play a role? *Suicide and Life-Threatening Behavior, 35*, 388–399.

Chen, E. Y., Matthews, L., Allen, C., Kuo, J. R., & Linehan, M. M. (2008). Dialectical behavior therapy for clients with binge-eating disorder or bulimia nervosa and borderline personality disorder. *International Journal of Eating Disorders, 41*, 505–512.

Corstorphine, E., Mountford, V., Tomlinson, S., Waller, G., & Meyer, C. (2007). Distress tolerance in the eating disorders. *Eating Behaviors, 8*, 91–97.

Evans, D. R., Baer, R. A., & Segerstrom, S. C. (2009). The effects of mindfulness and self-consciousness on persistence. *Personality and Individual Differences, 47*, 379–382.

Frankenburg, F. R., & Zanarini, M. C. (2004). The association between border-line personality disorder and chronic mental illnesses, poor health-related lifestyle choices, and costly forms of health care utilization. *Journal of Clinical Psychiatry, 65,* 1660–1665.

Glenn, C. R., & Klonsky, E. D. (2009). Emotion dysregulation as a core feature of borderline personality disorder. *Journal of Personality Disorders, 23,* 20–28.

Grant, B. F., Chou, P., Goldstein, R. B., Huang, B., Stinson, F. S., Saha, T. D., et al. (2008). Prevalence, correlates, disability, and comorbidity of DSM-IV borderline personality disorder: Results from the wave 2 national epidemiological survey on alcohol and related conditions. *Journal of Clinical Psychiatry, 69,* 533–545.

Gratz, K. L., Bornovalova, M. A., Delany-Brumsey, A., Nick, B., & Lejuez, C. W. (2007). A laboratory-based study of the relationship between childhood abuse and experiential avoidance among inner-city substance users: The role of emotional non-acceptance. *Behavior Therapy, 38,* 256–268.

Gratz, K. L., Breetz, A., & Tull, M. T. (2010). The moderating role of borderline personality in the relationships between deliberate self-harm and emotion-related factors. *Personality and Mental Health, 4,* 96–107.

Gratz, K. L., & Gunderson, J. G. (2006). Preliminary data on acceptance-based emotion regulation group intervention for deliberate self-harm among women with borderline personality disorder. *Behavior Therapy, 37,* 25–35.

Gratz, K. L., Hepworth, C., Tull, M. T., Paulson, A., Clarke, S., Remington, B., et al. (in press). An experimental investigation of emotional unwillingness and physical pain tolerance in deliberate self-harm: The moderating role of interpersonal distress. *Comprehensive Psychiatry.*

Gratz, K. L., & Roemer, L. (2004). Multidimensional assessment of emotion regulation and dysregulation: Development, factor structure, and initial validation of the Difficulties in Emotion Regulation Scale. *Journal of Psychopathology and Behavioral Assessment, 26,* 41–54.

Gratz, K. L., Rosenthal, M. Z., Tull, M. T., Lejuez, C. W., & Gunderson, J. G. (2006). An experimental investigation of emotion dysregulation in borderline personality disorder. *Journal of Abnormal Psychology, 115,* 850–855.

Gratz, K. L., Tull, M. T., & Gunderson, J. G. (2008). Preliminary data on the relationship between anxiety sensitivity and borderline personality disorder: The role of experiential avoidance. *Journal of Psychiatric Research, 42,* 550–559.

Gross, J. J., & Levenson, R. W. (1993). Emotional suppression: Physiology, self-report, and expressive behavior. *Journal of Personality and Social Psychology, 64,* 970–986.

Gross, J. J., & Levenson, R. W. (1997). Hiding feelings: The acute effects of inhibiting negative and positive emotion. *Journal of Abnormal Psychology, 106,* 95–103.

Gunderson, J. G. (2001). *Borderline personality disorder: A clinical guide.* Washington, DC: American Psychiatric Association.

Hayes, S. C., Strosahl, K. D., & Wilson, K. G. (1999). *Acceptance and commit-*

*ment therapy: An experiential approach to behavior change.* New York: Guilford Press.

Hayes, S. C., Strosahl, K. D., Wilson, K. G., Bissett, R. T., Pistorello, J., Toarmino, D., et al. (2004). Measuring experiential avoidance: A preliminary test of a working model. *Psychological Record, 54,* 553–578.

Hayes, S. C., Wilson, K. G., Gifford, E. V., Follette, V. M., & Strosahl, K. (1996). Experiential avoidance and behavioral disorders: A functional dimensional approach to diagnosis and treatment. *Journal of Consulting and Clinical Psychology, 64,* 1152–1168.

Heaton, R. K., Chelune, G. J., Talley, J. L., Kay, G. G., & Curtis, G. (1993). *Wisconsin Card Sort Test (WCST) manual revised and expanded.* Odessa, FL: Psychological Assessment Resources.

Karekla, M., Forsyth, J. P., & Kelly, M. M. (2004). Emotional avoidance and panicogenic responding to a biological challenge procedure. *Behavior Therapy, 35,* 725–746.

Lejuez, C. W., Kahler, C. W., & Brown, R. A. (2003). A modified computer version of the paced auditory serial addition task (PASAT) as a laboratory-based stressor. *The Behavior Therapist, 26,* 290–293.

Lenzenweger, M. F., Lane, M. C., Loranger, A. W., & Kessler, R. C. (2007). DSM-IV personality disorders in the National Comorbidity Survey replication. *Biological Psychiatry, 62,* 553–564.

Linehan, M. M. (1993). *Cognitive-behavioral treatment of borderline personality disorder.* New York: Guilford Press.

Linehan, M. M., Armstrong, H. E., Suarez, A., Allmon, D., & Heard, H. L. (1991). Cognitive-behavioral treatment of chronically parasuicidal borderline patients. *Archives of General Psychiatry, 48,* 1060–1064.

Linehan, M. M., Comtois, K. A., Murray, A. M., Brown, M. Z., Gallop, R. J., Heard, H. L., et al. (2006). Two-year randomized controlled trial and follow-up of dialectical behavior therapy vs. therapy by experts for suicidal behaviors and borderline personality disorder. *Archives of General Psychiatry, 63,* 757–766.

Linehan, M. M., Dimeff, L. A., Reynolds, S. K., Comtois, K. A., Welch, S. S., Heagerty, P., et al. (2002). Dialectical behavior therapy versus comprehensive validation therapy plus 12-step for the treatment of opioid dependent women meeting criteria for borderline personality disorder. *Drug and Alcohol Dependence, 67,* 13–26.

Linehan, M. M., Schmidt, H., Dimeff, L. A., Craft, J. C., Kanter, J., & Comtois, K. A. (1999). Dialectical behavior therapy for inpatients with borderline personality disorder and drug-dependence. *American Journal on Addictions, 8,* 279–292.

Lynch, T. R., Chapman, A. L., Rosenthal, M. Z., Kuo, J. R., & Linehan, M. M. (2006). Mechanisms of change in dialectical behavior therapy: Theoretical and empirical observations. *Journal of Clinical Psychology, 62,* 459–480.

Lynch, T. R., Cheavens, J. S., Morse, J. Q., & Rosenthal, M. Z. (2004). A model predicting suicidal ideation and hopelessness in depressed older adults: The impact of emotion inhibition and affect intensity. *Aging and Mental Health, 8,* 486–497.

Marx, B. P., & Sloan, D. M. (2005). Peritraumatic dissociation and experiential avoidance as predictors of posttraumatic stress symptomatology. *Behaviour Research and Therapy, 43,* 569–583.

Miller, A. L., Wyman, S. E., Huppert, J. D., Glassman, S. L., & Rathus, J. H. (2000). Analysis of behavioral skills utilized by suicidal adolescents receiving dialectical behavior therapy. *Cognitive and Behavioral Practice, 7,* 183–187.

Nock, M. K., & Mendes, W. B. (2008). Physiological arousal, distress tolerance, and social problem-solving deficits among adolescent self-injurers. *Journal of Consulting and Clinical Psychology, 76,* 28–38.

Plumb, J. C., Orsillo, S. M., & Luterek, J. A. (2004). A preliminary test of the role of experiential avoidance in post-event functioning. *Journal of Behavior Therapy and Experimental Psychiatry, 35,* 245–257.

Quinn, E. P., Brandon, T. H., & Copeland, A. L. (1996). Is task persistence related to smoking and substance abuse?: The application of learned industriousness theory to addictive behaviors. *Experimental and Clinical Psychopharmacology, 4,* 186–190.

Rosenthal, M. Z., Gratz, K. L., Kosson, D. S., Cheavens, J. S., Lejuez, C. W., & Lynch, T. R. (2008). Borderline personality disorder and emotional responding: A review of the research literature. *Clinical Psychology Review, 28,* 75–91.

Simons, J. S., & Gaher, R. M. (2005). The Distress Tolerance Scale: Development and validation of a self-report measure. *Motivation and Emotion, 29,* 83–102.

Skodol, A. E., Gunderson, J. G., Pfohl, B., Widiger, T. A., Livesley, W. J., & Siever, L. J. (2002). The borderline diagnosis: Psychopathology, comorbidity, and personality structure. *Biological Psychiatry, 51,* 936–950.

Stewart, S. H., Zvolensky, M. J., & Eifert, G. H. (2002). The relations of anxiety sensitivity, experiential avoidance, and alexithymic coping to young adults' motivations for drinking. *Behavior Modification, 26,* 274–296.

Strong, D. R., Lejuez, C. W., Daughters, S. B., Marinello, M., Kahler, C. W., & Brown, R. A. (2003). *The computerized mirror tracing task version 1.* Unpublished manual.

Torgersen, S., Kringlen, E., & Cramer, V. (2001). The prevalence of personality disorders in a community sample. *Archives of General Psychiatry, 58,* 590–596.

Trull, T. J., Sher, K. J., Minks-Brown, C., Durbin, J., & Burr, R. (2000). Borderline personality disorder and substance use disorders: A review and integration. *Clinical Psychology Review, 20,* 235–253.

Tull, M. T., Jakupcak, M., Paulson, A., & Gratz, K. L. (2007). The role of emotional inexpressivity and experiential avoidance in the relationship between posttraumatic stress disorder symptom severity and aggressive behavior among men exposed to interpersonal violence. *Anxiety, Stress, and Coping, 20,* 337–351.

Widiger, T. A., & Frances, A. J. (1989). Epidemiology, diagnosis, and comorbidity of borderline personality disorder. In A. Tasman, R. E. Hales, & A. J. Frances (Eds.), *American Psychiatric Press review of psychiatry* (Vol. 8, pp. 8–24). Washington, DC: American Psychiatric Press.

Widiger, T. A., & Weissman, M. M. (1991). Epidemiology of borderline personality disorder. *Hospital and Community Psychiatry, 42,* 1015–1021.

Zanarini, M. C., Frankenburg, F. R., Dubo, E. D., Sickel, A. E., Trikha, A., Levin, A., et al. (1998). Axis I comorbidity of borderline personality disorder. *American Journal of Psychiatry, 155,* 1733–1739.

Zanarini, M. C., Frankenburg, F. R., Khera, G. S., & Bleichmar, J. (2001). Treatment histories of borderline inpatients. *Comprehensive Psychiatry, 42,* 144–150.

Zvolensky, M. J., & Eifert, G. H. (2001). A review of psychological factors/processes affecting anxious responding during voluntary hyperventilation and inhalations of carbon dioxide-enriched air. *Clinical Psychology Review, 21,* 375–400.

Zvolensky, M. J., Marshall, E. C., Johnson, K., Hogan, J., Bernstein, A., & Bonn-Miller, M. O. (2009). Relations between anxiety sensitivity, distress tolerance, and fear reactivity to bodily sensations to coping and conformity: Marijuana use motives among young adult marijuana users. *Experimental and Clinical Psychopharmacology, 17,* 31–42.

# 10

## Chronic Musculoskeletal Pain and Related Health Conditions

Gordon J. G. Asmundson, Daniel L. Peluso,
R. Nicholas Carleton, Kelsey C. Collimore,
*and* Patrick G. Welch

In this chapter, we review the current state of knowledge regarding the distress tolerance construct in people with chronic musculoskeletal pain and, on that basis, attempt to provide evidence-based recommendations for clinical assessment and treatment. Where appropriate, we extend our analysis and recommendations to other related chronic health conditions (e.g., headache, irritable bowel syndrome, fibromyalgia). To accomplish these goals, we introduce and describe core features of chronic musculoskeletal pain, contextualize the current state of the field as it pertains to understanding distress tolerance in chronic pain, provide a review and critique of the extant literature relevant to the issue, and discuss theoretical implications and future research directions. We conclude the chapter by offering clinical recommendations for those treating people with chronic musculoskeletal pain or related chronic health conditions. These recommendations are predicated upon the current evidence base regarding distress tolerance in these populations.

## THE STATE OF THE FIELD

### Pain and Chronic Pain

We now understand that pain involves more than a pure sensory experience arising from noxious stimulation (e.g., physical injury or other pathology), as was once espoused by the medical model. The past four decades have yielded a variety of models that incorporate biological as well as psychological (e.g., perception, cognition, affect), behavioral (e.g., avoidance), and social (e.g., cultural) factors to explain pain. These biopsychosocial models, described in detail elsewhere (Asmundson & Wright, 2004), have dramatically improved our understanding of pain and our ability to effectively intervene in cases where it is unremitting. Today we understand pain as a complex perceptual phenomenon that involves a number of dimensions, including, but not limited to, intensity, quality, time course, and personal meaning (Merskey & Bogduk, 1994). We also understand that pain initiates short-term adaptive processes that facilitate the ability to identify, respond to, and resolve physical injury. There is, however, a significant proportion of the population who experience pain for periods that substantially exceed expected healing times for physical healing (e.g., Waddell, 1987).

Pain that persists 3 months or longer is, according to most authorities (e.g., Merskey & Bogduk, 1994), considered to be chronic pain. Chronic musculoskeletal pain, albeit not always maladaptive (Asmundson, Norton, Allerdings, Norton, & Larsen, 1998; Turk & Rudy, 1987), often leads to hypervigilance for pain, significant emotional distress, physical decline and deconditioning, and functional disability. It is also associated with inappropriate use of medical services and high-cost insurance claims (Nachemson, 1992; Spengler, Bigos, & Martin, 1986). Consequently, researchers and clinicians have focused considerable attention toward gaining a better understanding of the psychological processes by which musculoskeletal pain becomes chronic and, in cases where it does, how to intervene most effectively. Similar attention has been directed to understanding various chronic health conditions that are characterized, at least in part, by persistent pain, emotional distress, and reduced functioning, including chronic headaches (Kröner-Herwig, 2009; McFate & Scher, 2009), irritable bowel syndrome (Grossi, Goldberg, Locker, & Tenenbaum, 2008; Williams, Hartmann, Sandler, Miller, & Steege, 2004), and fibromyalgia (Arendt-Nielsen & Henriksson, 2007; Nijs, Meeus, & de Meirleir, 2006).

Over the past decade there have been numerous investigations of cognitive and affective aspects of the pain experience. One need only scan a few of the numerous reviews (e.g., Craig, 1994; Gatchel, Peng, Peters, Fuchs, & Turk, 2007; Kröner-Herwig, 2009; McFate & Scher, 2009; Thorn, Cross, & Walker, 2007; Vlaeyen & Linton, 2000) to gain an appreciation of the effort that has been put forth to understand the role that various forms of emotional distress play in chronic pain and its treatment. The distress tolerance construct—the capacity to experience and withstand negative psychological states (Simons & Gaher, 2005)—

as it pertains to chronic musculoskeletal pain and other chronic health conditions has not received much direct or otherwise focused empirical attention; however, there is a rich and well-developed literature on the seemingly overlapping construct of pain tolerance. Next, we compare and contrast the distress and pain tolerance constructs before highlighting major findings from the pain perception and pain tolerance evidence base as they pertain to chronic musculoskeletal pain, related conditions, and their assessment and treatment.

## Tolerance of Pain and Distress

The pain tolerance construct can be traced back to implicit narrative accounts of Homeric heroes as individuals who were capable of tolerating extreme amounts of pain (Homer, 2000). Likewise, the 1500 BCE Edwin Smith Papyrus suggests that relative failures to tolerate pain were used as indicators that one may have a significant medical issue (Waddell, 1992). Modern definitions of the construct are predicated on the current conceptualization of pain (as described previously) and require prolonged or exacerbated stimulation of specialized pain receptors beyond the pain threshold (i.e., the minimal intensity of a stimulus that is perceived as painful; Loeser & Treede, 2008). As such, pain tolerance is currently defined as "the maximum intensity of a stimulus that evokes pain and that a subject is willing to tolerate in a given situation" (Loeser & Treede, 2008, p. 47). Depending on the circumstances under which pain tolerance is being assessed, it might be operationalized as (1) the point at which an individual instructed to endure maximum pain reports a desire to have the stimulus discontinued or (2) the point at which an individual determines pain to be unbearable and acts to alleviate the experience.

Development of distress tolerance as a construct has followed a remarkably similar path as that of pain tolerance; indeed, the ability to tolerate distress has also been evangelized in classical text as a mark of heroics (Homer, 2000). Subsequent discussions of extreme distress as medical pathology were made in the now classical writings of Breuer and Freud (1974). Providing specific definitions of distress tolerance in the modern era began with early attempts to define distress itself. Distress has been described as an aversive state in which an animal is unable to adapt sufficiently to stressors and the associated stress, resulting in maladaptive behaviors (Institute for Laboratory Animal Research, 1992). The definition intentionally allowed for inclusion of a variety of phenomena, such as social interactions and taxing physical sensations, both of which can produce distress. The associated definition of distress tolerance originally described it as the ability to endure and accept intense negative affect so that problem solving can take place (Linehan, 1993). Most recently, distress tolerance has been described as a multimodal construct that denotes an individual's capacity—typically measured by elapsed time—to experience and withstand negative psychological states (Simons & Gaher, 2005).

There have, to date, been no direct empirical comparisons of the pain tolerance and distress tolerance constructs; however, they appear to be highly related if not parallel in nature. Pain tolerance does imply a specific focus on pain sensations, but, as described previously, the pain experience involves a negative affective component. Distress tolerance implies a focus on negative affect and related psychological states, but the experience of negative psychological states depends in part on somatic experiences interpreted to be unpleasant (Barlow, 2002; Mathews & MacLeod, 1994). Cognitive and behavioral components also overlap in that, for each, tolerance is measured via a subjective decision to act to attenuate or discontinue the aversive experience. Consequently, the experiences of pain and distress appear inextricably intertwined within a biopsychosocial context.

# RELEVANT EMPIRICAL LITERATURE

## Literature Review

Pain tolerance is typically measured in the laboratory setting using one of several pain induction procedures. Here we explain quantitative methodology used to assess pain tolerance, outline several common types of experimental methods of pain induction, and review key pain tolerance findings in samples from the general populations as well as from patients with chronic musculoskeletal pain and anxiety-related psychopathology.

## Definitions and Methods

Quantitative sensory testing (QST) is a quantitative method used to test somatosensory functioning of the nociceptive system or, in simpler terms, pain perception (Chong & Cros, 2004; Cruccu et al., 2004; Rolke et al., 2006; Shy et al., 2003). QST is conducted with active and willing participants using one or more of a wide variety of pain stimulation strategies. To illustrate, studies have used cold pain, heat pain, and ischemic pain (i.e., by artificially restricting blood flow to the target area), mechanical pain (i.e., by running a series of nylon filaments against the skin), pressure pain, and even rectal distension pain. Pain induction methods are disparate in terms of modality but nonetheless tend to be highly intercorrelated with respect to outcomes. For example, heat pain threshold and tolerance have demonstrated significant correlation with tolerance indexed by pressure tasks (Hastie et al., 2005; Petzke, Clauw, Ambrose, Khine, & Gracely, 2003). Although the nature of the painful stimuli is different, the phenomenological experience and tolerance of pain appear to be relatively comparable; consequently, findings from one modality of pain induction might be considered generalizable.

There are several outcome measures sought as feedback from participants in QST studies, including pain thresholds and pain tolerance as noted previously. From these outcome measures, researchers can make inferences regarding pain perception in individuals or groups. Reduced pain threshold and tolerance indicate heightened pain perception or hyperalgesia, whereas increased pain threshold and tolerance indicate attenuated pain perception or hypoalgesia/analgesia. Hyperalgesia is often referred to in the literature as increased pain sensitivity and hypoalgesia/analgesia as decreased pain sensitivity. Pain intensity ratings, which may reflect the cumulative distress of the pain experience, are also sometimes measured.

It is beyond the scope of this chapter to review the extant literature regarding general issues of pain perception; however, it is noteworthy that sex, menstrual cycle phase, age, and ethnicity have generally consistent associations with pain perception. The major findings can be summarized as follows:

1. Women typically exhibit greater sensitivity to experimentally induced pain across pain stimulation sites and experience greater pain-related distress than men (Paller, Campbell, Edwards, & Dobs, 2009). Meta-analytic findings suggest that effect sizes range from moderate to large, depending on the pain induction strategy used (e.g., larger effects for pressure and electrical pain induction and smaller effects for thermal pain induction) and whether pain threshold or tolerance were measured (i.e., effects more variable with threshold measures; Riley, Robinson, Wise, Myers, & Fillingim, 1998).

2. Women in the latter stages of the menstrual cycle exhibit greater sensitivity to experimentally induced pain (excluding electrical induction, which showed the reverse pattern) than do women in earlier stages of the menstrual cycle (Fillingim, 2004b). Meta-analytic findings suggest that effect sizes range from small to moderate, depending on stage in the menstrual cycle (e.g., effects were larger in the premenstrual phase), and are consistent for each of pain threshold and tolerance (Riley, Robinson, Wise, & Price, 1999).

3. Early theorists believed that pain tolerance increased with age (Critchley, 1931). In contrast, subsequent evidence quickly contrasted

such theories by demonstrating an inverse relationship between age and pain (Woodrow, Friedman, Siegelaub, & Collen, 1972). Indeed, there appears to be relatively robust evidence suggesting that older people actually demonstrate greater sensitivity to pain than younger people (Edwards & Fillingim, 2001; Gibson & Farrell, 2004). Accordingly, it appears that people become more vulnerable to pain and pain experiences as they age.

4. People of African American, Hispanic, and Asian descent demonstrate greater sensitivity to experimentally induced pain across pain induction strategies as well as to clinical (e.g., postsurgical) pain, and appear to experience greater pain-related distress and disability than non-Hispanic European Americans (Edwards, Fillingim, & Keefe, 2001). As noted by Edwards and colleagues (2001), there are a variety of biological, social, and psychological mechanisms that underlie these differences, many of which remain to be empirically appraised.

More germane to the present discussion is the growing body of literature regarding pain sensitivity in people with chronic musculoskeletal pain or related chronic health conditions and people exposed to trauma.

## Pain Sensitivity in Clinical Pain Samples

There is a sizable literature regarding pain perception among patients with chronic pain and related conditions. Some conditions are associated with increased pain sensitivity, both at condition-specific sites (e.g., the head and neck in chronic headache patients) as well as sites unrelated to the condition. These conditions include chronic primary headaches (i.e., tension-type, migraine, and cluster headaches) (Pielsticker & Lautenbacher, 2004), fibromyalgia (Kosek, 2004), and irritable bowel syndrome (Covelli, Price, & Verne, 2004). A number of other conditions have a less clear association with pain perception, with no systematic or generalized alterations in the way pain is perceived. Studies examining chronic musculoskeletal pain (e.g., back pain) have reported mixed findings, with evidence of increased pain sensitivity, decreased pain sensitivity, and normal pain sensitivity (Peters, 2004). Studies examining myofascial pain syndrome (Arendt-Nielsen, Graven-Nielsen, & Svensson, 2004) and temporomandibular pain syndrome (Rollman & Gillespie, 2004) have reported increased sensitivity to pain at condition-specific sites but mixed findings at sites unrelated to those conditions. To further complicate attempts to understand how the experience of chronic and unremitting pain impact pain perception, studies of patients with diabetes suggest that the sensory and pain perception alterations associated with diabetic neuropathy are dependent on the duration and severity of the disorder (Schepelmann & Lautenbacher, 2004).

The relationship between chronic musculoskeletal pain and related conditions and pain perception is clearly a complex one. This may be due, in part, to various individual-difference factors that influence the experience of pain and pain-related disability. Not all patients with chronic pain are disabled by their pain; however, it has been consistently shown that heightened emotional distress (e.g., negative affect, catastrophic thinking, fear of pain, pain-related anxiety, and anxiety sensitivity, or the fear of anxiety-related symptoms) is characteristic of those with significant functional limitations (e.g., Asmundson, Kuperos, & Norton, 1997; McCracken, Spertus, Janeck, Sinclair, & Wetzel, 1999; Turk & Rudy, 1988).

## Individual-Difference Variables and Pain Perception

Numerous studies in nonclinical and clinical pain samples have been conducted in an effort to understand the influence of individual-difference variables on pain perception. Depression (Dickens, McGowan, & Dale, 2003) and blood pressure (Duschek, Schwarzkopf, & Schandry, 2008; Fillingim, 2004a) have been associated with reduced pain sensitivity. On the other hand, state and trait anxiety (Carter et al., 2002; James, & Hardardottir, 2002; Jones, Zachariae, & Arendt-Nielsen, 2003), fear of pain (George, Dannecker, & Robinson, 2006; Hirsh, George, Bialosky, & Robinson, 2008), pain-related anxiety (Staats, Staats, & Hekmat, 2001), and heart rate (Lane, Lefebvre, Rose, & Keefe, 1995) have been associated with increased pain sensitivity. The picture for pain catastrophizing and anxiety sensitivity is less clear. Studies have shown pain catastrophizing (Heyneman, Fremouw, Gano, Kirkland, & Heiden, 1990; Sullivan, Bishop, & Pivik, 1995) and pain-related intrusive thoughts (Sullivan, Rouse, Bishop, & Johnston, 1997) to have positive association with pain severity ratings but not pain threshold or tolerance ratings for either heat or cold pain (Edwards, Haythornthwaite, Sullivan, & Fillingim, 2004; Hirsh et al., 2008; Roelofs, Peters, van der Zijden, & Vlaeyen, 2004). Likewise, anxiety sensitivity has been shown to have positive associations with pain severity ratings (Schmidt & Cook, 1999), particularly in women and for heat pain (Thompson, Keogh, French, & Davis, 2008), but appears unrelated to pain threshold and tolerance (Keogh & Birkby, 1999; Keogh & Mansoor, 2001; Roelofs et al., 2004).

A related line of inquiry has sought to determine whether cognitive control strategies can decrease pain sensitivity; that is, can cognitive control strategies promote hypoalgesia/analgesia? Despite the intuitive appeal of strategies such as distraction or suppression of pain-related thoughts as means for coping with pain, the evidence for their effectiveness is equivocal (Cioffi & Holloway, 1993; Harvey & McGuire, 2000; McCaul, Monson, & Maki, 1992; Sullivan et al., 1997). To illustrate, despite several laboratory and clinical studies showing distraction as an effective means of reducing pain sensitivity (Affleck, Urrows, Tennen, & Higgins, 1992; Brewer & Karoly, 1989; Jensen & Karoly, 1991), most studies suggest that directing attention away from pain is related to greater sensitivity to pain (i.e., lower pain tolerance, more severe pain) and greater pain-related disability (Buckelew et al., 1992; Goubert, Crombez, Eccleston, & Devulder, 2004; Keefe & Williams, 1990). Conversely, strategies that require direction of attention toward the sensory quality of pain (i.e., somatic focus) have generally proven effective in reducing pain sensitivity; but recent findings suggest that the effectiveness of these strategies may be dependent on the sex of the person experiencing pain (Keogh, Hatton, & Ellery, 2000).

Likewise, emerging evidence suggests that the effectiveness of distraction versus somatic focus may also depend on pain-related fear and related individual-difference variables. Distraction has been shown to be an ineffective strategy for dealing with pain in those with high anxiety sensitivity (Keogh & Mansoor, 2001) and who are fearful and/or catastrophize about their pain (Goubert, Crombez, & Van Damme, 2004; Hadjistavropoulos, Hadjistavropoulos, & Quine, 2000; Heyneman et al., 1990; Roelofs et al., 2004), whereas somatic focus is effective in reducing pain intensity (Keogh & Mansoor, 2001; Roelofs et al., 2004) as well as anxiety (Hadjistavropoulos et al., 2000). Few studies have examined acceptance-based strategies (i.e., wherein thoughts and emotions are fully experienced rather than avoided) for coping with experimentally induced pain, and none have considered these strategies with respect to pain-related fear and related individual-difference variables; however, the available evidence suggests that acceptance-based strategies are more effective than distraction in increasing pain tolerance (Feldner et al., 2006) and may (Masedo & Esteve, 2007) or may not (Gutiérrez, Luciano, Rodriguez, & Fink, 2004; Hayes, Strosahl, & Wilson, 1999;) reduce pain severity ratings.

The complexity of this literature, with differing patterns of findings for seemingly similar constructs and between pain induction strategies within the context of the same construct, makes difficult the task of disentangling the independent effects of mood, anxiety, and other individual-difference factors on pain perception and coping. Nevertheless, whether assessed in healthy controls or clinical participants, the findings to date are generally consistent in showing that anxious and fearful thinking are related to exacerbation of one or more aspects of the pain experience, and that coping strategies rooted in somatic focus (and possibly acceptance) may be most effective for reducing pain sensitivity in this context.

## Exposure to Trauma and Pain Perception

Investigations of pain perception among individuals exposed to trauma and those with posttraumatic stress disorder (PTSD) have been increasing in recent years and have the potential to inform our understanding of mechanisms responsible for alterations in pain tolerance. As with the literature pertaining to chronic pain and related conditions, the evidence is mixed as to whether traumatic stress and/or PTSD are related to systematic alterations in pain perception. Studies involving participants exposed to trauma have found evidence of increased sensitivity to pain (Scarinci, McDonald-Haile, Bradley, & Richter, 1994), decreased sensitivity to pain (Fillingim & Edwards, 2005; Fillingim, Maixner, Sigurdsson, & Kincaid, 1997; Kraus et al., 2009), and normal pain perception (Alexander et al., 1998; Whitehead, Crowell, Davidoff, Palsson, & Schuster, 1997). Similarly, studies involving patients with PTSD have found evidence of decreased sensitivity to pain (Geuze et al., 2007; Kraus et al., 2009) and normal pain perception (Pitman, van der Kolk, Orr, & Greenberg, 1990; Schmahl et al., 2008; van der Kolk, Greenberg, Orr, & Pitman, 1989). Defrin and colleagues (2008) reported that patients with PTSD, most of whom had chronic pain, but not healthy or clinical (i.e., having an anxiety disorder other than PTSD) controls, had reduced pain sensitivity to at-pain-threshold stimuli and increased pain sensitivity to stimuli above the threshold for pain.

For several reasons, this literature is, unfortunately, difficult to interpret. People exposed to experiences they would describe as traumatic and those with PTSD are more likely to have chronic musculoskeletal pain and related conditions (Asmundson, Coons, Taylor, & Katz, 2002); indeed, of the participants in the aforementioned studies, many had chronic musculoskeletal pain or a related condition (i.e., fibromyalgia, gastroesophageal reflux disease, irritable bowel syndrome, noncardiac chest pain, temporomandibular disorder). Moreover, these studies used inconsistent and restrictive operational definitions of traumatic stress, failed to consider or control for sex differences in pain perception, used a wide variety of pain induction strategies, and produced mixed findings using the same pain induction strategy. The studies do not, therefore, substantively improve our understanding of the independent effects of persistent pain versus trauma exposure or PTSD on pain perception.

## Summary

Studies investigating pain perception use a variety of pain stimulation strategies (e.g., thermal pain, pressure pain) and typically assess responses to the stimulation using one or more of several different outcome measures (e.g., pain threshold, pain tolerance, general pain severity ratings). Empirical evidence suggests consistent associations among sex, menstrual cycle phase, age, ethnicity, and pain perception. The relationship between pain perception and chronic health conditions is, on the other hand, less clear. The mixed findings may be due to various individual-difference characteristics (e.g., trait anxiety, fear of pain, anxiety sensitivity) that influence the experience of pain by either increasing or decreasing pain sensitivity. Emerging data suggest that traumatic event exposure and PTSD also alter pain perception; but here too the findings are mixed. Despite the complexity of the extant literature, the findings collectively suggest that anxious and fearful thinking are related to exacerbation of one or more aspects of the pain experience as well as the effectiveness of pain coping strategies. Additional investigation is needed to help delineate the complex relationships between chronic musculoskeletal pain and related chronic health conditions, individual-difference factors, traumatic event exposure, and pain perception and pain-related coping.

## Quality/Limitations of Extant Research

The literature on pain perception, both in patients with chronic musculoskeletal pain and related chronic health conditions and in healthy participants, is vast and replete with complexity. Within the scope of this review, we were limited to providing only an overview of major themes and complexities that have emerged from decades of investigation. We specifically sought to draw a link between this well-developed literature on pain perception, as well as the related issue of pain tolerance, and that of distress tolerance. We deemed this approach as both reasonable and necessary because of the dearth of empirical attention directed toward understanding distress tolerance in the context of chronic pain and related chronic health conditions. Indeed, a search of the terms *distress tolerance* and *pain* in the Key Concepts field of PsycInfo and Key Words field of ScienceDirect identified only one (DeBenedittis, Panerai, & Villamira, 1989) and four (Bruera, MacMillan, Hanson, & MacDonald, 1989; De Pascalis, Magurano, & Bellusci, 1999; De Pascalis & Perrone, 1996; Feldner et al., 2006) studies, respectively, that utilized these specific terms. We were unable to identify a single study regarding the pain experience that utilized a measure specifically designed to assess the distress tolerance construct (e.g., Distress Tolerance Scale; Simons & Gaher, 2005).

The study of Schmidt and Cook (1999), in which anxiety sensitivity was shown to be positively associated with pain severity ratings, included a measure of a construct seemingly related to distress tolerance; specifically, discomfort intolerance (i.e., an individual difference in the ability to tolerate uncomfortable physical sensations). Discomfort intolerance was found to be unrelated to ratings of pain severity. Despite the appearance of similarity, a study by Bernstein, Zvolensky, Vujanovic, and Moos (2009) suggests that discomfort tolerance is structurally distinct from distress tolerance. Bernstein and colleagues also demonstrated that anxiety sensitivity and distress tolerance share a common higher order factor accounting for individual differences in sensitivity to and (in)tolerance of negative affect and related emotional states. This latter finding is particularly relevant in the context of our decision to draw parallels between the investigation of pain tolerance and distress tolerance; indeed, despite the absence of studies directly assessing distress tolerance in the context of pain experiences, this finding adds substantively to the theoretical and empirical base from which we infer clinical recommendations and future research directions in this area.

There are several specific conceptual limitations that also warrant consideration in the context of studies of pain tolerance and their application to understanding distress tolerance. First, the various pain induction strategies described previously may not provide a valid test of the ability to tolerate emotional distress. We have assumed that pain tolerance and distress tolerance are inextricably linked; but this may not be the case. Future investigations may specifically address the issue of linkage between these constructs. On the other hand, it is well established that the pain experience involves not only physical sensation but affect, cognition, and behavior influenced by sociocultural context. As such, it seems reasonable that pain tolerance findings can be extrapolated to inform our understanding of distress tolerance. Second, it is possible that the motivation for persisting in pain induction tasks reflects experimental demand characteristics or other factors unrelated to pain tolerance per se (Arendt-Nielsen & Lautenbacher, 2004; Chapman, Schimek, Colpitts, Gerlach, & Dong, 1985). As noted in the distress tolerance literature, it is important to distinguish between distress tolerance and task persistence (Daughters, Lejuez, Kahler, Strong, & Brown, 2005), the latter denoting the behavioral propensity to persist toward a goal despite emotional distress. Because pain (and distress) induction tasks necessitate task persistence in order to derive measures of tolerance, it is difficult to determine the relative contribution of each to the measured outcome.

## THEORETICAL IMPLICATIONS
## AND FUTURE DIRECTIONS

The findings described previously hold several important implications for current distress tolerance theory in general, and with specific regard to fear-avoidance models and their application to chronic musculoskeletal pain and related chronic health conditions (Asmundson, Norton, & Norton, 1999; Asmundson, Wright, & Hadjistavropoulos, 2000; Vlaeyen & Linton, 2000). It is beyond the scope and space constraints of this chapter to provide a comprehensive agenda to guide future research efforts; however, several broad research directions can be derived from the noted theoretical implications. In a general sense, the findings illustrate that there exists a wide variety of factors that contribute to sensitivity to and (in)tolerance of noxious stimulation and associated negative emotional states. With respect to pain sensitivity, these factors range from gender and ethnicity to specific and potentially heritable individual differences. Future research specifically targeting the emergent distress tolerance construct will benefit from careful and comprehensive consideration of the role that such factors play and the influence they have on obtained results. In line with the notion that distress tolerance and anxiety sensitivity are lower order constructs of a higher order factor accounting for individual differences in sensitivity to and (in)tolerance of emotional states (Bernstein et al., 2009), the findings from the pain sensitivity literature imply that further exploration of the linkages between these and other related constructs in the broader context of emotion regulation is warranted.

More specific to chronic musculoskeletal pain and related chronic health conditions, continuing investigation of the complex interplay between individual-difference factors, with specific inclusion of the distress tolerance construct, may further inform our understanding of factors that contribute to the development and maintenance of persistent pain and its oft-accompanying emotional distress and functional limitations. Current understanding of the role of emotional distress in chronic musculoskeletal pain has been informed by detailed scrutiny of the role of fear of pain, pain-related anxiety, anxiety sensitivity, and related constructs (Asmundson et al., 1999; Asmundson, Vlaeyen, & Crombez, 2004; Vlaeyen & Linton, 2000). Given that the distress tolerance construct is related yet distinct for anxiety sensitivity, similarly detailed scrutiny of its role in the pain experience, perhaps alone and collectively with anxiety sensitivity (and related constructs), may yield information that will facilitate theoretical parsimony and identify new and potentially effective targets for intervention.

# CLINICAL IMPLICATIONS
# AND APPLICATIONS

## Clinical Implications

Clinical implications are described as they pertain to assessment and treatment. It is noteworthy that all aspects of clinical application that we describe warrant further empirical scrutiny and, as such, represent important future research directions.

### Clinical Conceptualization Illustration

In this section, we highlight issues pertinent to chronic musculoskeletal pain and related presentations that warrant consideration with respect to assessment and treatment of observed emotional distress. General conceptualization issues are discussed in detail elsewhere (e.g., Asmundson et al., 2004). It is important to note that we consider case formulation to be a conceptually driven process, placing empirically supported theoretical constructs and applications at the base of any decisions regarding assessment and treatment.

    We now know that pain is more than a purely sensory experience, and that persons with chronic musculoskeletal pain also experience difficulties in cognitive, affective, and behavioral domains. In recent years, it has become increasingly evident that a number of people with chronic musculoskeletal pain and related chronic health conditions frequently report significant expressions of emotional distress that warrant specific attention. These associated psychological factors may include Axis I or II conditions or subclinical syndromes (i.e., symptoms that do not reach the threshold for a disorder). Accordingly, a comprehensive assessment of pain requires exploring not only pain-specific factors (e.g., pain severity and/or intensity, pain location and distribution, attitudes and beliefs about pain, methods of coping with pain, pain-related functional impairment) but also pain-related emotional distress (e.g., fear of pain, pain-related anxiety, mood changes; Asmundson, 2002; Tait, 1999) and comorbid psychopathology (Asmundson & Katz, 2008).

## Clinical Techniques and Therapeutic Tactics

### Assessment

Assessment tools specifically designed for pain-related emotional distress are growing in number. Based on extant theory and research informing current understanding of distress tolerance in the context of pain experiences, as reviewed previously, it appears that anxious and fearful thinking are critical and generally well understood with respect to exacerbation of the pain experience and one's ability to tolerate distress and/or cope effectively. We recommend several self-report measures to aid in the assessment (and measurement of treatment progress and outcome) of emotional distress accompanying clinically significant pain, including the Pain Anxiety Symptoms Scale (PASS; McCracken, Zayfert, & Gross, 1992) and its short form (PASS-20; McCracken & Dhingra, 2002), Pain Catastrophizing Scale (Sullivan et al., 1995), Fear of Pain Questionnaire (FPQ; McNeil & Rainwater, 1998) and its short form (FPQ-SF; Asmundson, Bovell, Carleton, & McWilliams, 2008), and the Anxiety Sensitivity Index (Peterson & Reiss, 1992). It will be interesting to evaluate, both clinically and empirically, the unique value of adding measures of distress tolerance—the 15-item Distress Tolerance Scale (Simons & Gaher, 2005) and the identically named 20-item Distress Tolerance Scale (Corstorphine, Mountford, Tomlinson, Waller, & Meyer, 2007)—to the assessment (and treatment progress and outcome) package.

## Treatment/Prevention

Cognitive-behavioral therapy (CBT) is a highly effective treatment for chronic pain (Hadjistavropoulos & de Williams, 2004) and, relative to most other treatments and wait-list control conditions, produces significantly greater improvements in pain, pain behavior, affect, levels of activity, and ability to cope adaptively (Morley, Eccleston, & Williams, 1999). Generally, treating chronic musculoskeletal pain and related chronic health conditions with CBT implicitly recognizes that individuals with these conditions also experience other negative emotional states. CBT approaches to pain often address pain-related fear and anxiety as well as other forms of negative affect (e.g., depression) using some combination of psychoeducation, relaxation training, cognitive restructuring, graded activity or *in vivo* exposure techniques, and behavioral exposure techniques. Rooted in the extant theory and research that applies to distress tolerance in chronic musculoskeletal pain and related conditions are several promising treatment options. What we collectively refer to as active avoidance strategies (e.g., distraction, suppression) are generally ineffective methods for decreasing sensitivity to pain, whereas strategies requiring some form of approach toward pain (e.g., somatic focus, acceptance-based strategies) have proven generally effective under experimental conditions (as described previously) and in clinical settings (Dahl, Wilson, & Nilsson, 2004; McCracken & Vowles, 2006; Taylor & Asmundson, 2004).

## Clinical Future Directions

The literature regarding the aforementioned approach-based strategies has developed mostly in the context of studies that have utilized various pain induction procedures in nonclinical and clinical populations with or without consideration to the role of individual differences in anxious and fearful thinking to directed or spontaneous coping and observed outcomes. Further research utilizing somatic focus and acceptance-based strategies with clinical populations, and with attention to the aforementioned individual differences, may help disentangle the complexities of the mechanisms underlying pain perception and thereby provide additional evidence from which to base recommendation of one of these treatment approaches.

Another innovative approach strategy stemming from current understanding of anxiety sensitivity and its role in pain is the application of interoceptive exposure. This strategy, involving exposure to anxiety-provoking bodily sensations, is an empirically supported intervention that is often included as part of CBT for anxiety disorders (e.g., Taylor, 1999, 2000). Watt, Stewart, Lefaivre, and Uman (2006) provided preliminary evidence that interoceptive exposure is effective in reducing pain-related anxiety in female undergraduate participants with high and low levels of anxiety sensitivity. Most recently, Flink, Nicholas, Boersma, and Linton (2009) found that a combination of interoceptive exposure and a breathing-based technique were effective in improving pain acceptance and reducing pain-related distress among six individuals with chronic back pain. These findings provide a foundation from which to further explore the potential of interoceptive exposure as means of enhancing distress tolerance in people with conditions characterized by persistent pain.

## SUMMARY

The experience of pain is an extremely complex phenomenon, involving not only sensations of noxious stimulation but also psychological (e.g., perception, cognition, affect), behavioral (e.g., avoidance), and social (e.g., cultural) factors. Although adaptive in the short term, pain can become maladaptive when it is maintained over time by a complex reciprocal interplay among pain sensations, emotional distress (e.g., fear, anxiety, depressed mood), and disability. Working from the premise that chronic and unremitting pain is a significant source of emotional distress for many people with chronic musculoskeletal pain and related health conditions, and guided by the extant research on pain perception, future empirical inquiries of the emerging distress tolerance construct may build upon our understanding of this complex issue and how to most effectively intervene to reduce distress and disability. Strategies requiring some form of approach toward pain (e.g., somatic focus, acceptance-based strategies) have proven generally effective under experimental conditions and in clinical settings, whereas active avoidance strategies (e.g., distraction, suppression) are generally ineffective. The application of interoceptive exposure techniques to the reduction of pain and related distress represents a promising treatment consideration that warrants further investigation. Continued innovation in treatment techniques, perhaps guided by focused work on the emerging distress tolerance construct, will be decidedly important as we attempt to improve current understanding and identify additional effective treatments for chronic and disabling presentations of pain.

## REFERENCES

Affleck, G., Urrows S., Tennen, H., & Higgins, P. (1992). Daily coping with pain from rheumatoid arthritis: Patterns and correlates. *Pain, 51,* 221–229.

Alexander, R. W., Bradley, L. A., Alarcon, G. S., Triana-Alexander, M., Aaron, L. A., Alberts, K. R., et al. (1998). Sexual and physical abuse in women with fibromyalgia: Association with outpatient health care utilization and pain medication usage. *Arthritis Care and Research, 11,* 102–115.

Arendt-Nielsen, L., Graven-Nielsen, T., & Svensson, P. (2004). Disturbances of pain perception in myofascial pain syndrome and other musculoskeletal pains. In S. Lautenbacher & R. B. Fillingim (Eds.), *Plenum series in rehabilitation and health: Pathophysiology of pain perception* (pp. 93–106). New York: Kluwer Academic/Plenum Press.

Arendt-Nielsen, L., & Henriksson, K. (2007). Pathophysiological mechanisms in chronic musculoskeletal pain (fibromyalgia): The role of central and peripheral sensitization and pain disinhibition. *Best Practice and Research Clinical Rheumatology, 21,* 465–480.

Arendt-Nielsen, L., & Lautenbacher, S. (2004). Assessment of pain perception. In S. Lautenbacher & R. B. Fillingim (Eds.), *Plenum Series in Rehabilitation and Health: Pathophysiology of pain perception* (pp. 25–42). New York: Kluver Academic/Plenum Press.

Asmundson, G. J. G. (2002). Pain assessment: State-of-the-art applications from the cognitive-behavioural perspective. *Behaviour Research and Therapy, 40,* 547–550.

Asmundson, G. J. G., Bovell, C., Carleton, R. N., & McWilliams, L. A. (2008). The Fear of Pain Questionnaire—Short Form (FPQ-SF): Factorial validity and psychometric properties. *Pain, 134,* 51–58.

Asmundson, G. J. G., Coons, M. J., Taylor, S., & Katz, J. (2002). PTSD and the experience of pain: Research and clinical implications of shared vulnerability and mutual maintenance models. *Canadian Journal of Psychiatry, 47,* 930.

Asmundson, G. J. G., & Katz, J. (2008). Understanding pain and posttraumatic stress disorder comorbidity: Do pathological responses to trauma alter the perception of pain? *Pain, 138,* 247–249.

Asmundson, G. J. G., Kuperos, J. L., & Norton, G. R. (1997). Do patients with chronic pain selectively attend to pain-related information?: Preliminary evidence for the mediating role of fear. *Pain, 72,* 27–32.

Asmundson, G. J., Norton, G. R., Allerdings, M. D., Norton, P. J., & Larsen, D. K. (1998). Posttraumatic stress disorder and work-related injury. *Journal of Anxiety Disorders, 12,* 57–69.

Asmundson, G. J. G., Norton, P. J., & Norton, G. R. (1999). Beyond pain: The role of fear and avoidance in chronicity. *Clinical Psychology Review, 19,* 97–119.

Asmundson, J. G. J., Vlaeyen, J. W. S., & Crombez, G. (2004). *Understanding and treating fear of pain.* Oxford, UK: Oxford University Press.

Asmundson, G. J. G., & Wright, K. D. (2004). Biopsychosocial approaches to pain. In T. Hadjistavropoulos & K. D. Craig (Eds.), *Pain: Psychological perspectives* (pp. 35–57). Mahwah, NJ: Erlbaum.

Asmundson, G. J. G., Wright, K. D., & Hadjistavropoulos, H. D. (2000). Anxiety sensitivity and disabling chronic health conditions: State of the art and future directions. *Scandinavian Journal of Behaviour Therapy, 29,* 100–117.

Barlow, D. H. (2002). *Anxiety and its disorders: The nature and treatment of anxiety and panic* (2nd ed.). New York: Guilford Press.

Bernstein, A., Zvolensky, M. J., Vujanovic, A. A., & Moos, R. (2009). Integrating anxiety sensitivity, distress tolerance, and discomfort intolerance: A hierarchical model of affect sensitivity and tolerance. *Behavior Therapy, 40,* 291–301.

Breuer, J., & Freud, S. (1974). *Studies on hysteria* (J. Strachey, Trans.). New York: Basic Books.

Brewer, B. W., & Karoly, P. (1989). Effects of attentional focusing on pain perception. *Motivation and Emotion, 13,* 193–203.

Bruera, E., MacMillan, K., Hanson, J., & MacDonald, R. N. (1989). The Edmonton staging system for cancer pain: Preliminary report. *Pain, 37,* 203–209.

Buckelew, S. P., Conway, R. C., Shutty, M. S., Lawrence J. A., Grafing, M. R., Anderson, S. K., et al. (1992). Spontaneous coping strategies to manage acute pain and anxiety during electrodiagnostic studies. *Archives of Physical Medicine and Rehabilitation, 73,* 594–598.

Carter, L. E., McNeil, D. W., Vowles, K. E., Sorrell, J. T., Turk, C. L., Ries, B. J., et al. (2002). Effects of emotion on pain reports, tolerance and physiology. *Pain Research and Management, 7,* 21–30.

Chapman, C. R., Schimek, F., Colpitts, Y. H., Gerlach, R., & Dong, W. K. (1985). Peak latency differences in evoked potentials elicited by painful dental and cutaneous stimulation. *International Journal of Neuroscience, 27,* 1–12.

Chong, P. S. T., & Cros, D. P. (2004). Technology literature review: Quantitative sensory testing. *Muscle and Nerve, 29,* 734–747.

Cioffi, D., & Holloway, J. (1993). Delayed costs of suppressed pain. *Journal of Personality and Social Psychology, 64,* 274–282.

Corstorphine, E., Mountford, V., Tomlinson, S., Waller, G., & Meyer, C. (2007). Distress tolerance in the eating disorders. *Eating Behaviors, 8,* 91–97.

Covelli, C. R., Price, D. D., & Verne, G. N. (2004). Disturbances of pain perception in irritable bowel syndrome. In S. Lautenbacher & R. B. Fillingim (Eds.), *Plenum Series in Rehabilitation and Health: Pathophysiology of pain perception* (pp. 119–131). New York: Kluwer Academic/Plenum Press.

Craig, K. D. (1994). Emotional aspects of pain. In P. D. Wall & R. Melzack (Eds.), *The textbook of pain* (pp. 261–274). Edinburgh, UK: Churchill Livingstone.

Critchley, M. (1931). The neurology of old age. *Lancet, 1,* 1221–1230.

Cruccu, G., Anand, P., Attal, N., García-Larrea, L., Haanpaa, M., Jorum, E., et al. (2004). EFNS guidelines on neuropathic pain assessment. *European Journal of Neurology, 11,* 153–162.

Dahl, J., Wilson, K. G., & Nilsson, A. (2004). Acceptance and commitment therapy and the treatment of persons at risk for long-term disability resulting from stress and pain symptoms: A preliminary randomized trial. *Behavior Therapy, 35,* 785–802.

Daughters, S. B., Lejuez, C. W., Kahler, C. W., Strong, D. R., & Brown, R. A. (2005). Psychological distress tolerance and duration of most recent abstinence attempt among residential treatment-seeking substance abusers. *Psychology of Addictive Behaviors, 19,* 208–211.

DeBenedittis, G., Panerai, A. A., & Villamira, M. A. (1989). Effects of hypnotic analgesia and hypnotizability on experimental ischemic pain. *International Journal of Clinical and Experimental Hypnosis, 37,* 55–69.

Defrin, R., Ginzburg, K., Solomon, Z., Polad, E., Bloch, M., Govezensky, M., et al. (2008). Quantitative testing of pain perception in subjects with PTSD—Implications for the mechanism of the coexistence between PTSD and chronic pain. *Pain, 138,* 450–459.

De Pascalis, V., Magurano, M. R., & Bellusci, A. (1999). Pain perception, somatosensory event-related potentials and skin conductance responses to painful stimuli in high, mid, and low hypnotizable subjects: Effects of differential pain reduction strategies. *Pain, 83,* 499–508.

De Pascalis, V., & Perrone, M. (1996). EEG asymmetry and heart rate during experience of hypnotic analgesia in high and low hypnotizables. *International Journal of Psychophysiology, 21,* 163–175.

Dickens, C., McGowan, L., & Dale, S. (2003). Impact of depression on experimental pain perception: A systematic review of the literature with meta-analysis. *Psychosomatic Medicine, 65,* 369–375.

Duschek, S., Schwarzkopf, W., & Schandry, R. (2008). Increased pain sensitivity in low blood pressure. *Journal of Psychophysiology, 22,* 20–27.

Edwards, C. L., Fillingim, R. B., & Keefe, F. (2001). Race, ethnicity and pain. *Pain, 94,* 133–137.

Edwards, R. R., & Fillingim, R. B. (2001). Effects of age on temporal summation and habituation of thermal pain: Clinical relevance in healthy older and younger adults. *Journal of Pain, 2,* 307–317.

Edwards, R. R., Haythornthwaite, J. A., Sullivan, M. J., & Fillingim, R. B. (2004). Catastrophizing as a mediator of sex differences in pain: Differential effects for daily pain versus laboratory-induced pain. *Pain, 111,* 335–341.

Feldner, M. T., Hekmat, H., Zvolensky, M. J., Vowles, K. E., Secrist, Z., & Leen-Feldner, E. W. (2006). The role of experiential avoidance in acute pain tolerance: A laboratory test. *Journal of Behavior Therapy and Experimental Psychiatry, 37,* 146–158.

Fillingim, R. B. (2004a). Alterations in pain perception in cardiovascular disease. In S. Lautenbacher & R. B. Fillingim (Eds.), *Plenum Series in Rehabilitation and Health: Pathophysiology of pain perception* (pp. 185–197). New York: Kluwer Academic/Plenum Press.

Fillingim, R. B. (2004b). Disturbances of pain perception in menstrual cycle-related disorders. In S. Lautenbacher & R. B. Fillingim (Eds.), *Plenum Series in Rehabilitation and Health: Pathophysiology of pain perception* (pp. 133–140). New York: Kluwer Academic/Plenum Press.

Fillingim, R. B., & Edwards, R. R. (2005). Is self-reported childhood abuse history associated with pain perception among healthy young women and men? *Clinical Journal of Pain, 21,* 387–397.

Fillingim, R. B., Maixner, W., Sigurdsson, A., & Kincaid, S. (1997). Sexual and physical abuse history in subjects with temporomandibular disorders: Relationship to clinical variables, pain sensitivity, and psychologic factors. *Journal of Orofacial Pain, 11,* 48–57.

Flink, I. K., Nicholas, M. K., Boersma, K., & Linton, S. J. (2009). Reducing the threat value of chronic pain: A preliminary replicated single-case study of interoceptive exposure versus distraction in six individuals with chronic back pain. *Behaviour Research and Therapy, 47,* 721–728.

Gatchel, R. J., Peng, Y. B., Peters, M. L., Fuchs, P. N., & Turk, D. C. (2007). The biopsychosocial approach to chronic pain: Scientific advances and future directions. *Psychological Bulletin, 133,* 581–624.

George, S. Z., Dannecker, E. A., & Robinson, M. E. (2006). Fear of pain, not pain catastrophizing, predicts acute pain intensity, but neither factor predicts tolerance or blood pressure reactivity: An experimental investigation in pain-free individuals. *European Journal of Pain, 10,* 457–465.

Geuze, E., Westenberg, H. G. M., Jochims, A., de Kloet, C. S., Bohus, M., Vermetten, E., et al. (2007). Altered pain processing in veterans with posttraumatic stress disorder. *Archives of General Psychiatry, 64,* 76–85.

Gibson, S. J., & Farrell, M. (2004). A review of age differences in the neurophysiology of nociception and the perceptual experience of pain. *Clinical Journal of Pain, 20,* 227–239.

Goubert, L., Crombez, G., Eccleston, C., & Devulder, J. (2004). Distraction from chronic pain during a pain-inducing activity is associated with greater port-activity pain. *Pain, 110,* 220–227.

Goubert, L., Crombez, G., & Van Damme, S. (2004). The role of neuroticism, pain catastrophizing and pain-related fear in vigilance to pain: A structural equations approach. *Pain, 107,* 234–241.

Grossi, M. L., Goldberg, M. B., Locker, D., & Tenenbaum, H. C. (2008). Irritable bowel syndrome patients versus responding and nonresponding temporomandibular disorder patients: A neuropsychologic profile comparative study. *International Journal of Prosthodontics, 21*, 201–209.

Guttiérrez, O., Luciano, C., Rodriguez, M., & Fink, B. C. (2004). Comparison between an acceptance-based protocol and a cognitive control-based protocol for coping with pain. *Behavior Therapy, 35*, 767–783.

Hadjistavropoulos, H., & de Williams, A. C. C. (2004). Psychological interventions and chronic pain. In T. Hadjistavropoulos & K. D. Craig (Eds.), *Pain: Psychological perspectives* (pp. 271–301). Mahwah, NJ: Erlbaum.

Hadjistavropoulos, H. D., Hadjistavropoulos, T., & Quine, A. (2000). Health anxiety moderates the effects of distraction versus attention to pain. *Behaviour Research and Therapy, 38*, 425–438.

Harvey, A. G., & McGuire, B. E. (2000). Suppressing and attending to pain-related thoughts in chronic pain patients. *Behaviour Research and Therapy, 38*, 1117–1124.

Hastie, B. A., Riley, J. L., III, Robinson, M. E., Glover, T., Campbell, C. M., Staud, R., et al. (2005). Cluster analysis of multiple experimental pain modalities. *Pain, 116*, 227–237.

Hayes, S. C., Strosahl, K. D., & Wilson, K. G. (1999). *Acceptance and commitment therapy: An experiential approach to behavior change*. New York: Guilford Press.

Heyneman, N. E., Fremouw, W. J., Gano, D., Kirkland, F., & Heiden, L. (1990). Individual differences and the effectiveness of different coping strategies for pain. *Cognitive Therapy and Research, 14*, 63–77.

Hirsh, A. T., George, S. Z., Bialosky, J. E., & Robinson, M. E. (2008). Fear of pain, pain catastrophizing, and acute pain perception: Relative prediction and timing of assessment. *Journal of Pain, 9*, 806–812.

Homer. (2000). *The essential Homer* (S. Lombardo, Trans.). Indianapolis, IN: Hackett.

Institute for Laboratory Animal Research. (1992). *Recognition and alleviation of pain and distress in laboratory animals*. Washington, DC: National Academy Press.

James, J. E., & Hardardottir, D. (2002). Influence of attention focus and trait anxiety on tolerance of acute pain. *British Journal of Health Psychology, 7*, 149–162.

Jensen, M. P., & Karoly, P. (1991). Control beliefs, coping efforts, and adjustment to chronic pain. *Journal of Consulting and Clinical Psychology, 59*, 431–438.

Jones, A., Zachariae, R., & Arendt-Nielsen, L. (2003). Dispositional anxiety and the experience of pain: Gender-specific effects. *European Journal of Pain, 7*, 387–395.

Keefe, F. J., & Williams, D. A. (1990). A comparison of coping strategies in chronic pain patients in different age groups. *Journal of Gerontology, 45*, 161–165.

Keogh, E., & Birkby, J. (1999). The effect of anxiety sensitivity and gender on the experience of pain. *Cognition and Emotion, 13*, 813–829.

Keogh, E., Hatton, H., & Ellery, D. (2000). Avoidance versus focused attention and the perception of pain: Differential effects for men and women. *Pain, 85*, 225–230.

Keogh, E., & Mansoor, L. (2001). Investigating the effects of anxiety sensitivity and coping on the perception of cold pressor pain in healthy women. *European Journal of Pain, 5*, 11–22.

Kosek, E. (2004). Disturbances of pain perception in fibromyalgia. In S. Lautenbacher & R. B. Fillingim (Eds.), *Plenum Series in Rehabilitation and Health: Pathophysiology of pain perception* (pp. 77–91). New York: Kluwer Academic/Plenum Press.

Kraus, A., Geuze, E., Schmahl, C., Grefffrath, W., Treede, R. D., Bohus, M., et al. (2009). Differentiation of pain ratings in combat-related posttraumatic stress disorder. *Pain, 143*, 179–185.

Kröner-Herwig, B. (2009). Chronic pain syndromes and their treatment by psychological interventions. *Current Opinion in Psychiatry, 22*, 200–204.

Lane, J. D., Lefebvre, J. C., Rose, J. E., & Keefe, F. J. (1995). Effects of cigarette smoking on perception of thermal pain. *Experimental and Clinical Psychopharmacology, 3*, 140–147.

Linehan, M. M. (1993). *Cognitive-behavioural treatment of borderline personality disorder*. New York: Guilford Press.

Loeser, J. D., & Treede, R. (2008). The Kyoto protocol of IASP basic pain terminology. *Pain, 137*, 473–477.

Masedo, A. I., & Esteve, M. R. (2007). Effects of suppression, acceptance and spontaneous coping on pain tolerance, pain intensity and distress. *Behaviour Research and Therapy, 45*, 199–209.

Mathews, A., & MacLeod, C. (1994). Cognitive approaches to emotion and emotional disorders. *Annual Review of Psychology, 45*, 25–50.

McCaul, K. D., Monson, N., & Maki, R. H. (1992). Does distraction reduce pain produced distress among college students? *Health Psychology, 11*, 210–217.

McCracken, L. M., & Dhingra, L. (2002). A short version of the Pain Anxiety Symptoms Scale (PASS-20): Preliminary development and validity. *Pain Research and Management, 7*, 45–50.

McCracken, L. M., Spertus, I. L., Janeck, A. S., Sinclair, D., & Wetzel, F. T. (1999). Behavioral dimensions of adjustment in persons with chronic pain: Pain-related anxiety and acceptance. *Pain, 80*, 283–289.

McCracken, L. M., & Vowles, K. E. (2006). Acceptance of chronic pain. *Current Pain and Headache Reports, 10*, 90–94.

McCracken, L. M., Zayfert, C., & Gross, R. T. (1992). The Pain Anxiety Symptoms Scale: Development and validation of a scale to measure fear of pain. *Pain, 50*, 67–73.

McFate, T., & Scher, A. I. (2009). Chronic pain disorders and headache chronification. *Current Pain and Headache Reports, 13*, 308–313.

McNeil, D. W., & Rainwater, A. J. (1998). Development of the Fear of Pain Questionnaire—III. *Journal of Behavior Medicine, 21*, 389–410.

Merskey, H., & Bogduk, N. (1994). *Classification of chronic pain: Descriptions of chronic pain syndromes and definitions of pain terms* (2nd ed.). Seattle, WA: IASP Press.

Morley, S., Eccleston, C., & Williams, A. (1999). Systematic review and meta-analysis of randomized controlled trials of cognitive behaviour therapy and behaviour therapy for chronic pain in adults, excluding headache. *Pain, 80,* 1–13.

Nachemson, A. L. (1992). Newest knowledge of low back pain: A critical look. *Clinical Orthopaedics and Related Research,* 8–20.

Nijs, J., Meeus, M., & de Meirleir, K. (2006). Chronic musculoskeletal pain in chronic fatigue syndrome: Recent developments and therapeutic implications. *Manual Therapy, 11,* 187–191.

Paller, C. J., Campbell, C. M., Edwards, R. R., & Dobs, A. S. (2009). Sex-based differences in pain perception and treatment. *Pain Medicine, 10,* 289–299.

Peters, M. (2004). Disturbances of pain perception in chronic back pain. In S. Lautenbacher & R. B. Fillingim (Eds.), *Plenum Series in Rehabilitation and Health: Pathophysiology of pain perception* (pp. 59–75). New York: Kluwer Academic/Plenum Press.

Peterson, R. A., & Reiss, S. (1992). *Anxiety Sensitivity Index manual* (2nd ed.). Worthington, OH: International Diagnostic Systems.

Petzke, F., Clauw, D. J., Ambrose, K., Khine, A., & Gracely, R. H. (2003). Increased pain sensitivity in fibromyalgia: Effects of stimulus type and mode of presentation. *Pain, 105,* 403–413.

Pielsticker, A., & Lautenbacher, S. (2004). Disturbances of pain perception in primary headache: Migraine, tension-type, and cluster headaches. In S. Lautenbacher & R. B. Fillingim (Eds.), *Plenum Series in Rehabilitation and Health: Pathophysiology of pain perception* (pp. 42–57). New York: Kluwer Academic/Plenum Press.

Pitman, R. K., van der Kolk, B. A., Orr, S. P., & Greenberg, M. S. (1990). Naloxone-reversible analgesic response to combat-related stimuli in posttraumatic stress disorder: A pilot study. *Archives of General Psychiatry, 47,* 541–544.

Riley, J. L., III, Robinson, M. E., Wise, E. A., Myers, C. D., & Fillingim, R. B. (1998). Sex differences in the perception of noxious experimental stimuli: A meta-analysis. *Pain, 74,* 181–187.

Riley, J. L., III, Robinson, M. E., Wise, E. A., & Price, D. D. (1999). A meta-analytic review of pain perception across the menstrual cycle. *Pain, 81,* 225–235.

Roelofs, J., Peters, M. L., van der Zijden, M., & Vlaeyen, J. W. (2004). Does fear of pain moderate the effects of sensory focusing and distraction on cold pressor pain in pain-free individuals? *Journal of Pain, 5,* 250–256.

Rolke, R., Baron, R., Maier, C., Tölle, T. R., Treede, R. D., Beyer, A., et al. (2006). Quantitative sensory testing in the German research network on neuropathic pain (DFNS): Standardized protocol and reference values. *Pain, 123,* 231–243.

Rollman, G. B., & Gillespie, J. M. (2004). Disturbances of pain perception in tempormandibular pain syndrome. In S. Lautenbacher & R. B. Fillingim (Eds.), *Plenum Series in Rehabilitation and Health: Pathophysiology of pain perception* (pp. 107–118). New York: Kluwer Academic/Plenum Press.

Scarinci, I. C., McDonald-Haile, J., Bradley, L. A., & Richter, J. E. (1994). Altered pain perception and psychosocial features among women with gastrointestinal disorders and history of abuse: A preliminary model. *American Journal of Medicine, 97,* 108–118.

Schepelmann, K., & Lautenbacher, S. (2004). Disturbances of pain perception in disorders of the peripheral nervous system. In S. Lautenbacher & R. B. Fillingim (Eds.), *Plenum Series in Rehabilitation and Health: Pathophysiology of pain perception* (pp. 141–154). New York: Kluwer Academic/Plenum Press.

Schmahl, C., Meinzer, M., Zeuch, A., Fichter, M., Cebulla, M., Kleindienst, N., et al. (2008). Pain sensitivity is reduced in borderline personality disorder, but not in posttraumatic stress disorder and bulimia nervosa. *World Journal of Biological Psychiatry, 29,* 1–8.

Schmidt, N. B., & Cook, J. H. (1999). Effects of anxiety sensitivity on anxiety and pain during a cold pressor challenge in patients with panic disorder. *Behaviour Research and Therapy, 37,* 313–323.

Shy, M. E., Frohman, E. M., So, Y. T., Arezzo, J. C., Cornblath, D. R., Giuliani, M. J., et al. (2003). Quantitative sensory testing: Report of the Therapeutics and Technology Assessment Subcommittee of the American Academy of Neurology. *Neurology, 60,* 898–904.

Simons, J. S., & Gaher, R. M. (2005). The Distress Tolerance Scale: Development and validation of a self-report measure. *Motivation and Emotion, 29,* 83–102.

Spengler, D. M., Bigos, S. J., & Martin, N. A. (1986). Back injuries in industry: A retrospective study. 1. Overview and cost analysis. *Spine, 11,* 241–245.

Staats, P. S., Staats, A., & Hekmat, H. (2001). The additive impact of anxiety and a placebo on pain. *Pain Medicine, 2,* 267–279.

Sullivan, M. J. L., Bishop, S. R., & Pivik, J. (1995). The Pain Catastrophizing Scale: Development and validation. *Psychological Assessment, 7,* 524–532.

Sullivan, M. J. L., Rouse, D., Bishop, S., & Johnston, S. (1997). Thought suppression, catastrophizing, and pain. *Cognitive Therapy and Research, 21,* 555–568.

Tait, R. (1999). Evaluation of treatment effectiveness in patients with intractable pain: Measures and methods. In R. J. Gatchel & D. C. Turk (Eds.), *Psychosocial factors in pain: Critical perspectives* (pp. 457–480). New York: Guilford Press.

Taylor, S. (1999). *Anxiety sensitivity: Theory, research, and treatment of the fear of anxiety.* Mahwah, NJ: Erlbaum.

Taylor, S. (2000). *Understanding and treating panic disorder: Cognitive-behavioural approaches.* New York: Wiley.

Taylor, S., & Asmundson, G. J. G. (2004). *Treating health anxiety: A cognitive-behavioral approach.* New York: Guilford Press.

Thompson, T., Keogh, E., French, C. C., & Davis, R. (2008). Anxiety sensitivity and pain: Generalisability across noxious stimuli. *Pain, 134,* 187–196.

Thorn, B. E., Cross, T. H., & Walker, B. B. (2007). Meta-analyses and systematic reviews of psychological treatments for chronic pain: Relevance to an evidence-based practice. *Health Psychology, 26,* 10–12.

Turk, D. C., & Rudy, T. E. (1987). IASP taxonomy of chronic pain syndromes: Preliminary assessment of reliability. *Pain, 30,* 177–189.

Turk, D. C., & Rudy, T. E. (1988). Toward an empirically derived taxonomy of chronic pain patients: Integration of psychological assessment data. *Journal of Consulting and Clinical Psychology, 56,* 233–238.

van der Kolk, B. A., Greenberg, M. S., Orr, S. P., & Pitman, R. K. (1989). Endogenous opioids, stress induced analgesia, and posttraumatic stress disorder. *Psychopharmacology Bulletin, 25,* 417–421.

Vlaeyen, J. W. S., & Linton, S. J. (2000). Fear-avoidance and its consequences in chronic musculoskeletal pain: A state of the art. *Pain, 85,* 317–332.

Waddell, G. (1987). A new clinical model for the treatment of low back pain. *Spine, 12,* 623–644.

Waddell, G. (1992). Biopsychosocial analysis of low back pain. *Bailliere's Clinical Rheumatology, 6,* 523–557.

Watt, M. C., Stewart, S. H., Lefaivre, M. J., & Uman, L. S. (2006). A brief cognitive-behavioral approach to reducing anxiety sensitivity decreases pain-related anxiety. *Cognitive Behaviour Therapy, 35,* 248–256.

Whitehead, W. E., Crowell, M. D., Davidoff, A. L., Palsson, O. S., & Schuster, M. M. (1997). Pain from rectal distension in women with irritable bowel syndrome: Relationship to sexual abuse. *Digestive Diseases and Sciences, 42,* 796–804.

Williams, R. E., Hartmann, K. E., Sandler, R. S., Miller, W. C., & Steege, J. F. (2004). Prevalence and characteristics of irritable bowel syndrome among women with chronic pelvic pain. *Obstetrics and Gynecology, 104,* 452–458.

Woodrow, K. M., Friedman, G. D., Siegelaub, A. B., & Collen, M. F. (1972). Pain tolerance: Differences according to age, sex and race. *Psychosomatic Medicine, 34,* 548–556.

# 11

# Eating Disorders

Michael D. Anestis, Erin L. Fink,
April R. Smith, Edward A. Selby,
*and* Thomas E. Joiner

$A$lthough research on eating disorders has focused on dysregulated emotions for quite some time, the scope of this focus has narrowed somewhat in recent years to examine more closely several specific factors relevant to the broader construct of emotion regulation. One such factor garnering consistent support is distress tolerance, defined as the degree to which an individual deems the subjective experience of negative affect to be unbearable (Simons & Gaher, 2005), which has been implicated in both the cause and maintenance of dysregulated eating behaviors, such as those present in bulimia nervosa (BN) and binge-eating disorder (BED).

In 2007, Corstorphine, Mountford, Tomlinson, Waller, and Meyer developed a measure of distress tolerance, the Distress Tolerance Scale, and validated it using both a clinical and a nonclinical sample of women with dysregulated eating behaviors. They found a general pattern indicating that avoidance of affect was related to unhealthy attitudes about eating. Additionally, women in the clinical sample displayed significantly higher scores on the Avoidance of Affect subscale. This suggests that dysregulated eating is a potential maladaptive outcome for those who have low tolerance for negative affect and, as such, avoid actively facing and remediating negative emotional states. In another study that elaborated on these findings, Anestis, Selby, Fink, and Joiner (2007) found that distress tolerance predicted bulimic symptoms even when controlling for a host of other variables, including depressive symptoms and impulsivity. Furthermore, distress tolerance displayed a significant interaction with negative urgency, or the tendency to act rashly in an effort to immediately reduce negative affect (Whiteside & Lynam, 2001), such that those scoring high on negative urgency and low on distress tolerance were more likely to display bulimic behaviors. This indicates that those who have problems tolerating distress and who are also prone to act rashly in the face of negative emotions are particularly likely to engage in dysregulated eating behaviors.

The theoretical implications of research on distress tolerance in those with BN and BED are important for understanding the cause and treatment of both disorders. Although research has consistently demonstrated a relationship between disordered eating and maladaptive coping with negative affect, there remains a lack of knowledge about the mechanisms by which some individuals become more susceptible to the negative effects of distress. To be certain, all individuals experience distress throughout their lives. However, vast individual differences exist not only in the ability to cope with negative affect but also in determining appropriate strategies for remediating such emotional states when they are encountered. Some newer types of psychotherapy have addressed this question. For example, dialectical behavior therapy (DBT; Linehan, 1993a, 1993b), which has been successfully used to treat borderline personality disorder (BPD; Linehan, 1998), seeks to teach individuals effective ways to manage aversive emotional states. Such types of therapy may prove invaluable in the treatment of disorders such as BN, which display a strong relationship with difficulties tolerating distress. A number of studies have confirmed the potential utility of DBT for both BN and BED (Telch, Agras, & Linehan, 2000, 2001).

Although the theoretical implications of the relationship between distress tolerance and anorexia nervosa (AN) are less understood, it stands to reason that emotion regulation is no less important in this disorder. In contrast to BN and BED, AN is characterized by extreme control of food intake and restriction of calories. Numerous studies have shown a relationship between restrictive eating habits and alexithymia (e.g., de Zwaan, Biener, Bach, Wiesnagrotzki, & Stacher, 1996), defined as difficulty in identifying and describing one's emotions and in recognizing emotional states in others. At present, it is somewhat unclear how alexithymia, which is present in many individuals who restrict their eating (de Zwann et al., 1996; Nkam, Langlois-Thery, Dollfus, & Petit, 1997), relates to distress tolerance, but it may be that the inability to identify and describe emotions can lead to significant difficulties for these individuals when faced with distressful situations. Theoretically, if individuals are unsure of what emotion it is that they are feeling when under stress, it would likely be more difficult to alleviate their feelings of distress through adaptive means. As such, it is probable that distress tolerance plays a key role in the destructive behaviors present in AN, albeit most likely through different means than that observed in BN and BED. Future research would benefit from an exploration of the potential relationship between AN and distress tolerance.

## REVIEW OF EXTANT LITERATURE

The link between distress tolerance and eating pathology has been investigated with increasing regularity in recent years. Initially, evidence supporting this link was fairly indirect, with empirical work focusing on a variety of emotional processes only tangentially related to and theoretically consistent with distress tolerance. More recently, however, several studies have directly measured distress tolerance in an effort to understand whether this particular variable might serve as a pivotal mechanism in numerous components of eating pathology.

### Initial Research

Early research on the relationship between distress tolerance and eating pathology was, in large part, theoretical. Heatherton and Baumeister (1991), for instance, proposed a model of binge eating that conceptualized bingeing as an attempt to focus attention toward a physical sensation so as to facilitate an escape from aversive self-awareness. This escape model was founded on the idea that, at times, an individual's awareness of his or her own internal state was a source of immense discomfort that required immediate regulation. The authors argued that intense negative affect might be the driving force behind the need to escape and the willingness to utilize maladaptive behaviors to attain such means. Subsequent work examining this model provided compelling evidence of an important role for negative affect in eating disorder symptoms.

Along these lines, several studies have found that individuals who binge eat experience high levels of negative affect immediately before binge episodes. Arnow, Kenardy, and Agras (1995), for instance, found that women with bulimia nervosa (BN) reported experiencing negative affective states such as depression and anxiety before engaging in binge eating. Such studies were subject to the limitations inherent in retrospective self-report studies, however, and as such, newer methodologies were developed in an attempt to mitigate such problems.

Ecological momentary assessment (EMA; Smyth et al., 2001), which typically involves having participants carry hand-held computers for a period of time and completing questionnaires in response to a series of prompts, has been a particularly commonly used approach toward further examination of the link between negative affect and eating disorder symptoms. Stein and colleagues (2007) reported that both hunger and negative affect were higher immediately before binge episodes than at non-binge times. They also reported, however, that negative affect was even higher post–binge episodes. Similarly, Hilbert and Tuschen-Caffier (2007) found that both individuals with BN and those with BED experienced heightened levels of negative affect before bingeing, and that mood further deteriorated post-binge. Individuals with BED, however, experienced less negative affect prior to binge episodes than did individuals with BN, an interesting consideration with respect to distress tolerance because it may indicate that such individuals find even moderate levels of negative affect unbearable and thus require less antecedent stress to precipitate a binge episode. Contrary to the these findings, Smyth and colleagues (2007) indicated that individuals not only reported higher levels of negative affect before binge episodes but also reported immediate, significant decreases in negative affect post-binge. In this particular sample, all participants were women diagnosed with BN, so the degree to which the findings generalize across eating disorders and eating disorder symptom severity is unclear. Although numerous studies utilizing EMA approaches have found that individuals experience significantly greater levels of negative affect before binge episodes, it is important to note that this is not a universal finding. Wegner and colleagues (2002), for instance, found that although negative affect was higher on binge days than on non-binge days, there was no difference in mood immediately before and after binge episodes.

Despite some inconsistencies across these studies, the general consensus from the just-mentioned findings is that negative affect plays an important role in eating disorder symptoms, particularly with respect to binge eating. Given the presence of inconsistencies, however, the question then becomes whether the mere presence of negative affect is the pivotal variable to consider or whether differences in the manner in which particular individuals experience negative affect might serve as a more robust predictor of eating disorder symptoms. Along these lines, a significant amount of research has examined whether emotion regulation is the more important variable to consider.

Emotion regulation is a fairly broad construct encompassing a variety of individual-difference variables, but the larger category can be reasonably defined as the manner in which individuals attempt to modulate or maintain current affective states (Thompson, 1994). Whiteside and colleagues (2007) reported that difficulty identifying and making sense of emotions as well as limited access to emotion regulation strategies predicted binge eating above and beyond the effects of biological sex, restriction of food, and overvaluation of body weight and shape. Therefore, it might be that individuals who binge eat do so in response to negative affect because of a deficiency in emotion regulation skills. Other studies have reported findings that indicate that, in addition to a general lack of skills for regulating negative affect, individuals who binge eat do so in part because of a failure to inhibit behaviors in the face of negative emotions. Specifically, Fischer, Smith, and Anderson (2003) found that negative urgency, the tendency to act rashly specifically in response to negative affect (Whiteside & Lynam, 2001), predicted bulimic symptoms. Additionally, Fischer, Anderson, and Smith (2004) reported that expectancies moderated the relationship between negative urgency and bulimic symptoms, such that a stronger belief that eating will diminish negative emotions in combination with greater levels of negative urgency conferred the greatest risk for bulimic behaviors. Anestis, Selby, and Joiner (2007) reported that residual change in levels of negative urgency over the course of 4 to 6 weeks was positively correlated with residual change in dysregulated eating behaviors. Anestis, Smith, Fink, and Joiner (2009) built upon these findings, reporting that in an outpatient community clinic negative urgency predicted dysregulated eating behaviors above and beyond biological sex and other components of impulsivity. Taken together, these findings indicate that individuals who find negative affect particularly aversive and feel compelled to utilize behaviors to quickly attenuate such feelings are vulnerable to engaging in dysregulated eating behaviors, particularly binge eating. Such findings are consistent with a distress tolerance model of eating disorders but still rely upon indirect evidence.

## Distress Tolerance in the Treatment of Eating Disorders

Although a substantial proportion of the empirical support for a distress tolerance model of eating disorders lacks direct measurement of distress tolerance, this weakness in the literature is not universal. The first studies that directly linked distress tolerance with eating disorders were treatment oriented. Specifically, a series of articles have examined the efficacy of DBT (Linehan, 1993a, 1993b) for both BED and BN. DBT, an empirically supported treatment for BPD (Linehan, 1998), teaches clients a variety of skills, many of which center on the effective management of emotions. One of the four modules of DBT focuses specifically on distress tolerance. In a theoretical report, Wiser and Telch (1999) considered the potential utility of DBT in BED, positing that individuals who frequently binge eat do so in part because of an inability to tolerate distress. In a case study with one female client diagnosed with BN, Safer, Telch, and Agras (2001) demonstrated that a modified DBT protocol significantly decreased eating disorder symptomatology. Similarly, Safer, Lock, and Coutourier (2007) demonstrated that a modified DBT protocol for adolescent BED that included family sessions successfully reduced eating disorder symptomatology. In an uncontrolled trial of DBT for BED, a substantial majority (82%) of clients reported zero objective binges 4 weeks after participating in a modified DBT protocol consisting of 20 sessions (Telch et al., 2000). Additionally, in a controlled trial of the revised DBT protocol, 89% of clients reported no objective binge-eating episodes after 20 sessions compared with only 12.5% of wait-list controls (Telch et al., 2001). In two separate studies examining the efficacy of DBT in treating individuals with an eating disorder (BED or BN) and comorbid BPD, substantial symptom reduction and treatment retention were reported, again offering empirical support for a treatment approach to eating disorders based heavily on the need to address low levels of distress tolerance (Chen, Matthews, Allen, Kuo, & Linehan, 2008; Palmer et al., 2003).

## Distress Tolerance and Symptoms of Eating Disorders

Not all of the literature linking distress tolerance to eating disorder symptomatology has been treatment oriented. Using their self-report Distress Tolerance Scale, Corstorphine and colleagues (2007) found that individuals diagnosed with an eating disorder exhibited significant difficulties tolerating distress. Specifically, women with eating disorders scored more highly on the Avoidance of Affect subscale and lower on the Accept and Manage subscale than did controls with no eating disorder. This finding indicates that women with eating disorders are likely to avoid emotional experiences and experience difficulties effectively regulating their affective states. In this particular study, the eating-disordered group consisted of women diagnosed with AN, BN, and eating disorder not otherwise specified. Building off this finding, Mountford, Corstorphine, Tomlinson, and Waller (2007) found that difficulties tolerating distress partially mediated the relationship between females' perceived invalidation by their fathers and eating disorder symptoms.

Utilizing a different questionnaire also entitled the Distress Tolerance Scale (Simons & Gaher, 2005), Anestis and colleagues (2007) found that distress tolerance moderated the previously reported relationship between negative urgency and dysregulated eating behaviors (Anestis et al., 2007; Fischer et al., 2003, 2004). In this sample, individuals with low distress tolerance and high negative urgency exhibited the greatest levels of dysregulated eating behaviors. The authors posit that this indicates that individuals who have difficulty tolerating distress and are motivated to utilize behaviors capable of offering immediate relief from such experiences are prone to utilizing dysregulated eating behaviors, particularly binge eating. Additionally, they found that distress tolerance mediated the previously reported relationship between anxiety sensitivity—the fear of anxiety-related sensations (e.g., accelerated heart rate)—and dysregulated eating behaviors (Anestis, Holm-Denoma, Gordon, Schmidt, & Joiner, 2008). These findings indicate that a lack of skills in effectively regulating negative affect may not fully account for behavioral dysregulation that occurs explicitly within the context of negative affective states. Instead, individuals' subjective evaluation of the magnitude of that affective state and beliefs regarding their ability to withstand it may play a pivotal role. As such, what might be perceived as minor affective discomfort to some, unlikely to trigger a dysregulated behavioral response, may be evaluated as intolerable to others.

Given these findings, a distress tolerance model for eating disorders, particularly with respect to binge eating and purging, appears to fit well within a framework of negative reinforcement. Because individuals with low distress tolerance are overwhelmed by less severe experiences of negative affect than people with moderate or high levels of distress tolerance, they are likely to encounter overwhelming states of negative affect with a greater frequency. Constantly faced with emotional states they find extremely aversive, such individuals are then likely to quickly turn to behaviors capable of offering immediate, even if fleeting, relief.

Although the growing base of evidence supporting a significant relationship between distress tolerance and eating disorders is compelling, there are several limitations that must be considered that may have significant impact on the nature of the relationship. First, none of the research specifically measuring distress tolerance has included longitudinal analyses. As such, the theorized direction of the relationship—low distress tolerance leading to the development of eating disorder symptoms—relies on assumptions that could prove to be incorrect. Second, although behavioral measures of distress tolerance exist, all of the research examining the relationship between distress tolerance and eating disorders has used self-report questionnaires. Such methodology relies on participants to be accurate and honest and assumes that they understand the questions as worded. Although there is no reason to believe that the measures used in these studies are inadequate measures of the construct, a multimethod approach toward measurement would increase confidence in the results. Finally, although a multitude of studies have reported results consistent with a distress tolerance model for binge eating and purging, no studies have examined any potential relationship between distress tolerance and AN. Given the pain involved in restricting food intake, it seems theoretically plausible that individuals with the restricting subtype of AN would exhibit extremely high elevations on measures of distress tolerance. This would indicate that distress tolerance operates quite differently in AN than it does in BN and BED. If this is the case, distress tolerance would then serve as an important variable capable of indicating the degree to which individuals are vulnerable to particular eating disorder symptoms. As of now, however, such evidence is lacking.

Despite these limitations, the rapid growth in empirical studies examining the relationship between distress tolerance and eating disorders is impressive. Current studies have helped delineate potential mechanisms driving binge eating and purging and have provided evidence for the efficacious treatment of both BN and BED. Future work on this topic is necessary, but a strong foundation has been created.

## THEORETICAL IMPLICATIONS AND FUTURE DIRECTIONS

The research on the relationship between distress tolerance and eating disorders mentioned previously has several important theoretical implications. Primarily, it offers support for a model of binge eating and purging based in large part on affect regulation. It appears that negative affect serves as a pivotal antecedent to binge-eating behavior, and that individuals who have difficulties inhibiting behavior in the context of negative affect are prone to binge eating and purging. Additionally, it appears that individuals who are able to tolerate only minimal levels of negative affect are at particularly high risk for utilizing dysregulated eating behaviors. As such, the manner in which certain eating disorders, particularly BED and BN, are conceptualized may need to be altered. If low distress tolerance serves as a primary risk factor for BN and BED, then these disorders may be better classified as relating closely to non-eating disorders such as BPD than to AN. Such a shift in conceptualizations would not be intended to minimize the frequency with which AN and other eating disorders co-occur; however, such a shift would serve to emphasize common risk factors across disorders.

Future work utilizing longitudinal data accumulated through both behavioral and self-report measures of distress tolerance will serve to answer many of these questions. Additionally, studies that examine distress tolerance in AN as well as BED and BN will not only help to clarify the relationship between distress tolerance and eating disorders but will add potential insight into the mechanisms that differentiate one eating disorder from another. A clearer understanding of how individuals' subjective experience of emotions impacts vulnerabilities to eating disorder behaviors could prove invaluable. If individuals with low distress tolerance report being overwhelmed by negative emotions more frequently than others even without experiencing a greater amount of negative affect, this would impact how researchers and clinicians conceptualize antecedents to binge episodes and other eating disorder behaviors. In this scenario, environmental stress would become entirely relative and the importance of teaching individuals with low distress tolerance skills to increase their ability to withstand negative affect would become impossible to overstate.

## CLINICAL IMPLICATIONS AND APPLICATIONS

Cognitive-behavioral therapy (CBT) has been found to be an effective treatment for BN and BED (e.g., Fairburn, 2002) and is often considered to be the best first choice for treatment. However, given rates of CBT treatment failure and relapse (e.g., Wilfley & Cohen, 1997), it appears that additional treatment strategies are needed. One such strategy, with growing empirical and theoretical support, is to increase patients' distress tolerance (Corstorphine et al., 2007). Many individuals with BN and BED report considerable difficulties regulating their emotions, and they often use maladaptive coping strategies, such as binge eating and vomiting, in order to reduce their emotional turmoil (e.g., Stice, Nemeroff, & Shaw, 1996). Thus, teaching patients how to accept and tolerate their emotional distress may be an important treatment intervention. As discussed earlier, one promising approach to increasing distress tolerance among individuals with an eating disorder is DBT, which specifically targets distress tolerance, along with mindfulness, emotion regulation, and interpersonal effectiveness.

As mentioned earlier in the chapter, traditional DBT, as developed by Marsha Linehan, has received growing support for the treatment of both BED and BN. Wisniewski and Kelly (2003) have proposed a framework for adapting traditional DBT to target some of the specific issues that patients with eating disorders experience; we briefly describe their adaptations here. Standard DBT operates with the assumption that the primary conflict, or dialectic, for patients is between acceptance and change. However, according to the adapted approach for eating disorders, the main aim of treatment is to "resolve the dialectical dilemma between rigid, overcontrolled eating and the absence of eating structure or plan" (Wisniewski & Kelly, 2003). Similar to standard DBT, in order to resolve this conflict, patients are taught skills to increase goal-directed behavior and decrease non-goal-directed behavior. Wisniewski and Kelly suggest that, as with standard DBT, at treatment initiation all patients must freely commit to therapy and create a hierarchy of treatment targets, with life-threatening behaviors (e.g., suicide, nonsuicidal self-injury) placed at the top. Additional life-threatening conditions that may occur in people with eating disorders (e.g., bradychardia, electrolyte imbalances) should also be targeted. Next on the hierarchy are therapy-interfering behaviors, which for patients with eating disorders may include refusal to be weighed or inability to fully participate in therapy because of an impoverished physical state. Following therapy-interfering behaviors are those that interfere with quality of life, which may include restricting, bingeing, purging, overexercising, and counting calories. Aside from focusing on treatment targets that are more likely to be endorsed by individuals with eating disorders, Wisniewski and Kelly also suggest expanding the weekly homework, or "diary card," to allow for patients to log food consumption, eating disorder behaviors, and difficulties following their food plan. The adaptation also calls for the addition of a nutrition module, which provides psychoeducational material on nutrition and dieting. Finally, the authors advise expanding the mindfulness module to include mindful eating, mindful attention to one's body, and mindful acceptance of one's body.

For many disorders, comorbidities tend to be the rule rather than the exception, and eating disorders are no different. For instance, researchers have found that up to 50% of women with BN have co-occurring alcohol use disorders (Dansky, Brewerton, & Kilpatrick, 2000). Moreover, almost half of those with BN meet criteria for at least one Axis II diagnosis (Carroll, Touyz, & Beumont, 1996), and more than 80% of women with BN have a lifetime mood disorder (Bushnell et al., 1994). Comorbidity among individuals with eating disorders further suggests the use of DBT because it has been found to be an effective treatment for many of the disorders that are often comorbid with BN and BED. Specifically, DBT has been found to be more effective than treatment as usual in the treatment of BPD and comorbid substance abuse (Harned et al., 2008; Linehan et al., 1999); has been found to be effective in the treatment of comorbid personality disorders (Lynch & Cheavens, 2008); and was successfully used to treat co-occurring depression and personality disorders in older adults (Lynch, Cheavens, Cukrowicz, Thorp, & Bronner, 2007).

Another treatment approach that could potentially address distress tolerance in clients with eating disorders is acceptance and commitment therapy (ACT; Hayes, Strosahl, & Wilson, 1999). ACT encourages clients to accept unpleasant thoughts and emotions and to avoid utilizing control strategies. Distress in the form of negative emotions and thoughts is conceptualized as a natural part of goal-directed behavior rather than an obstacle impeding progress. By reframing the nature of distress, this therapeutic approach can potentially offer a path toward increasing distress tolerance. Very little research has been conducted testing the efficacy of ACT in the treatment of eating disorders, however, so this is purely speculative. Heffner, Sperry, Eifert, and Detweiler (2002) published a case study in which they successfully utilized ACT to treat an adolescent female diagnosed with AN; thus, preliminary evidence is promising, but additional research is needed before this technique can be considered a front-line approach for addressing difficulties with distress tolerance.

If distress tolerance becomes a treatment target, it will be important for the mental health professional providing treatment to measure continuously not only distress tolerance but also facets that are believed to be affected by distress tolerance. Corstorphine and colleagues' (2007) Distress Tolerance Scale was developed specifically for use with eating disorder populations and would likely be useful in this regard. Their Distress Tolerance Scale consists of three subscales: Accepting and Managing Emotion, which measures the degree to which the presence of negative affect impacts problem-solving abilities; Avoidance of Affect, which assesses emotional avoidance; and Anticipate and Distract, which reflects an ability to manage emotional vulnerability proactively. Corstorphine and colleagues found that women with eating disorders had elevated Avoidance of Affect scores compared with a nonclinical sample of women, suggesting that those with eating disorders are more likely to avoid their emotions than those without an eating disorder. Thus, if using this scale to measure distress tolerance over the course of treatment, one would hope to see a decrease on the Avoidance of Affect subscale and increases on the Accepting and Managing Emotion and Anticipate and Distract subscales.

Additionally, because binge eating and purging are believed to be manifestations of poor distress tolerance (e.g., Corstorphine et al., 2007; Heatherton & Baumeister, 1991; McManus & Waller, 1995), it would be important to measure these behaviors over the course of treatment as well. As individuals become better able to accept and regulate their emotions, they should be less likely to engage in eating disorder behaviors.

Thus far, there are no specific treatments for targeting and preventing distress tolerance for people with eating disorders; however, a review of available research provides some suggestions. A potentially direct approach would be to teach patients the skills involved in the distress tolerance module of DBT. Once these skills have been learned, patients can be encouraged to participate in in-session eating exposures, in which they are asked to use distress tolerance skills in the moment. Because our culture tends to invalidate realistic standards of beauty (Wisniewski & Kelly, 2003), helping patients understand the consequences of internalizing the "thin ideal," as well as teaching them strategies to refute this ideal, may also be useful treatment interventions. Patients could be encouraged to accept their own bodies rather than looking to outside sources for comparisons. Along these lines, media literacy programs, which teach people to evaluate media images and messages critically, have been found to reduce thin-ideal internalization (Piran, Levine, & Irving, 2000) and weight concern (Wade, Davidson, & O'Dea, 2003).

Instructing patients in how to reduce emotional avoidance and increase emotional problem solving might also be helpful in increasing their distress tolerance (Corstorphine et al., 2007). Additionally, teaching them how to interpret and respond to hunger and satiety cues may make them less likely to binge eat, restrict, and/or purge in response to negative affect. There is evidence that individuals with eating disorders have nutrition-related vulnerability; in other words, they have biologically dysregulated hunger and satiety cues (Wisniewski & Kelly, 2003). Thus, helping them learn to interpret these cues accurately could reduce this vulnerability.

Overall, evidence that targeting distress tolerance is a worthwhile intervention for those with either BN or BED continues to grow. Multiple studies have found DBT, which targets distress tolerance, to be an effective treatment for people with BN and BED (e.g., Chen et al., 2008; Palmer et al., 2003; Safer et al., 2001; Telch et al., 2001). However, continued research is needed to answer important remaining questions. For example, studies comparing standard DBT with the modified version for patients with eating disorders (as suggested by Wisniewski and Kelly, 2003) are needed to determine whether the modified version results in significant improvements over and above the standard version. Moreover, to date it is unclear what role distress tolerance may play in the development and maintenance of AN, although there is increasing evidence that people with AN exhibit alexithymia, or difficulty identifying and expressing emotions (de Zwann et al., 1996; Nkam, et al., 1997). Moreover, another study found that recovering patients with AN reported more psychological distress than controls in response to both a speech and free-association task (Miller, Erickson, Branom, & Steiner, 2009). Furthermore, these recovered patients scored above the 80th percentile on a distress measure, indicating that they were still experiencing clinically significant amounts of stress despite being in the recovery process. Future research should more closely examine how distress tolerance operates within AN and whether or not treatments that prioritize distress tolerance skills are effective with this population. Given the discomfort inherent in restricting food intake, it may also be that individuals with AN exhibit abnormally high levels of distress tolerance. If this is the case, interventions that aim to teach them to better attend to affective cues may be important. Finally, DBT can be costly and difficult to administer; thus, dismantling studies are needed to determine whether specific modules, like distress tolerance, could be taught in isolation with equal effectiveness as the standard DBT treatment package.

## SUMMARY

Current research indicates that distress tolerance serves as an important factor in eating disorders. The degree to which individuals are capable of tolerating negative affect may have important influences on a variety of dysregulated eating behaviors, particularly binge eating and purging. Future research to determine whether particular negative affective states are more important than others in driving dysregulated eating behaviors would be invaluable. Additionally, future research examining the role of distress tolerance in AN should serve to clarify a potentially pivotal difference among eating disorders: Should individuals with AN exhibit high levels of distress tolerance, subjective evaluations of affective experiences may prove to be a key marker determining which dysregulated eating behavior vulnerabilities they possess even before such behaviors begin.

Distress tolerance may also be an important area for developing treatments of eating disorders. Although some ways of incorporating distress tolerance into treating eating disorders have been discussed, such as with therapies like DBT, there may be additional strategies to address distress tolerance that have yet to be identified. This could potentially be done with cognitive restructuring, building up patients' distress threshold by examining evidence of strength and forbearance. Alternatively, if individuals are prone to experiencing more distress as a result of neurobiological factors, treatments may focus on ways to help them tolerate distress through activities that help them distract from upsetting emotions, such as mindfulness. The research on distress tolerance in eating disorders is still young, but distress tolerance appears to be a very promising mechanism to explore in eating disorder psychopathology and treatment.

## REFERENCES

Anestis, M. D., Holm-Denoma, J. M., Gordon, K. H., Schmidt, N. B., & Joiner, T. E. (2008). The role of anxiety sensitivity in eating pathology. *Cognitive Therapy and Research, 32,* 370–385.

Anestis, M. D., Selby, E. A., Fink, E., & Joiner, T. E. (2007). The multifaceted role of distress tolerance in dysregulated eating behaviors. *International Journal of Eating Disorders, 40,* 718–726.

Anestis, M. D., Selby, E. A., & Joiner, T. E. (2007). The role of urgency in maladaptive behaviors. *Behaviour Research and Therapy, 45,* 3018–3029.

Anestis, M. D., Smith, A. R., Fink, E. L., & Joiner, T. E. (2009). Dysregulated eating and distress: Examining the specific role of urgency in a clinical population. *Cognitive Therapy and Research, 33,* 390–397.

Arnow, B., Kenardy, J., & Agras, W. S. (1995). The Emotional Eating Scale: The development of a measure to assess coping with negative affect by eating. *International Journal of Eating Disorders, 18,* 79–90.

Bushnell, J. A., Wells, J. E., McKenzie, J. M., Hornblow, A. R., Oakley-Browne, M. A., & Joyce, P. R. (1994). Bulimia comorbidity in the general population and in the clinic. *Psychological Medicine, 24,* 605–611.

Carroll, J. M., Touyz, S. W., & Beumont, P. (1996). Specific comorbidity between bulimia nervosa and personality disorders. *International Journal of Eating Disorders, 19,* 159–171.

Chen, E. Y., Matthews, L., Allen, C., Kuo, J. R., & Linehan, M. M. (2008). Dialectical behavior therapy for clients with binge eating disorder or bulimia nervosa and borderline personality disorder. *International Journal of Eating Disorders, 41,* 505–512.

Corstorphine, E., Mountford, V., Tomlinson, S., Waller, G., & Meyer, C. (2007). Distress tolerance in the eating disorders. *Eating Behaviors, 8,* 91–97.

Dansky, B. S., Brewerton, T. D., & Kilpatrick, D. G. (2000). Comorbidity of bulimia nervosa and alcohol use disorders: Results from the National Women's Study. *International Journal of Eating Disorders, 27,* 180–190.

de Zwaan, M., Biener, D., Bach, M., Wiesnagrotzki, S., & Stacher, G. (1996). Pain sensitivity, alexithymia, and depression in patients with eating disorders: Are they related? *Journal of Psychosomatic Research, 41,* 65–70.

Fairburn, C. G. (2002). Cognitive-behavioral therapy for bulimia nervosa. In C. G. Fairburn & K. D. Brownell (Eds.) *Eating disorders and obesity* (2nd ed., pp. 302–307). New York: Guilford Press.

Fischer, S., Anderson, K. G., & Smith, G. T. (2004). Coping with distress by eating or drinking: Role of trait urgency and expectancies. *Psychology of Addictive Behaviors, 18,* 269–274.

Fischer, S., Smith, G. T., & Anderson, K. G. (2003). Clarifying the role of impulsivity in bulimia nervosa. *International Journal of Eating Disorders, 33,* 406–411.

Harned, M. S., Chapman, A. L., Dexter-Mazza, E. T., Murray, A., Comtois, K., & Linehan, M. M. (2008). Treating co-occurring axis I disorders in recurrently suicidal women with borderline personality disorder: A 2-year randomized trial of dialectical behavior therapy versus community treatment by experts. *Journal of Consulting and Clinical Psychology, 76,* 1068–1075.

Hayes, S. C., Strosahl, K. D., & Wilson, K. G. (1999). *Acceptance and commitment therapy: An experimental approach to behavior change.* New York: Guilford Press.

Heatherton, T. F., & Baumeister, R. F. (1991). Binge eating as escape from self-awareness. *Psychological Bulletin, 110,* 86–108.

Heffner, M., Sperry, J., Eifert, G. H., & Detweiler, M. (2002). Acceptance and commitment therapy in the treatment of an adolescent female with anorexia nervosa: A case example. *Cognitive and Behavioral Practice, 9,* 232–236.

Hilbert, A., & Tuschen-Caffier, B. (2007). Maintenance of binge eating through

negative mood: A naturalistic comparison of binge eating disorder and bulimia nervosa. *International Journal of Eating Disorders, 40,* 521–530.

Linehan, M. M. (1993a). *Cognitive-behavioral treatment of borderline personality disorder.* New York: Guilford Press.

Linehan, M. M. (1993b). *Skills training manual for treating borderline personality disorder.* New York: Guilford Press.

Linehan, M. M. (1998). An illustration of dialectical behavior therapy. *In Session, 4,* 21–44.

Linehan, M. M., Schmidt, H., Dimeff, L. A., Kanter, J. W., Craft, J. C., Comtois,
K. A., et al. (1999). Dialectical behavior therapy for patients with borderline
personality disorder and drug-dependence. *American Journal on Addiction,
8,* 279–292.

Lynch, T. R., & Cheavens, J. S. (2008). Dialectical behavior therapy for comorbid personality disorders. *Journal of Clinical Psychology, 64,* 154–167.

Lynch, T. R., Cheavens, J. S., Cukrowicz, K. C., Thorp, S. R., & Bronner, L.
(2007). Treatment of older adults with co-morbid personality disorder and
depression: A dialectical behavior therapy approach. *International Journal
of Geriatric Psychiatry, 22,* 131–143.

McManus, F., & Waller, G. (1995). A functional analysis of binge-eating. *Clinical
Psychology Review, 8,* 845–863.

Miller, S. P., Erickson, S. J., Branom, C., & Steiner, H. (2009). Habitual response
to stress in recovering adolescent anorexic patients. *Child Psychiatry and
Human Development, 40,* 43–54.

Mountford, V., Corstorphine, E., Tomlinson, S., & Waller, G. (2007). Development of a measure to assess invalidating childhood environments in the eating disorders. *Eating Behaviors, 8,* 45–58.

Nkam, I., Langlois-Thery, S., Dollfus, S., & Petit, M. (1997). Alexithymia in
negative symptoms and non-negative symptoms. *Encephale, 23,* 358–363.

Palmer, R. L., Birchall, H., Damani, S., Gatward, N., McGrain, L., & Parker,
L. (2003). A dialectical behavior therapy program for people with an eat-
ing disorder and borderline personality disorder: Description and outcome.
*International Journal of Eating Disorders, 33,* 281–286.

Piran, N., Levine, M. P., & Irving, L. M. (2000). Go girls! Media literacy, activ-
ism, and advocacy project. *Healthy Weight Journal, 14,* 89–90.

Safer, D. L., Lock, J., & Coutourier, J. L. (2007). Dialectical behavior therapy
modified for adolescent binge eating disorder: A case report. *Cognitive and
Behavioral Practice, 14,* 157–167.

Safer, D. L., Telch, C. F., & Agras, W. S. (2001). Dialectical behavior therapy
adapted for bulimia: A case report. *International Journal of Eating Disorders, 30,* 101–106.

Simons, J. S., & Gaher, R. M. (2005). The Distress Tolerance Scale: Development and validation of a self-report measure. *Motivation and Emotion, 29,*
83–102.

Smyth, J., Wonderlich, S., Crosby, R., Miltenberger, R., Mitchell, J., & Rorty, M.
(2001). The use of ecological momentary assessment approaches in eating
disorder research. *International Journal of Eating Disorders, 30,* 83–95.

Smyth, J. M., Wonderlich, S. A., Heron, K. E., Sliwinski, M. J., Crosby, R. D.,

Mitchell, J. E., et al. (2007). Daily and momentary mood and stress are associated with binge eating and vomiting in bulimia nervosa patients in the natural environment. *Journal of Consulting and Clinical Psychology, 75*, 629–638.

Stein, R. I., Kenardy, J., Wiseman, C. V., Zoler Dounchis, J., Arnow, B. A., & Wilfley, D. E. (2007). What's driving the binge in binge eating disorder?: A prospective examination of precursors and consequences. *International Journal of Eating Disorders, 40*, 195–203.

Stice, E., Nemeroff, C., & Shaw, H. E. (1996). Test of the dual pathway model of bulimia nervosa: Evidence for dietary restraint and affect regulation mechanisms. *Journal of Social and Clinical Psychology, 15*, 340–363.

Telch, C. F., Agras, W. S., & Linehan, M. M. (2000). Group dialectical behavior therapy for binge eating disorder: A preliminary, uncontrolled trial. *Behavior Therapy, 31*, 569–582.

Telch, C. F., Agras, W. S., & Linehan, M. M. (2001). Dialectical behavior therapy for binge eating disorder. *Journal of Consulting and Clinical Psychology, 69*, 1061–1065.

Thompson, R. A. (1994). The development of emotion regulation: Biological and behavioral considerations. *Monographs of the Society for Research in Child Development, 59*, 25–52.

Wade, T. D., Davidson, S., & O'Dea, J. A. (2003). A preliminary controlled evaluation of a school-based media literacy program and self-esteem program for reducing eating disorder risk factors. *International Journal of Eating Disorders, 33*, 371–383.

Wegner, K. E., Smyth, J. M., Crosby, R. D., Wittrock, D., Wonderlich, S. A., & Mitchell, J. E. (2002). An evaluation of the relationship between mood and binge eating in the natural environment using ecological momentary assessment. *International Journal of Eating Disorders, 32*, 352–361.

Whiteside, S. P., & Lynam, D. R. (2001). The five factor model and impulsivity: Using a structural model of personality to understand impulsivity. *Personality and Individual Differences, 30*, 669–689.

Whiteside, U., Chen, E., Neighbors, C., Hunter, D., Lo, T., & Larimer, M. (2007). Difficulties regulating emotions: Do binge eaters have fewer strategies to modulate and tolerate negative affect? *Eating Behaviors, 8*, 162–169.

Wilfley, D. E., & Cohen, L. R. (1997). Psychological treatment of bulimia nervosa and binge eating disorder. *Psychopharmacology Bulletin, 33*, 437–454.

Wiser, S., & Telch, C. F. (1999). Dialectical behavior therapy for binge-eating disorder. *Journal of Clinical Psychology, 5*, 755–768.

Wisniewski, L., & Kelly, E. (2003). The application of dialectical behavior therapy to the treatment of eating disorders. *Cognitive and Behavioral Practice, 10*, 131–138.

# PART III

## Future Directions

# 12

# Research Synthesis and the Future

Amit Bernstein, Anka A. Vujanovic,
Teresa M. Leyro, *and* Michael J. Zvolensky

The overarching aim of the present volume was to provide a field-wide conceptual and methodological review of the theoretical and empirical literature on distress tolerance. Special attention was paid to elucidating the nature of the distress tolerance construct(s), illuminating its nomological network, reviewing its potential role(s) in psychopathology, and articulating its demonstrated and potential clinical implications for treatment and prevention of various types of psychopathology.

Research evaluating the theoretical and clinical importance of the distress tolerance construct(s) for vulnerability to, and maintenance of, psychopathology is in the early stages of development. Indeed, as highlighted throughout this volume, extant work has often involved extrapolation from various areas of research theoretically relevant to distress tolerance (e.g., anxiety sensitivity, emotion regulation). Thus, the primary means by which to address our limited empirical knowledge of this construct is to call attention to the fact that we have much to learn with respect to the nature of distress tolerance, its relations to psychopathology, its measurement, and its utility in the prevention and treatment of psychopathology. The purpose of the present chapter is to consider a selection of broad-based gaps in the literature noted across chapters in the present volume, thereby highlighting promising future directions in the area of distress tolerance research.

Specifically, in the present chapter, we focus on six key domains of interest, corresponding to gaps in the extant knowledge base, that may serve as a framework for guiding future distress tolerance-related research: (1) conceptual and definitional precision of the construct, (2) operational definition(s) and measurement development and evaluation, (3) phenomenology of the construct, (4) relations to other constructs and processes, (5) relations to psychopathology, and (6) therapeutic change and intervention research. The following is a summary of these domains and their implications for future directions for research on distress tolerance and related processes, putatively linked to vulnerability for the development and maintenance of various forms of psychopathology.

## CONCEPTUAL AND DEFINITIONAL PRECISION OF THE CONSTRUCT(S)

### Heterogenity in Conceptual Perspectives of "Distress"

As highlighted throughout chapters in the present volume, distress tolerance research has been characterized by a great degree of conceptual heterogenity. For example, some distress tolerance-related constructs relate to aversive physical sensations (Schmidt & Cook, 1999) or pain (e.g., Burns, Bruehl, & Caceres, 2004; Hines & Brown, 1932; Rhudy & Meagher, 2003, Willoughby, Hailey, Mulkana, & Rowe, 2002), others are focused more generally on noxious affective or emotional states (Simons & Gaher, 2005), others are related to psychological or cognitive frustration (e.g., Gronwall & Sampson, 1974; Matthews & Stoney, 1988; Quinn, Brandon, & Copeland, 1996), and yet others more specifically focus on specific contexts such as those involving ambiguous (Furnham & Ribchester, 1995) or uncertain (Dugas, Gagnon, Ladouceur, & Freeston, 1998) life events. Although there is some natural degree of overlap between various distress tolerance constructs or conceptualizations, each also has been studied within the context of, and in relation to, relatively specific clinical problems. However, despite the noted heterogeneity, these various conceptual perspectives on distress tolerance commonly pertain to tolerance of (various types of) *experiential distress* (Zvolensky, Leyro, Bernstein, & Vujanovic, Chapter 1, this volume). This is thus the consistent and common conceptual link across these various perspectives and the basis for defining distress tolerance as a single, albeit multifaceted, umbrella construct.

For the purpose of elucidating the nature(s) of distress tolerance and advancing its operationalization, as well as its relations with various other constructs and psychopathology, it is important that future work theoretically and empirically focus systematically on the nature of *distress* within the distress tolerance construct. For example, although distress tolerance research broadly has involved study of affective and nonaffective (somatic) processes, these lines of research have historically remained largely independent. Integrative and arguably fundamental theoretical and methodological work may be an important first step in advancing this construct. Furthermore, research to date has not systematically evaluated whether there is a common, underlying affective element across various forms of distressing experiences that have been the focus of distress tolerance conceptualizations, such as those related to thoughts, physical sensations, and contextual events. Study of this common affective experience or interpretive bias of distress may be a fruitful means of unifying heterogenous theory and empirical study of distress tolerance and its relations (see also Asmundson, Peluso, Carleton, Collimore, & Welch, Chapter 10, this volume, for further discussion).

Another related core issue centers on the lack of specificity with respect to the nature or forms of distress key to conceptual and operational definitions of distress tolerance. For example, tolerance of distressing affective states and its measurement have not been clearly linked to specific forms of affective or psychological distress. A significant contribution to the literature may result from study of individual differences with respect to tolerance of various, specific (distressing) affective states, such as anxiety, fear, sadness, disgust, and anger. It is noteworthy that such specificity has been incorporated with respect to the study of certain facets of distress tolerance (e.g., Weems, Chapter 2, this volume), such as tolerance of uncertainty (e.g., Schmidt, Mitchell, Keough, & Riccardi, Chapter 5, this volume). Importantly, as noted in the review of the intolerance of uncertainty literature and its relations to specific anxiety disorders, increased specificity may help not only to advance our theoretical understanding of the phenomenological nature of distress tolerance and its facets but also to clarify the linkages of such tolerance variables to specific forms of psychopathology. That is, more precise theoretical models and assessment tools may help illuminate the nature of distress tolerance and psychopathology relations.

## Nature of Tolerance

Just as with the conceptualization of distress within the distress tolerance construct(s), there is heterogeneity and lack of clarity in the conceptual (and operational) definition(s) of the term *tolerance* in the existing literature. Various conceptual perspectives on tolerance of distress broadly denote individual differences in the extent to which a person withstands a certain form and degree of experiential distress (Otto, Powers, & Fischmann, 2005; Simons & Gaher, 2005). Conceptually and operationally, however, distress tolerance can and has been used to refer both to (1) an individual's perceived capacity to withstand negative affective or other aversive states and (2) behavioral acts of withstanding negative emotional states. Accordingly, there have been two methodological literatures focused on distress tolerance. Reviews within the present volume demonstrate that this has occurred as much or more as a function of a methodological artifact (e.g., nature of self-report vs. non-self-report or behavioral indices of distress tolerance) as opposed to an explicit conceptual perspective on the nature of distress tolerance.

The self-report literature often has oriented to the perceived capacity to withstand aversive states. The non-self-report (behavioral or biobehavioral) literature, on the other hand, has tended to be oriented to the actual behavioral ability to tolerate (or rather avoid) specific types of aversive states in real time. There likely are differences between the *perceived* element of distress tolerance capacity and *actual* behavioral tolerance of distress, although direct study of this relatively central conceptual and methodological issue is lacking.

## Context and Flexibility in Tolerance of Distress

Because contextual flexibility in the regulation of emotion has been shown to be associated with reduced psychopathology and more adaptive functioning (Eftekhari, Zoellner, & Vigil, 2009), there is a need to consider the role(s) of contextual flexibility in distress tolerance processes and in vulnerability and resilience to psychopathology. Although the current review has largely focused on psychopathological sequelae of limited or low levels of distress tolerance, it should not be lost that the flexibility in use of distress tolerance skills may play a central role in its adaptive/maladaptive features. For example, to the extent that individuals maintain rigid beliefs about their inability to tolerate negatively perceived emotional experiences like sadness, they may thereby paradoxically amplify or facilitate the chance of experiencing greater or ongoing negative mood states and depressive symptoms. Thus, perhaps low levels of distress tolerance, and specifically the intolerance of negative affective states, may be particularly linked to vulnerability when such intolerance is demonstrated across contexts and over time. In contrast, individuals who are able to adjust their tolerance of distress in a contextually sensitive manner, and thereby adaptively cope with various distressing experiences (e.g., daily hassles, traumatic stress, interpersonal conflict), may be less prone to develop or maintain psychopathology. Context-sensitive regulation of distress tolerance may represent an important dimension of this construct and its role in psychopathology. In other words, rigidly using the same cognitive or behavioral skill set regarding tolerance for distress across contexts and in response to diverse types of emotional experiences (e.g., sadness, anxiety, anger) may in part account for its role in psychopathology, in contrast to the simpler conceptual argument that more tolerance is better and less is worse. Existing work on distress tolerance has not yet directly addressed this central issue of flexibility and contextual sensitivity of distress tolerance and its correlates.

Relatedly, Lynch and Mizon (Chapter 3, this volume) argued compellingly that greater scientific and clinical attention should be focused on individual tendencies to manifest exceedingly high levels of distress tolerance. These authors argue that an especially heightened perceived ability to tolerate distress, or a heightened actual behavioral tolerance of distress, may facilitate situations in which an individual tolerates a high degree of distress despite the fact that such tolerance may be maladaptive and lead to unwanted outcomes. For example, an individual may manifest an especially high tolerance of protracted mistreatment by a loved one, although the ongoing suffering does not necessarily lead to positive or valued emotional or life circumstances, perhaps even predisposing the individual to clinical symptoms or syndromes.

One potential focus of study with respect to distress under- and over-tolerance might be the evaluation of contextually appropriate and inappropriate *or* flexible and inflexible tolerance of distress, wherein either especially low or high levels of tolerance are particularly maladaptive if applied rigidly across emotional and situational contexts. This multidimensional approach to conceptualizing and studying distress tolerance may offer a clinically meaningful line of inquiry with the potential to better understand distress tolerance and psychopathology relations as well as to advance intervention efforts for various clinical populations.

## OPERATIONAL DEFINITION(S) AND MEASUREMENT

### Construct–Method Synthesis

Another fundamental aspect of the distress tolerance literature, which relates closely to the conceptual definitional issues discussed previously, involves the approach to operationalization and measurement of distress tolerance. Method and measurement perspectives directly inform what we learn about the theoretical meaning of the construct and vice versa. Accordingly, all indices of distress tolerance are a product of a construct-method composition. In this capacity, there should be an increased focus on evaluation of theory in the context of the measurement methodology used.

For example, extant studies using self-report and behavioral methods to operationalize distress tolerance illustrate an "accident" of the literature, a seldom regarded construct-method confound. Specifically, self-report measures of distress tolerance not only differ from behavioral measures of distress tolerance methodologically but, moreover, index perceived capacity to tolerate various forms of distress. In contrast, behavioral measures of distress tolerance not only differ from self-report measures methodologically, but they also assess acts of withstanding distress in real-time experimental paradigms. Thus, our inferences and understanding of this construct may be the result of the methods used to index the construct and/or confounds related to the measurement tools employed to index the construct. Empirical study thus far has not expressly attempted to disentangle the current construct-method confound in distress tolerance research. Advancing such research will help to clarify and broaden our knowledge of distress tolerance and its relations to psychopathology in a number of ways. For example, such construct-method study may help to explicate whether perceived capacity to tolerate and behavioral capacity to tolerate are similarly clinically important and whether these conceptual facets of distress tolerance are unique or common elements of vulnerability to psychopathology. As another example, such work may help to elucidate whether and how these conceptual facets of distress tolerance shape one another as well as how psychopathology may affect each of these conceptual and operational facets of distress tolerance.

## Construct Validity of Biobehavioral Indices

The inclusion of biobehavioral or non-self-report measures of distress tolerance and self-report measures, in some respects, reflects an apparent methodological strength of this literature (i.e., multimeasure and multimethod). However, it is not clear how these various self- and non-self-report measures relate to one another. As one initial example of such study, Gratz, Rosenthal, Tull, Lejuez, & Gunderson (2006) found evidence of a strong relationship between latency to terminate the computerized paced serial auditory addition task (PASAT-C) and a measure of experiential avoidance (i.e., the Acceptance and Action Questionnaire; Hayes et al., 2004). This highlights the importance of more systematic study to develop multimethodological measurement of a common distress tolerance construct, or some specific facet(s) of this construct, for the purpose of more rigorously measuring individual differences in the variable, thereby facilitating more internally valid study of the role of the construct in vulnerability for psychopathology (see also Richards, Daughters, Bornovalova, Brown, & Lejuez, Chapter 8, this volume, for further discussion).

Key areas of importance with regard to further empirical and theoretical development involve the examination of the construct validity of various distress tolerance indices. For example, are behavioral tasks, such as the cognitive frustration tasks (e.g., anagram, PASAT, mirror tracing), valid indices of distress tolerance (perceived or behavioral)? Furthermore, do indices of persistence (i.e., propensity to maintain a behavior related to reward contingencies; Cloninger, Przybeck, & Švrakic, 1991) correspond to willingness and ability to tolerate unwanted or distressing states elicited by these behavioral tasks (e.g., frustration)? How might reward components of these tasks affect the measurement of the construct? (See also Asmundson et al., Chapter 10, this volume, for a discussion of this limitation of extant research in the context of distress broadly and pain tolerance specifically.) As one illustrative example, because of the standard contingencies in studies utilizing these biobehavioral methods (specifically, cognitive frustration tasks), performance on these tasks is typically contingent or positively reinforced (e.g., solving anagrams and accurate mirror tracing is rewarded). Consequently, performance and persistence/tolerance on these tasks may be partially confounded. Namely, persistence on these tasks may be a result of greater distress tolerance and also a by-product of reward seeking (i.e., performance on tasks may improve as a function of the time that a participant is willing to persist in completing each task in order to receive task reward). An alternative perspective is that these behavioral tasks do index distress tolerance insofar as they reflect individual differences in motivation to seek negative reinforcement relative to motivation to seek positive reinforcement. Conceptual clarity within this domain of distress tolerance research may be clarified by theoretical models of the basic behavioral and neurobiological processes underlying distress tolerance and persistence (Trafton & Gifford, Chapter 4, this volume). Future research may also usefully begin to clarify these questions by experimentally manipulating contingencies in these tasks to understand their role on persistence/tolerance as well as including and manipulating reward contingencies in testing other indices of perceived capacity and behavioral tolerance of distress. Delay discounting theory and method may be particularly relevant to understanding these distress tolerance–reward contingencies (e.g., Bickel & Marsch, 2001).

## Latent Structure

Researchers have operated from the perspective that specific types of distress tolerance are dimensional in structure and trait-like in nature, and operational definitions and measures of the construct have followed suit. Yet the latent structural nature of distress tolerance, as well as its putative facets, has yet to be tested beyond factor analytic modeling of specific measures. Indeed, latent structural study has not yet been conducted to evaluate a broad-based model of distress tolerance that may incorporate the various first-order factors or dimensions of the putative higher order construct. Furthermore, the construct has been studied under the implicit assumption that it is continuous or dimensional. Yet no test of this assumption has been completed. Such latent structural study has proven important in advancing our understanding of related constructs (Bernstein, Zvolensky, Vujanovic, & Moos, 2009; Taylor, Jang, Stewart, & Stein, 2008). One particularly promising data analytic approach for studying various (competing) putative latent structural models of distress tolerance may be factor mixture modeling (e.g., Lubke & Muthén, 2005). FMM integrates mixture modeling and factor analysis for the purpose of concurrently modeling the fit of various competing, latent structural models composed of categorical and/or continuous forms of variability.

## PHENOMENOLOGY OF CONSTRUCT AND RELATED PROCESSES

### Expression of Intolerance and Tolerance

Inspection of the knowledge base reviewed in the chapters of the present volume indicates that we know little about the means by which individuals express tolerance or intolerance to unwanted or distressing affective states or the automatic or effortful strategies used to respond to tolerance/intolerance. For example, individuals who are intolerant of certain distressing affective states may express such intolerance behaviorally in a variety of ways, including cognitive or affective suppression, avoidant coping, and so on. Likewise, individuals who are tolerant of unwanted or distressing affective states may express such tolerance behaviorally in a variety of ways, including acceptance, approach-oriented coping, and so on. To understand the nature of distress tolerance, it is important to study these basic processes between individuals (i.e., differences in expression of and response strategies to distress in/tolerance between individuals) and within individuals (i.e., variety of means of expression of and response strategies to distress in/tolerance within individuals). This information may be clinically useful because it may guide therapeutic change in distress tolerance by targeting processes related to its expression.

### Trait or Context-Sensitive State

The chapter authors in the present volume also make clear that there is limited theory and data regarding a fundamental, but implicit, assumption underlying much extant work on distress tolerance: its presumed trait-like stability over time and across contexts. Specifically, there is emerging, albeit limited, research that has expressly evaluated the degree to which distress tolerance may be characterized by a context-sensitive/dependent expression as opposed to a context-insensitive, more rigid trait-like expression (e.g., Bernstein, Trafton, Ilgen, & Zvolensky, 2008). Initial studies in the area of tolerance of pain, for example, highlight that affective distress may result in reduced levels of pain tolerance (Jones, Spindler, Jorgensen, & Zachariae, 2002; Rhudy & Meager, 2003; Willoughby et al., 2002; Zelman, Howland, Nichols, & Cleeland, 1991), consistent with the hypothesis that distress tolerance may be context sensitive. Future research may focus on understanding this core aspect of the nature of this construct(s) (for a discussion of this issue, see also Trafton & Gifford, Chapter 4, and Vujanovic, Bernstein, & Litz, Chapter 6, this volume).

## RELATIONS TO OTHER RISK
## AND PROTECTIVE FACTORS AND PROCESSES
### Distress Tolerance and Its Nomological Network

An important gap in the distress tolerance literature involves theory and empirical tests of the linkages among the distress tolerance construct(s), related measures, and the variety of other variables that may compose its nomological network. Theory and empirical data are specifically lacking with regard to the relations of distress tolerance with a variety of potentially overlapping and related risk and protective factors and processes. Such research will advance understanding of the nature of distress tolerance construct(s) and the larger processes within which distress tolerance may operate in regard to vulnerability for psychopathology. The lack of theory and empirical study focused on the putative nature of distress tolerance further highlights the limited study of distress tolerance in relation to the variety of existing and well-documented variables reviewed in the present volume, as articulated by Lynch and Mizon (Chapter 3, this volume; see also Clen, Mennin, & Fresco, Chapter 7, this volume). It is important that studies of distress tolerance empirically evaluate these relations and the unique and overlapping associations between distress tolerance and these conceptually related, more well-established constructs. Such research will presumably facilitate more conclusive evaluation of the conceptual and explanatory uniqueness of the construct and thereby elucidate its potentially specific role(s) with regard to psychopathology relative to other risk and resilience factors.

In this domain, it may be beneficial for future study to examine distress tolerance with respect to the variety of factors and processes that have been theorized to structurally and functionally relate to distress tolerance. Such variables could include, but are not limited to, experiential avoidance (Hayes, Strosahl, & Wilson, 1999), emotional suppression (Richards & Gross, 2000) and avoidant (Folkman & Lazarus, 1986) or disengagement coping (Compas, Connor-Smith, Saltzman, Thomsen, & Wadsworth, 2001), emotion dysregulation (Kashdan & Steger, 2006; Linehan, 1993; Rottenberg & Gross, 2003), anxiety sensitivity (Bernstein & Zvolensky, 2007; McNally, 2002; Taylor, 1999), and personality-based perspectives on persistence (Barkley, 1997; Cloninger et al., 1991). In such work, it may be important to evaluate structural and functional uniqueness, relatedness, and overlap between the constructs. For example, factor analytic and other emerging latent structural variable modeling methods may be particularly promising tools for explicating the latent structural topography of the nomological network of distress tolerance (e.g., Bernstein et al., 2009).

It may be particularly useful to evaluate the nature of the relations between distress tolerance and its theoretically related factors with respect to one another in regard to the development and maintenance of psychopathology. Such study will serve to inform an additional area of needed work evaluating the incremental validity of the construct(s) relative to other risk/resilience factors as well as tests of potential mediating and moderating mechanisms underlying vulnerability to psychopathology within which distress tolerance operates. As one example, it may be useful to evaluate what factors moderate (e.g., contextual factors) or mediate (e.g., chronic avoidance) associations between distress tolerance and various forms of psychopathology and whether distress tolerance moderates or mediates other processes underlying psychopathology development or maintenance.

## Mechanisms Underlying Distress Tolerance

As noted by several chapter authors in the present volume, the broad literature on distress tolerance lacks theory and empirical study of mechanisms underlying the construct(s). Chapter authors discussed a variety of ideas regarding such mechanisms (e.g., Gratz & Tull, Chapter 9, and Clen et al., Chapter 7). Work contributed to the present volume, namely related to neurobiolgoical and behavioral theory involving reinforcement processes, may be particularly useful in addressing this core theoretical issue. Various theoretical perspectives on mechanisms underlying distress tolerance may be forwarded, although, as the chapters in this volume illustrate, this has not been done in a systematic manner to date within the distress tolerance literature.

One promising proposal may involve theorizing by Trafton and Gifford (Chapter 4, this volume), related to context, intraperson individual differences, and neurobiological and behavioral processes related to pursuit of negative reinforcement opportunities. Specifically, Trafton and Gifford assert that (1) behaviorally, distress tolerance involves inhibiting or not responding to a negative reinforcement opportunity (see also Richards et al., Chapter 8, this volume); (2) distress tolerance reflects one specific type or example of control over responding to immediate reward opportunities (relief from distress as a negative reinforcement); (3) distress intolerance may, therefore, be understood as a facet of impulsivity to respond to immediate (negative) reinforcement or reward as opposed to pursuing alternative reinforcers that may be accessible if immediate negative reinforcement is inhibited or not pursued; (4) consequent to this behavioral conceptualization, neurobiological substrates underlying and modulating reward learning and response may mediate tolerance to distress; and thus (5) if this is an accurate portrayal, then a number of neurobiological processes may be identified that may underlie and modify the expression of distress tolerance. Trafton and Gifford (Chapter 4, this volume) further argue that if this behavioral and neurobiological model is accurate, then it follows that a variety of interrelated processes may shape the development, maintenance, and expression of distress tolerance, including "assigning value to context-specific opportunities based on experience and cognitions, learning from experienced behavioral consequences, adaptation to the environment at a rate determined by genetics, and executive functions." A focused program of study explicating these foundational elements and processes underlying distress tolerance may be a particularly fruitful and clinically significant area of future study.

## Developmental Origins

We also lack study and knowledge regarding factors related to the development and maintenance of distress tolerance (e.g., Weems, Chapter 2, this volume; Gratz & Tull, Chapter 9, this volume). Few factors beyond psychopathology or mood have been explored empirically in relation to the development or change in distress tolerance, such as learning history, genetic or biological factors, environmental stressors or traumatic stress, and other emotion regulation or coping strategies such as acceptance.

Furthermore, limited research has explored the temporal order or the impact of change in distress tolerance on psychopathology on the one hand, and change in psychopathology on distress tolerance on the other. Such developmentally informed research is central to understanding whether distress tolerance and related factors among adults may indeed function as risk factors for psychopathology (e.g., Kraemer, Kazdin, Offord, & Kessler, 1997). For example, it may be useful to evaluate whether distress tolerance and psychopathology development and maintenance influence one another transactionally over time (e.g., Weems, Chapter 2, this volume). Although the current body of research has not directly evaluated such possibilities, it may theoretically be likely that distress intolerance or contextually insensitive applications of distress tolerance are associated with psychopathology vulnerability, and that greater levels of psychopathology, in turn, may potentiate greater intolerance of such (chronic and severe) distress.

## NATURE OF VULNERABILITY/RESILIENCE AND RELATIONS WITH PSYCHOPATHOLOGY

### Determination of Status as Specific versus Common (Transdiagnostic) Risk Marker or Factor

As illustrated by chapter authors in the present volume, the degree to which distress tolerance is related to specific or to multiple forms of psychopathology represents an important area of research. This knowledge is central to guiding intervention and prevention strategies focused on distress tolerance and related processes. Furthermore, it is important to explore the possibility that although certain facets of distress tolerance may have common or transdiagnostic relevance, others may be more narrowly related to vulnerability for specific disorders. For example, intolerance of uncertainty may have greater specificity with respect to certain forms of psychopathology (e.g., generalized anxiety disorder), whereas other conceptual and operational measures of distress tolerance of negative affective states, broadly speaking, may be more universally or transdiagnostically linked to psychopathology.

## THERAPEUTIC CHANGE AND INTERVENTION RESEARCH ISSUES

### Therapeutic Mechanisms

It is striking that there is limited study of change or malleability of distress tolerance in the context of intervention programs. This gap in the empirical literature is unexpected, particularly considering that distress tolerance has been a focus of the theoretical basis of a number of widely disseminated clinical interventions as noted across the chapters in the present volume (e.g., Barlow, Allen, & Choate, 2004; Brown et al., 2008; Linehan, 1993). One exception in this domain has been the important work by Dugas, Ladouceur, and colleagues (Dugas & Ladouceur,

**TABLE 12.1. Future Directions for Distress Tolerance Research**

I. *Conceptual and definitional precision of the construct*
   • Heterogenity in conceptual perspectives of "distress"
   • Nature of tolerance
   • Context and flexibility in tolerance of distress

II. *Operational definitions and measurement development and evaluation*
   • Construct-method synthesis
   • Construct validity of behavioral indices
   • Latent structure

III. *Phenomenology of the construct*
   • Expression of intolerance and tolerance
   • Trait or context-sensitive state

IV. *Relations to other constructs and processes*
   • Distress tolerance and its nomological network
   • Mechanisms underlying distress tolerance
   • Developmental origins

V. *Relations to psychopathology*
   • Determination of status as specific versus common (transdiagnostic) risk marker or factor

VI. *Therapeutic change and intervention research*
   • Therapeutic mechanism
   • Intervention development and evaluation

2000; Dugas et al., 2003; Ladouceur, Gosselin, & Dugas, 2000), who have found that a change in intolerance uncertainty is related to positive treatment outcome in generalized anxiety disorder (Dugas & Ladouceur, 2000; Dugas et al., 2003; Ladouceur, Dugas, et al., 2000). This work indicates that at least this particular distress tolerance-related construct is malleable and related to therapeutic change for one type of anxiety psychopathology. In another study, Miller, Wyman, Huppert, Glassman, and Rathus (2000) found that perceived helpfulness of the dialectical behavior therapy distress tolerance skills were positively associated with improvements in interpersonal problems among a sample of suicidal adolescents. Outside of these (limited) empirical findings, there is a need for more direct support for distress tolerance as a mechanism of clinical change. Here, it would be useful to examine empirically whether changes in distress tolerance precede (temporally) and/or mediate changes in psychopathology and related problems from pre- to posttreatment. Such study would provide valuable insight into the utility of distress tolerance in the prevention and treatment of psychopathology. Research in this area also is necessary to test whether distress tolerance may be a causal risk factor in regard to a given form(s) of psychopathology.

## Intervention Development and Evaluation

A related knowledge deficit involves testing and developing therapeutic interventions that may be effective and efficient in engendering change in distress tolerance (e.g., greater tolerance or greater contextual flexibility in tolerance). Multiple chapter authors in this volume discussed this issue (e.g., Gratz & Tull, Chapter 9; Lynch & Mizon, Chapter 3; Richards et al., Chapter 8). Promising therapeutic approaches may involve, for example, techniques such as interoceptive exposure and mindfulness skills training. Future work may contribute to this facet of the distress tolerance literature by explicitly measuring change in distress tolerance and the nature of such change (e.g., overall levels, contextual flexibility in its expression) in response to various intervention techniques. Various promising therapeutic approaches merit focused study, such as dialectical behavior therapy (Linehan, 1993) and acceptance-based emotion regulation group therapy (Gratz & Gunderson, 2006).

## SUMMARY

Distress tolerance may be an important construct(s) related to the onset and maintenance of many forms of psychopathology as well as their prevention and treatment. As highlighted in the present chapter, a number of fundamental questions remain regarding the conceptual and operational definition(s) of the construct(s), its phenomenology, its relations to other constructs and processes, its relations to psychopathology vulnerability and resilience, and its role as a treatment and preventive intervention target. Future research will make important contributions to our understanding of distress tolerance(s) and its role(s) in psychopathology vulnerability and resilience.

## REFERENCES

Barkley, R. (1997). Attention-deficit/hyperactivity disorder, self-regulation, and time: Toward a more comprehensive theory. *Journal of Developmental and Behavioral Pediatrics, 18,* 271–279.

Barlow, D., Allen, L., & Choate, M. (2004). Toward a unified treatment for emotional disorders. *Behavior Therapy, 35,* 205–230.

Bernstein, A., Trafton, J., Ilgen, M., & Zvolensky, M. J. (2008). An evaluation of the role of smoking context on a biobehavioral index of distress tolerance. *Addictive Behaviors, 33,* 1409–1415.

Bernstein, A., & Zolensky, M. J. (2007). Anxiety sensitivity: Selective review of promising research and future directions. *Expert Review of Neurotherapeutics, 7,* 97–101.

Bernstein, Z., Zvolensky, M. J., Vujanovic, A. A., & Moos, R. (2009). Anxiety sensitivity, distress tolerance, and discomfort intolerance: A hierarchical model of affect sensitivity and tolerance. *Behavior Therapy, 40,* 291–301.

Bickel, W., & Marsch, L. (2001). Toward a behavioral economic understanding of drug dependence: Delay discounting processes. *Addiction, 96,* 73–86.

Brown, R., Palm, K., Strong, D., Lejuez, C., Kahler, C., Zvolensky, M., et al. (2008). Distress tolerance treatment for early-lapse smokers: Rationale, program description, and preliminary findings. *Behavior Modification, 32,* 302–332.

Burns, J., Bruehl, S., & Caceres, C. (2004). Anger management style, blood pressure reactivity, and acute pain sensitivity: Evidence for "trait × situation" models. *Annals of Behavioral Medicine, 27,* 195–204.

Cloninger, C., Przybeck, T., & Švrakic, D. (1991). The Tridimensional Personality Questionnaire: U.S. normative data. *Psychological Reports, 69,* 1047–1057.

Compas, B., Connor-Smith, J., Saltzman, H., Thomsen, A., & Wadsworth, M. (2001). Coping with stress during childhood and adolescence: Problems, progress, and potential in theory and research. *Psychological Bulletin, 127,* 87–127.

Dugas, M. J., Gagnon, F., Ladouceur, R., & Freeston, H. (1998). Generalized anxiety disorder: A preliminary test of a conceptual model. *Behaviour Research and Therapy, 36,* 215–226.

Dugas, M. J., & Ladouceur, R. (2000). Treatment of GAD: Targeting intolerance of uncertainty in two types of worry. *Behavior Modification, 24,* 635–657.

Dugas, M., Ladouceur, R., Léger, E., Freeston, M., Langolis, F., Provencher, M., et al. (2003). Group cognitive-behavioral therapy for generalized anxiety disorder: Treatment outcome and long-term follow-up. *Journal of Consulting and Clinical Psychology, 71,* 821–825.

Eftekhari, A., Zoellner, L. A., & Vigil, S. A. (2009). Patterns of emotion regulation and psychopathology. *Anxiety, Stress, and Coping, 22,* 571–586.

Folkman, S., & Lazarus, R. (1986). Stress processes and depressive symptomatology. *Journal of Abnormal Psychology, 95,* 107–113.

Furnham, A., & Ribchester, T. (1995). Tolerance of ambiguity: A review of the concept, its measurement and applications. *Current Psychology, 14,* 179–199.

Gratz, K. L., & Gunderson, J. G. (2006). Preliminary data on an acceptance-based emotion regulation group intervention for deliberate self-harm among women with borderline personality disorder. *Behavior Therapy, 37,* 25–35.

Gratz, K. L., Rosenthal, M., Tull, M., Lejuez, C., & Gunderson, J. (2006). An experimental investigation of emotion dysregulation in borderline personality disorder. *Journal of Abnormal Psychology, 115,* 850–855.

Gronwall, D., & Sampson, H. (1974). *The psychological effects of concussion.* Oxford, UK: Auckland University Press.

Hayes, S. C., Strosahl, K. D., & Wilson, K. G. (1999). *Acceptance and commitment therapy: An experiential approach to behavior change.* New York: Guilford Press.

Hayes, S. C., Strosahl, K., Wilson, K., Bissett, R., Pistorello, J., Toarmino, D., et al. (2004). Measuring experiential avoidance: A preliminary test of a working model. *Psychological Record, 54,* 553–578.

Hines, E. A., & Brown, G. E. (1932). A standard stimulus for measuring vasomotor reactions: Its application in the study of hypertension. *Proceedings of the Staff Meeting of the Mayo Clinic, 7,* 332–335.

Jones, A., Spindler, H., Jorgensen, M., & Zachariae, R. (2002). The effect of situation-evoked anxiety and gender on pain report using the cold pressor test. *Scandinavian Journal of Psychology, 43,* 307–313.

Kashdan, T., & Steger, M. (2006). Expanding the topography of social anxiety: An experience-sampling assessment of positive emotions, positive events, and emotion suppression. *Psychological Science, 17,* 120–128.

Kraemer, H., Kazdin, A., Offord, D., & Kessler, R. (1997). Coming to terms with the terms of risk. *Archives of General Psychiatry, 54,* 337–343.

Ladouceur, R., Dugas, M. J., Freeston, M. H., Leger, E., Gagnon, F., & Thibodeau, N. (2000). Efficacy of a cognitive-behavioral treatment for generalized anxiety disorder: Evaluation in a controlled clinical trial. *Journal of Consulting and Clinical Psychology, 68,* 957–964.

Ladouceur, M. J., Gosselin, P., & Dugas, M. J. (2000). Experimental manipulation of intolerance of uncertainty: A study of the theoretical model of worry. *Behaviour Research and Therapy, 38,* 933–941.

Linehan, M. M. (1993). *Skills training manual for treating borderline personality disorder.* New York: Guilford Press.

Lubke, G., & Muthén, B. (2005). Investigating population heterogeneity with factor mixture models. *Psychological Methods, 10,* 21–39.

Matthews, K. A., & Stoney, C. M. (1988). Influences of sex and age on cardiovascular responses during stress. *Psychosomatic Medicine, 50,* 46–56.

McNally, R. (2002). Anxiety sensitivity and panic disorder. *Biological Psychiatry, 52,* 938–946.

Miller, A., Wyman, S., Huppert, J., Glassman, S., & Rathus, J. (2000). Analysis of behavioral skills utilized by suicidal adolescents receiving dialectical behavior therapy. *Cognitive and Behavioral Practice, 7,* 183–187.

Otto, M., Powers, M., & Fischmann, D. (2005). Emotional exposure in the treatment of substance use disorders: Conceptual model, evidence, and future directions. *Clinical Psychology Review, 25,* 824–839.

Quinn, E. P., Brandon, T. H., & Copeland, A. L. (1996). Is task persistence related to smoking and substance abuse: The application of learned industriousness theory to addictive behaviors. *Experimental and Clinical Psychopharmacology, 4,* 186–190.

Rhudy, J., & Meagher, M. (2003). Negative affect: Effects on an evaluative measure of human pain. *Pain, 104,* 617–626.

Richards, J., & Gross, J. (2000). Emotion regulation and memory: The cognitive costs of keeping one's cool. *Journal of Personality and Social Psychology, 79,* 410–424.

Rottenberg, J., & Gross, J. (2003). When emotion goes wrong: Realizing the promise of affective science. *Clinical Psychology: Science and Practice, 10,* 227–232.

Schmidt, N. B., & Cook, J. H. (1999). Effects of anxiety sensitivity on anxiety and pain during a cold pressor challenge in patients with panic disorder. *Behaviour Research and Therapy, 37,* 313–323.

Simons, J., & Gaher, R. (2005). The Distress Tolerance Scale: Development and validation of a self-report measure. *Motivation and Emotion, 29,* 83–102.

Taylor, S. (1999). *Anxiety sensitivity: Theory, research, and treatment of the fear of anxiety.* Mahwah, NJ: Erlbaum.

Taylor, S., Jang, K., Stewart, S., & Stein, M. (2008). Etiology of the dimensions of anxiety sensitivity: A behavioral-genetic analysis. *Journal of Anxiety Disorders, 22,* 899–914.

Willoughby, S., Hailey, B., Mulkana, S., & Rowe, J. (2002). The effect of laboratory-induced depressed mood state on responses to pain. *Behavioral Medicine, 28,* 23–31.

Zelman, D., Howland, E., Nichols, S., & Cleeland, C. (1991). The effects of induced mood on laboratory pain. *Pain, 46,* 105–111.

Zvolensky, M., & Otto, M. (2007). Affective intolerance, sensitivity, and processing: Advances in clinical science introduction. *Behavior Therapy, 38,* 228–233.

# Index

281